Doubling Farmers Income Through Animal Husbandry

Co-Editors

Dr. Amit Singh
Assistant Professor
Department of Veterinary & Animal Husbandry Extension
College of Veterinary Sciences & Animal Husbandry
Uttar Pradesh Pandit Deen Dayal Upadhyaya Pashu Chikitsa Vigyan
Vishwavidyalaya Evam Go-Anusandhan Sansthan, Mathura–281 001

Dr. Madhu Tiwari
Assistant Professor
Department of Animal Genetics & Breeding
College of Veterinary Sciences & Animal Husbandry
Uttar Pradesh Pandit Deen Dayal Upadhyaya Pashu Chikitsa Vigyan
Vishwavidyalaya Evam Go-Anusandhan Sansthan, Mathura–281 001

Dr. Daya Shankar
Professor
Department of Veterinary Parasitology
College of Veterinary Sciences & Animal Husbandry
Uttar Pradesh Pandit Deen Dayal Upadhyaya Pashu Chikitsa Vigyan
Vishwavidyalaya Evam Go-Anusandhan Sansthan, Mathura–281 001

Doubling Farmers Income Through Animal Husbandry

Dr. Sanjeev Kumar Singh
Associate Professor & Incharge
Department of Veterinary & Animal Husbandry Extension
College of Veterinary Sciences & Animal Husbandry
Uttar Pradesh Pandit Deen Dayal Upadhyaya Pashu Chikitsa
Vigyan Vishwavidyalaya Evam Go-Anusandhan Sansthan
Mathura-281 001

Prof. Satish Kumar Garg
Dean, College of Veterinary Sciences & Animal Husbandry
Uttar Pradesh Pandit Deen Dayal Upadhyaya Pashu Chikitsa
Vigyan Vishwavidyalaya Evam Go-Anusandhan Sansthan
Mathura–281 001

SSPH

SATISH SERIAL PUBLISHING HOUSE
403, Express Tower, Commercial Complex
Azadpur, Delhi-110033 (India)
Phone : 011-27672852, Fax : 91-11-27672046
e-mail : info@satishserial.com, hkjain1975@yahoo.com
Website : www.satishserial.com

Published by :

SATISH SERIAL PUBLISHING HOUSE
403, Express Tower, Commercial Complex, Azadpur, Delhi-110033 (INDIA)
Phone : 011-27672852 Fax : 91-11-27672046
E-mail : info@satishserial.com, hkjain1975@yahoo.com

ISBN 978-93-88020-20-6

Composed, Designed & Printed in India

Preface

Indian farmers have remained a deprived community in the society, since times immemorial and poverty has come to be symbolized with Indian farming community. Although, farmers had been the force behind green-revolution, white-revolution, yellow-revolution, blue-revolution and several others, that had made the country not only self-sufficient but also nutritionally-secured. However, even after almost seventy years of independence, farmers are struggling to meet their both ends meet and ironically, still remain poor and deprived. They are dependent on the unpredictable weather, fluctuating market, lower minimum support price for their produce and many more unpredictable matters. They have to constantly worry about the re-payment of loans, education of children and even feeding their family. Looking at the plight of the farmers, Govt. of India has initiated certain farmers-friendly policies and undertook appropriate measures including scientific and technological interventions, assured market, assured minimum support price, e-marketing, etc. apart from assuring supply of quality seeds, fertilizers and addressing the soil-health issues. All the efforts are being directed towards "doubling the farmer's income" which in fact is a very challenging task.

Crop-science alone will not be sufficient to achieve the target set by Govt. of India. Our agricultural practices should be inclusive of animal husbandry, poultry, fish farming, bee-keeping and other agri-practices along with crop science and we also need to strengthen our value addition chain and evolve awareness and entrepreneurship amongst farming community. Farmers have to be educated in scientific and integrated farming, judicious use of resources on one hand to reduce their inputs, value addition and utilization of e-marketing for better returns. Accordingly, extension personnels and ground level-workers have to be educated and armed with newer and time-tested technologies to help out the farmers. It is an attempt of the authors to bring out the relevant information on different aspects of livestock keeping, dairy farming, poultry farming, hatchery establishment and maintenance, piggery, etc. to strengthen the animal husbandry practices in commonman's language. This book is also dealing with the role of women in Indian economy, especially livestock-keeping, who are half the population, and are equally involved in production yet largely ignored. Emphasis has been given on scientific methods of animal husbandry farming practices for sustainable source of income for farmers through value addition and also using livestock by-products.

Based on the impact of cross-breeding programme in animal husbandry, especially cattle, we have also reviewed our animal breeding policy and today, we are convinced to stop cross-breeding programme in cattle. Efforts are being made on conservation and propagation of native breeds as our native-breeds, are climate-change resilient. The authors have also made efforts to focus on augmentation of assisted reproductive techniques as well as selection and breeding strategies along with emphasis on integrated farming system coupled with low-input managemental practices. We hope that this book will be of immense use to its readers and in fulfilling the aspiration of "Doubling the Farmers Income".

Editors

Contents

Chapter 1

Role of ICT in Doubling Farmer's Income

Jitendra Chauhan[1], Amit Singh[2] and Sanjeev Kumar Singh[3]

[1] Coordinator, Agriculture Education and Extension Affairs, Office of Union Minister of Agriculture, Krishi Bhawan, New Delhi

[2] Food Safety Officer, Noida, [3] Departyment of Veterinary and Animal Husbandry Extension, College of Veterinary Science and Animal Husbandry, Uttar Pradesh Pandit Deen Dayal Upadhyaya Pashu Chikitsa Vigyan Vishwavidhyalaya Evam Go Anusandhan Sansthan, Mathura

Introduction

"If farmers give up farming, even the Rishis (Sages) cannot afford to survive."- Thirukkural (300 BCE)

The above sacred verse from an ancient Indian literary text opines that no living person, however, minimal his worldly needs be, could think of leading their lives without farming. The same condition continues to be applicable to the present days as well and whatever may be the per-capita income levels, the food cannot be simply downloaded from the internet. Though farming is the backbone of Indian economy, it is still intractably dependent on the vagaries of monsoons and dotted with small and fragmented holdings, which in turn, are run by resource poor farmers. Agricultural practices and advancements differ globally, since plants have their own differences and the location plays a role on their development as well. But through the exchange of knowledge from different agriculturally-involved individuals from all over the world, improvement of techniques can be experienced as well. It has made an impact on how information is shared, and being able to use for the advancement of the agricultural sector. Agriculture in India is the core sector for food security, nutritional security, and sustainable development & for poverty alleviation. It contributes approximately 16% of GDP. Milestones in agriculture development in India includes green revolution, evergreen revolution, blue revolution, white revolution, Yellow revolution, bio-technology revolution and the most recent one is Information and communication technology revolution. Information & communication technologies play a crucial role in disseminating information to farmers enabling them to decide on the nutrition diet of livestock but flow of AR, cropping pattern, use of high-yielding seeds, fertilizer application, pest management, marketing, etc. Traditionally, Indian farmers have been following indigenous production methods and rely upon friends, relatives, fellow farmers and input dealers to get information regarding agriculture and animal husbandry. With advancement of science and technology, multiple options to access modern technologies have become available. It is evident from the replacement of indigenous varieties of seeds by high-yielding varieties and traditional equipment and practices by power tillers, tractors and others machines.

Information and Communication Technology (ICT) in Agriculture & Animal Husbandry

Information and Communication Technology (ICT) is used as an overarching term incorporating all modes of transmission, like electronic devices, networks, mobiles, services and applications which help to disseminate information with the help of technology. In the recent years, ICT has proved to be extremely beneficial for farmers including small land holders, marginalized and poor farmers, and helped them in marketing, precision farming and improved profits. Through ICT, farmers have been empowered to exchange their opinions, experiences and ideas. It has given farmers more exposure and allowed them to use science that looks at agriculture from an integrated perspective. Also, e-Agriculture is one of the action lines identified in the declaration and plan of action of the World Summit on the Information Society. E-agriculture has the potential to put India on the higher pedestal of 'Second Green Revolution' by making Indian agricultural sector self-sufficient. Availability of timely information and technology has proved very crucial in areas, like disease prevalence and drought management thereby helping the farmers not only in avoiding crop and livestock loss but also thwarting economic loss, this raised the demand of planning and making strategies that could equip farmers with various information rights from sowing seeds to harvesting. ICT has now become a reliable instrument for improving the quantity and quality of the agricultural production. The efforts of the government in the area of ICT have escalated the living standard of Indian farmers and made them ICT-friendly, which has resulted in increased penetration of useful information about livestock, crops, soils, climate and cultivation processes. Several measures have been taken for encouraging Indian farmers to be more ICT–friendly, which include e-choupal, e–krishi, e-aid and many more. Numerous mobile applications have also been launched by the Government of India for the same including Mandi trades, M-power social, Kisan suvidha, Crop insurance, Agri market and m–Kisan application. The need of marketing agricultural produce at competitive prices will change the farmers' attitude towards ICT. Thus, this new technology will help and contribute more in sustaining the Indian agriculture.

Application of ICT in Agriculture

Access to markets and marketing information by smallholder farmers depending on agriculture in developing countries have always been challenging. Factors, such as poor road infrastructure, illiteracy, financial constraints, poor communication means and lack of access to information, all limited their access to markets. These smallholders depend on traditional means of communication and sell their produce at the farm gate and local markets. This has not been fruitful for these poor farmers as traders, intermediaries and other stakeholders in the chain take a large share of their produce. As a result, rural farmers remain poor and agriculture contributes little to their income, economy and welfare. The use of information and communication technologies (ICTs) is one approach to linking smallholder farmers to markets and aware them with current marketing information, i.e., the basic aim is to increase farmers' income and improve productivity. Some of the common agriculture and animal husbandry oriented get applications are discussed as hereunder.

Websites/Portals

In order to meet the information needs of the farmer, Ministry of Agriculture and Farmers' Welfare has developed different websites and web portals that allows farmers to access the information using Internet. Information on Market Price, Soil Health Card, Crop Insurance, government schemes, etc. is available to farmers through websites. These websites also aim at enhancing communication between the research institutions and the farmers, thereby increase the communication and knowledge sharing between researchers and subject-matter experts. Farmers' Portal, Agmarknet, Soil Health Card Portal, e-NAM, Crop Insurance, etc. are the web portals developed for farmers by the government of India.

E-Sagu

E-Sagu is a web-based personalized agro-advisory system, which uses Information Technology (digital photo based) to help farmers adopt better/scientific management practices in agriculture and animal husbandry. In e-Sagu, rather than visiting the crop in person, the agricultural or livestock expert delivers the expert advice at regular intervals (once in one or two weeks) to each farm by getting the status in the form of digital photographs or any other information.

Use of Mobile Apps

Spreading agricultural related information to farmers in the poorest communities are made easier by proliferation of mobile phones. Today, mobile apps and services are being designed and released in different parts of the world. Mobile apps help to fulfill the larger objective of farmers' empowerment and facilitates in extension services which can address the global food security issues. Few mobile apps developed for farmers are:

Kisan Suvidha mobile app provides information on five critical parameters - weather, input dealers, market price, plant protection and expert advisories. An additional tab directly connects the farmer with the Kisan Call Centre, where agriculture experts answer their queries. Unique features, like extreme weather alerts and market prices of commodity in nearest area and the maximum price in state as well as India, have been added in the app to empower farmers in the best possible manner.

Pusa Krishi app helps farmers to get information about latest technologies developed in research labs. This app is actually transferring the technologies from "LAB to LAND".

Agrimarket mobile app can be used to get the market price of crops in market within 50 km of the devices location. This app automatically captures the location of person using mobile GPS and fetches the market price.

Crop Insurance mobile app can be used to calculate the Insurance Premium for notified crops based on area, coverage amount and loan amount.

I-kisan It is a Nagarjuna group initiative, and encompasses comprehensive agri-portal addressing the information, knowledge and business requirements of various players in the agri arena viz., farmers, trade channel partners and agri input / output companies. Leveraging information technology and extensive field presence, i–kisan is positioned as an information/knowledge exchange platform and an e-marketplace.

Use of basic mobile telephony

Mobile telephony has transformed the tenor of our lives. In India, increased penetration of mobile handsets, large number of potential users, increased spread of communication, and low cost of usage lead to growth of large number of mobile based information delivery models for the agricultural sector. SMS, IVRS, OBD, USSD, etc. are the few modes used to meet the information needs of the farmer. In m-kisan (mkisan.gov. in), around 2 crore farmers are registered and experts/ scientists of different departments, like IMD, ICAR, State Government, State Agriculture Universities send information to farmers. Weather information about likelihood of rainfall, temperature, etc. enables farmers to make informed decision in choice of seed varieties, decide on timing of sowing and harvesting. Information on occurrence of rainfall and other climatic uncertainties help in organizing better storage facilities. With market information, farmers get better information about markets to sell produce, prevailing market prices and quantity demanded in the market. Thus, they are able to take decisions to sell produce at the right price and right time in the nearby markets. This helps in reducing distress sales by farmers due to market supply fluctuations.

Green SIM : This programme is implemented by IFFCO Kisan Sanchar Limited (IKSL). The features of IKSL services include delivering up to four free voice messages on areas of interest, and have a helpline services managed by experts and organize phone-in programmes and mobile-based quizzes. Farmers' queries are answered in 22 local languages.

Kisan Call Centres (KCC)

To harness the potential of ICT in Agriculture, Ministry of Agriculture took a new initiative by launching the scheme "Kisan Call Centres (KCCs)" on January 21, 2004 aimed at answering farmers queries on a telephone call in farmers own dialect. These call Centers are working in 14 different locations covering all the States and UTs. This Scheme provides agriculture related information to the farming community through toll free telephone lines. A countrywide common eleven digit number has been allotted for Kisan Call Centre. Kisan call centre 18001801551 (from any landline/mobile) and 1551 (from BSNL landline). The number is accessible through all mobile phones and landlines of all telecom networks including private service providers. In case, if the operator at the call centre is notable to address the farmers query immediately, them the call will be forwarded to identified agricultural/animal husbandry specialists.

The agricultural advisory sensices have largely followed vertical models of information transfer to the farmer clientele. However social made tools enables such as whats app greater use participation & feedback in extension activities. It has wide popularity even in moral India due to its too interval requirements. It's potential can be seen through shering of relevant farm information as well as offring timely advise to farmers. The group managing directly of what app in the form of phorus profermes and vides make it one of the cheapest multimedia messaging platforms.

Facebook

The social media platform, such as Facebook is being effectively used in Kerala for reaching out to farmers and extension workers. Based on the success of using Facebook by the Vattamkulam Krishi Bhavan (Malappuram, District, Kerala), the Government of Kerala has decided to officially include Facebook as an important tool to strengthen the extension activities of the Department of Agriculture. The state agriculture department has urged all the officials under it to extend the activities of the department through the social media to enhance the productivity and profitability of farming. All the farmers registered with the department will have to maintain a social media account to be in touch with the local Krishi Bhavan. The government has mandated that all agricultural officers should have active Facebook accounts.

Whats App

Thus ICT can play critical role in strengthening the capacities of not only farmers but also for the field level functionaries and intermediaries. The use of information and communication technologies (ICTs) is to link farmers to markets as well as for delivery of extenure services in rural India. Application of ECT in various cooperatives & milk collection centres helps in measurement of butter fat context of milk, test the milk quality as well as simultaneous identification of adulterated mlk makes their functioning feasible. Thus the only alternative to empower Indian villages is to use ECT tools to bridge gaps in the adoption of recommended new techniques in a cost-effective.

References

ICT in agriculture national round table conference, 2017.

Magesa M., 2015 Technical Centre for Agricultural and Rural Cooperation (CTA) working paper on Linking Rural Farmers to Markets Using ICTs.

Strategies for doubling farmer's income in Gujarat by 2022. Report of state level co-ordination committee to develop strategies and road map to double the farmer's income by 2022. (2017).

Thematic background note 2018, national conference agriculture, 2022 doubling farmers income, ministry of agriculture and farmers welfare.

Thakur, D., Chander, M. and Katoch, V. (2018). What app model for farmer led extension: Linking Actors & Generally localised information for farmers. Asian Journal of Agricultural extension, Economics and Sociology 26(4): 1-4.

□□□

Chapter 2

Role of Women in Livestock Sector

Madhu Tiwari, Deepak Sharma and Avneesh Kumar

Department of Animal Genetics & Breeding, College of Veterinary Science and Animal Husbandry, Uttar Pradesh Pandit Deen Dayal Upadhyaya Pashu Chikitsa Vigyan Vishwavidhyalaya Evam Go Anusandhan Sansthan, Mathura

Livestock sector, a key asset for rural livelihoods, is an integral component of agriculture based countries, such as India. The capacity of livestock systems to provide protein-rich food to billions of smallholder rural food producers and urban consumers, generate income and employment, reduce vulnerabilities in pastoral systems is commendable. It can immensely improve small-scale mixed farming with crop and livestock component systems and support livelihood opportunities to millions of livestock farmers and make them an appealing vehicle for pro-poor development. Increased consumption of livestock products, particularly in the fast-growing economies of the developing world, has been an important determinant of rising prices for meat and milk. These price surges provide new incentives and opportunities for using livestock as an instrument to help poor people escape poverty due to the multiple benefits that they offer and the multiple roles that they play in different production systems. Livestock provide income, creates employment opportunities and provide food and nutrition security across different production systems and along different value chains. It offers numerous advantages over other agricultural sectors and is considered an entry point for promoting gender balance in rural areas. It also plays important roles in securing household food security. This happens through various pathways: (i) in times of food shortages, households sell livestock to purchase other food, such as cereals and legumes; (ii) income from regular livestock and livestock product sales is used for food purchases to supplement household food production and to diversify diets; (iii) livestock and livestock products are consumed and provide a protein diet for households.

Animal husbandry expands and maintains three major pathways out of poverty: (1) Securing the assets of the poor, (2) Improving smallholder and pastoral productivity and (3) Increasing market participation by the poor. Poverty and hunger in rural areas can be ex-terminated easily by promoting small scale livestock enterprises by creating additional source of income and job opportunities. In rural livestock based countries two-third portion of low income livestock keepers are constituted by rural women, especially the activities related to small livestock production (poultry, sheep, goats), milking and processing of milk are carried out primarily by women. In fact, the major share of the credit for India's position as largest milk producing country in the world and the significant increase in the per capita availability of milk in the country has to go to the largely illiterate rural women dairy farmers. Dairy co-operatives have been chief means of bringing women in poor areas successfully into the cash economy along with sheep, goats and poultry rearing.

In developing countries, women's role in livestock production varies from no role at all to a very high level of responsibility. Underestimating their contribution can jeopardize the success of development initiatives. A IFAD (Niamir-Fuller, 1994) publication on women as livestock managers in developing countries classifies the division of labour by gender and age into ***four categories, representing a range of women's responsibility***:

- Men are completely responsible for livestock, with no involvement of women.
- Men are responsible for managing all livestock, and women are responsible for processing livestock products.
- Women are responsible for managing and processing small stock and any other animals kept near the homestead, whereas men are responsible for other animals.
- Women are responsible for managing and herding large stock and other animals and for processing livestock products.

In transhumant systems, women typically have complete responsibility for animals that are kept close to the homestead, such as poultry, calves and other small livestock, and for sick animals. Women rarely have major herding and management responsibilities for large stock and herd cattle, sheep and goats, while men take care of the camels.

In agropastoral systems, women also generally manage and control the animals that remain around the homestead. In most traditional Asian agropastoral societies, for instance, women manage water and feed small ruminants and other small livestock near their homesteads, whereas men herd the other animals. But there can be variations on this pattern. Situations do exist, however, in which women are completely prohibited from having anything to do with livestock, as in the Great Lakes region of Central Africa. Cultural differences in women's roles can even exist within large tribes. For instance, the Fulani of Benin allow women to raise and sell hens and guinea-fowls, but the Fulani of Niger do not. In some societies, such as the Maasai in East Africa, women may even slaughter sheep and goat, although this is considered men's exclusive responsibility. Women may also market larger livestock, when men are absent, for instance, during the seasonal outmigration of men.

In animal husbandry women play multiple roles. Most of the animal farming activities, such as fodder collection, feeding, watering, and health care management, household-level processing, value addition and marketing are performed by women. It is a common practice by rural women to prepare dungcakes by mixing twigs and crop residues which is then utilized as a fuel for cooking. They are well aware of each animal's behaviour, their production characteristics, knowledgeable about local feed resources and are able to identify beneficial grasses, weeds and fodder trees for feeding of dairy animals. Women know the feeding behaviour of each animal and prepare feed mixtures accordingly. As men are leaving rural areas to urban areas for employment, the responsibilities to look after livestock in households come on the shoulders of women. In tribal areas also men leave for working as laboures and the women take the leading role in livestock keeping. Verma and Goldey (2007) reported that on an average, a woman devoted 3.5 hours/day towards animal husbandry activities against only 1.6 hours/day devoted by men. Even if income is not the only factor that determines the socio-economic position of women, it greatly influences their status and well-being. Increasing women's income through improved livestock production would, therefore, also increase their status.

Gender-blindness is the result partly of a paternalistic bias, and partly due to the attitudes of the women themselves, who may be conditioned by their culture and society to underestimate the value of their work. Access, control and management of resources such as small ruminants, grazing areas and feed resources empower women and lead to an overall positive impact on the welfare of the household. In urban Indian society, gender roles are getting faded as women are also steeping out for work. There are many hurdles laid by societies in form of social and cultural taboos in accessing natural resources, extension services, marketing opportunities and financial services as well as in exercising their decision-making powers. These barriers lead to stopping women to achieve their full potential in all sectors, like agriculture or animal husbandry which affect the overall income of the household even the food security and nutrition of whole family gets compromised.

In a household kitchen, the role of women is significant, as they are responsible for decision-making of cooking. They look after the nutritional requirements of family members specially kids. This makes them an overall influencer in promoting a healthy well-balanced diet for every individual of household. Thus, in rural household where milk and eggs are usually found in one's backyard because of backyard poultry rearing and livestock keeping the women are in a decisive role of nutrition of family with a positive impact on trend of livestock keeping to promote a healthy diet. But as gender roles are more stringent in rural society, it affects the income generation and getting better payment for livestock produce of livestock maintained by women as compared to men.

Issues faced by women while working in livestock sector

- *Ownership of land* - Rural women faces severe challenges to hold land tenure in rural area because of village patriarchal system. Land tenure are certain rights which a person hold in order to own and have access to use land for desired purposes. Tenure provides the owner to make short term and long term decision to make the livestock or agriculture enterprise sustainable. As women have to manage a certain project the terms and condition of the land tenure should be designed in such a way to guarantee a smooth and tension free operation of the project. In ideal conditions, when the common land is converted to state ownership and then to private ownership, the women should not loose their traditional rights. The new law should ensure that the women got to keep their traditional right in case of property transfer. Culturally, women's access to land involved right of use, but not ownership. Conversion of common land to state ownership and then to private land, men often get upper hand and try to surpass women for their traditional rights. It would be ideal if both men and women get equal consideration for new laws related to land tenure. In addition, women are rarely aware of their rights. Though with changing time, a strong gender equality concern in the land tenure legislation need to be considered and implemented. Farmers with land tenure security are more readily to accept new technologies or interventions.

- *Access to capital and knowledge* : Women generally lack collateral, decision- making power in the household and control over loans. Ensuring women's access to extension services, knowledge, credit and technologies is, therefore, critical. Project experiences show that special credit lines for women are successful if these are made transparent and adapted to the cultural and social reality of the concerned families.

- *Ownership of livestock* : For women, purchase or receipt of a cow does not necessarily imply ownership. Analysis of the specific conditions of the project area and target households and monitoring of change are important to formulate and achieve realistic project goals.

- *Responsibilities and division of labour* : Including women in project activities does not automatically benefit them. Periodic analysis of labour, with corresponding adjustments to the time spent by women on the different tasks, or introduction of labour-reducing measures could diminish the risk of overwork.

- *Role of livestock in household nutrition* : Due to differences in the ways in which men and women have outlook towards utilization of income, if men are getting better return from animal husbandry practices, it will not automatically reflect into improved household nutrition, but it is seen that when women takes up an enterprise which causes increased monetary return, they tend to prioritize household well-being more as compared to men. Moreover, project designers should be aware that if the project objective is to increase the income of small farmers, the nutritional and social needs of vulnerable groups will need to be met through special programmes.

- *Influence of processing and marketing of livestock products on household economy* : The division of work between men and women in processing and marketing needs to be analysed and project activities adapted accordingly.

- *Role of farmers' organizations* : An important function of well-organized farmers' groups is to represent the interests of their members. Therefore, specific measures should be included at design to guarantee women's participation in such organizations (or create organizations specifically for women, if needed).
- *Information and relevant indicators* : What animals to be reread and what kind of production system is to be followed; mixed farming with livestock as a component; good land availability inputs proper utilization of natural resources involvement of technology; animal husbandry complemented with other activities; seasonal occupations and sources of income, etc. should be examined from a gender perspective.

Various benefits for Women engaged in livestock sector

- *Enhanced skills and knowledge :* Identifying and supporting women's role as livestock owners, processors and users of livestock products while strengthening their decision-making power and capabilities, are key aspects in promoting women's economic and social empowerment and consequently provides a way to enable rural women to break the cycle of poverty. With adequate support in training, integration of good practices, up-gradation of knowledge and skills in livestock management could improve women capabilities leading to higher productivity and well-being of poorer households. A Participatory Action Research (PAR) design can be adopted for improving women capabilities in scientific livestock management. It is based on need assessment, self-reflective and critical inquiry into their own problems of livestock rearing. According to Devendra and Chatalakhana, (2002), participatory research, a problem-oriented approach mainly responds to needs, resource availability, capabilities and opportunities of small farmers for developing viable strategies. Multiple techniques, such as participatory rural appraisal, focused discussions, training, demonstrations, field visits are included in PAR. PAR need to be designed to ensure empowering stakeholders, building collaborative efforts and capabilities enhancement through knowledge acquisition and skill development (Nirmala *et al.*, 2012).

- *Decision-making and empowerment* : Livestock ownership is increasing women's decision-making and economic power within both the household and the community. It is also a source of cash and/or can open up access to credit (the sale of small ruminants can provide an emergency source of cash for medical treatment or school fees, while daily milk provides a regular flow of cash income often used to purchase food and household items).
- *Household welfare* : The management, processing and marketing of livestock products generate more income than most of the activities women tend to be involved in, and bring benefits for the whole family (for instance, by increasing food security at the household level: small ruminants provide food products, such as milk, butter, cheese and meat, all of which are a source of protein, minerals and vitamins).
- *Income generation* : Animals provide raw material, such as wool, skins, and bones used by women to make clothes, or as fuel for home consumption and for sale. Processing of these materials can be an important source of additional employment and income for poor rural women.
- *Self-esteem* : It is well said that a person can be fed only for a day by giving him one fish to cook but the person can be fed for life-time, if you teach them fishing. Similarly if women themselves are owning, operating and earning their livelihood by themselves, it is certainly going to enhance their self-esteem.
- *Access to credit* : Livestock ownership increases the likelihood of gaining access to credit.

Suggestions to empower women for active participation in livestock sector

- Policy-makers should seriously recognize the women's role in livestock sector. Women should be incorporated in overall development process like more women should be employed in agricultural extension and in policy-making as well.
- Proper education is a very important factor. She should be educated about the opportunity in the growing livestock sector of India to become an entrepreneur or a worker.
- Gender issues must be covered under the curriculum in agricultural universities to make more gender sensitive policies and programmes in livestock and agricultural sector.

- Rural women should be given enough access to financial, extension services, new technologies with collaboration with traditional practices and markets so that her potential can be optimized.
- Women livestock workers form a heterogeneous group, so the policy framed for the whole country may prove ineffective, when there are distinct differences among rural women based on caste, geographical area, type of livestock reared and livestock products.
- Generally, women own more poultry around the world and they have more decision-making power with regard to poultry and small ruminants, so these small ruminants and poultry sector can be served as niche to empower rural women. Moreover, small animals, like sheep, goats, pigs and poultry have low initial investment and operational costs, so they can be easily kept by the land scarce poor households and women for commercial purposes. Similarly different livestock products are also to be identified which can especially serve women (Khan and Gupta, 2016).
- Measures to improve productivity and production will only succeed, if additional income can be generated by selling products outside the home. Women's access to markets, mobility and control over the proceeds of the sale are important considerations in this respect.
- Although income is not the only factor that determines women's socio-economic position, it greatly influences their status and living conditions. Increasing women's income by boosting livestock production, therefore, strengthens their position. As men may feel exposed by this process, projects must involve men and women in all negotiations to bring about equitable and sustainable changes.
- Efforts are needed to increase the capacity of women to negotiate with confidence and meet their strategic needs (Patel et al., 2016).

Few success stories of women involved in livestock sector

- Amul, managed by the Gujarat Cooperative Milk Marketing Federation (GCMMF), is owned by more than 3 million small farmers in the state of Gujarat. At the end of the transaction, more than 80 per cent of profits are received directly by farmers.

Where the whole region has been benefitted from the co-operative, women have especially profited from the venture. Most of the dairy-related activities are usually taken care of by the women of the state. They are involved mainly in the primary production stage of the chain and men mostly take care of marketing and processing. Working at the ground level, women are the sole reasons for the success of this business model. The co-operative movement has resulted in several women entrepreneurs empowering them to be equally contributive financially in their families. This also resulted in the improvement of the status of women, and the male female ratio.

- A woman entrepreneur, Smt. Chitra. M, 41 year old, B.A graduate runs a successful sheep and goat farm with the name "Samrudhi sheep and goat farm" which is 14 km away from Shivamogga city. The owner resides in the premises of the farm to overlook the farm activities. The land holding is 9 acres, out of which 2 acres used for shed construction, owner's house and garden, another 3 acres for maize or grass cultivation and remaining land is used for the cultivation of sugarcane. The entrepreneur owned 200 sheep (190 females, 10 males) and 10 goats which were purchased by the financial support from her family. The breed reared were Deccani, Kenguri sheep and Osmanbadi and Sirohi goat breed. This unit generated income and provided employment and food security. Two labourers were appointed to look after the animal and these workers were provided with good wages, quarters and groceries. She took active participation in care of pregnant animals, care at lambing, providing special feeding during fattening process and care of young ones. She was also involved in health care activities, decision-making and marketing related activities. The dung was collected at the ground level which was sold as the manure later on. Initially, her expenditure on education for children was less but after starting this enterprise, her disposal of expenditure on education improved i.e., the children were sent to residency schools for their higher education to the city, purchased land, has renovated her house and achieved better social recognition. The farming also had some constraints, like grazing land, problem of theft and unfair price competition from surrounding sheep farmers during the peak period. But these constraints were taken care by cultivating their own pasture, CCTV cameras were fixed to overcome theft and sale of animal in peak and non-peak season compensated the loss during peak season. The entrepreneur has attended training programs conducted by many government sheep farm and also in Veterinary colleges to get updated with the latest technologies. By seeing her persistent improvement in sheep farming, she was recognized and selected as president for sheep and wool co-operative society in Shivamogga district. She also acts as role model for neighbouring women farmers and motivated them to venture in sheep farming sector (Malagittimath *et al.*, 2017).

- One of the shining examples of a self-sufficient farmer is Rita Kamila, she was able to achieve a manageable source of livelihood. She has worked almost single-handedly on her land to achieve the right mix of farming and animal husbandry. Her enterprise is located in Sunderbans, West Bengal. She is popularly known as a model farmer in local, she identified the current scenario trend of organic farming and started producing various organic produce under her farm. Going a step beyond, she went for mixed farming model with fish culture and livestock components. Livestock manure and fish waste produced in the farm was sent to biogas plant to produce fuel for cooking and electricity and the remains of digested waste used as manure in farmlands. By having these innovative practices, she not only ensured food and nutritional security to her family but also she became center of attraction and a light bearer for fellow farmers community.
- A successful dairy entrepreneur, Mrs. Anusayabai Raghunath Shinde from Tadborgaon village of Pathri block, Parbhani district, Maharashtra State. She worked on her own farm, other's farm and also engaged in dairy entrepreneurship. Due to economic crises, her brother suggested her to do dairy enterprise, because she had experience of this enterprise in her father's house. From her savings and borrowing some money from a moneylender, she purchased two buffaloes in the year 2000 and a year later, she purchased a cow which had calves in next few years. She through her own efforts, succeeded in dairy production. She had 2 acres of land on which she produced green fodder to feed milch animals. She was the only person in her family who looked after all the animal management and cared to prepare dairy products, sale and marketing. One boy was employed for grazing the animals on fixed amount per year. She had been shouldering

responsibilities of marketing dairy products, borrowing loan and refunding it. She was not only taking care of animals but also performing all activities related to child and home care. She was involved in fodder management, purchase of fodder, feeding of animals, sale of produce, pre and post-natal management of animals, consultation with veterinarians regarding sick animals. She daily spent 4-5 hours in this enterprise. Her son helped to sell the products (Ekale *et al.*, 2006).

These entrepreneurs are the amazing examples of women success in livestock sector, wherein they not only had economic stability but also acquired entrepreneurship skills, like self-confidence, creativity, calculated risk taking capacity, determination, need for achievement, individuality, leadership and optimism.

Conclusions

In India, livestock production is largely in the hands of women. Most of the agriculture workers in rural areas (approx. 70 %) are women. They play role as food producers (approx. 80%), and processor of basic foodstuffs (approx. 10%). Not only this,it is estimated that 60 -90 % rural marketing is done by women. It is evident from above contribution of women that they make up more than two-third of the work power in agricultural production. Various farming activities related to animal husbandry, such as feeding, watering, fodder collection, and health care, management, milking are performed by women. Having this much contribution in rural economy still women face gender biasness in all aspect of work and social life. The essential point is that women usually do a great deal of the work in livestock management, a fact that development initiatives frequently ignore or underestimate. This can result in information being channeled to men only, inadequate consideration of the demands that new technologies or breeds might make on women's time and labour, and other similar mistakes that can threaten the initiative's success. Despite their considerable involvement and contribution, significant gender inequalities also exist in access to technologies, credit, information, inputs and services probably because of inequities in ownership of productive assets including land and livestock. The rapidly increasing demand for livestock products creates opportunities for empowerment of women. Therefore, there is a need to correct gender bias in livestock sector, veterinary education, research and service delivery systems as to enhance the effectiveness of women-oriented livestock development programs. When women control additional income, they spend more of it than men do on food, health, clothing and education for their children. Enabling and empowering rural women, therefore, translates into improved overall well-being for children, households and communities, which in turn, contribute to building human capital for future generations and to long-term social and economic growth. Therefore, there is a need to correct gender unfairness in livestock sector. Efforts are needed to increase the capacity of women to negotiate with confidence and meet their strategic needs.

References

1. Khan, A.A. and Gupta, S. (2016). Role of Indian livestock sector in rural women empowerment. Int. J. Agric.Sc & Vet.Med.4(2): 30-41.
2. Devendra. C. and Chantalakhana (2002). Animals, poor people and food security: Opportunities for improved livelihoods through efficient natural resource management. Outlook On Agriculture. 31(3): 161-175.
3. Ekale, J.V.; Bellurkarand C. M. and Jadhav, D.L. (2006). Case Study of a successful dairy woman entrepreneur. Dairying, Foods & H.S. 25(3/4): 248-250.
4. Niamir-Fuller, M. (1994). Women Livestock Managers in the Third World: Focus on Technical Issues Related to Gender Roles in Livestock Production, Staff Working Paper 18, Rome: IFAD, December.
5. Nirmala, G.; Ramana, D.B.V. and Venkateswarlu, B., (2012) Women and Scientific livestock management: improving capabilities through particioatory action research in semi-arid areas of South India. APCBEE Procedia, 4: 152–157.
6. Malagittimath, P.G.; Veeranna, K.C.; Harisha, M. And, Gopala. G. T. (2017). Case Study on a Successful Woman Livestock Entrepreneur in Shivamogga District of Karnataka. International Journal of Livestock Research. Vol 7(5): 284-289.
7. Patel, S.J.; Patel, M.D.; Patel, J.H.; Patel, A.S. and Gelani, R.N. (2016). Role of women gender in livestock sector: A review. J. Livestock Sci., 7: 92-96.
8. Verma, S. K. and Goldey, P. (2007). Gender roles in farming systems in Haryana state, India. http://www.ucc.ie/famine/conference/papers/varma.pdf.

❑❑❑

Chapter 3

Integrated Farming System (IFS): An Innovative and Unique Approach for Upliftment of Livestock Owners

Vijay Kumar[1] and Sanjeev Kumar Singh[2]

[1] ICAR-Central Institute of Research on Goats, Makhdoom, Farah, Mathura,
[2] Department of Veterinary and Animal Husbandry Exstension, College of Veterinary Science and Animal Husbandry, Uttar Pradesh Pandit Deen Dayal Upadhyaya Pashu Chikitsa Vigyan Vishwavidhyalaya Evam Go Anusandhan Sansthan, Mathura

The goal of reading this chapter is to understand:

1. Role of agriculture and livestock in India
2. Challenges before Indian Agriculture
3. Integrated farming system (IFS) approaches
4. IFS model developed for Uttar Pradesh
5. Integrated livestock – fish culture
6. SWOT analysis of small landholding farmers in India

Livestock production plays a crucial role in livelihood of people living in rural part of India. Common property resources, pastures and water are used to keep the animals, but the great concern is that there is a decrease in overall availability switch from communal grazing to mixed farming systems. With population growth, the crop encroachment disrupts pastoral areas, causing artificially local grazing pressure. To achieve sustainable increase of productivity and management, integrated approaches are recommended and in this regard, livestock should be systematically included for better socio-economic status of the community. At present in India, 63 per cent holdings are below 1 ha accounting for 19% of the operated area, while over 86% of holdings are less than 2 ha account for nearly

40 per cent of the area (APCAS, 2010). As per estimates, more than 95% of the holdings will be under the category of small and marginal holders in 2050. The small landholders are better contributors to the total production (78%) but weak in terms of generating adequate income and sustaining their own livelihood. Small holdings (below 0.8 ha) generate insufficient income to keep a farm family out of poverty despite high productivity (Chand *et al.*, 2011). India is facing some challenges which are given below:

Challenge	Current status	Rate of changes (per year)
India Population	1.2 billion	+ 1.95%
Food insecure population	194 million	1.0%
Soil degradation	120.40mha	5-10 mha
Desertification	105.19 mha	6 Mha
Irrigated area per person	0.245 ha	-1.3%
Grain harvested area per person	0.22 ha	-0.55%
Forested area per capita	0.59 ha	-0.78%
Atmospheric concentration of GHGs		
CO_2	370 ppm	+0.5%
CH_4	1.74 ppm	+0.75%
N_2O	311 ppb	+0.25%

Holding size (ha) and number of farm families in India (as per 2010-11 Agricultural censuses)

Parameters	Marginal	Small	Semi -medium	Medium	Large	All size
Average size of operational Holding (ha)	0.38	1.42	2.71	5.76	17.37	1.16
% farm holding	67.04	17.93	10.05	4.25	0.73	100
% area operated	22.24	22.07	23.59	21.18	10.92	100

85% of total holdings are under small and marginal farmer having the operational area of 44% Marginal farmers have no marketable surplus due to their holding and family size http://agcensus.dacnet.nic.in/NL/nationalt1sizetable4.aspx

Requirement by 2020 to meet the balanced diet as per norms prescribed by ICMR

Food items	Crops/item Requirement (gm/capita/day)	Requirement in million tons	
		Year 2010	Year 2020
Cereals and millets	420	234.40	280.99
Pulses and legumes	70	22.61	26.76
Fats and oils	22	12.44	14.72
Vegetables	125	109.52	129.62
Roots and tubers	75	42.39	50.18
Fruits	50	43.81	51.85
Milk	250	84.79	100.35
Sugar	30	16.36	20.07
Egg	45	25.44	30.11
Fish	25	14.13	16.73

http://www.icmr.nic.in/

Present agriculture is facing many problems, as given below:

- Decline in agriculture growth rate
- Decline in factor productivity
- Static or decline in food production
- Increasing malnutrition
- Shrinkage in net cultivable area
- Increasing environmental pollution
- Depleting ground water table
- Increasing cost of production
- Low farm income
- Problems of Farm labours due to large scale migration

(http://planningcommission.nic.in/plans/planrel/fiveyr/1st/1planch18.html)

Now, question comes, what is the solution of these problems? The simple answer would be "Integrated Farming System".

In the "Integrated Farming Systems" nothing is wasted, the by-product of one system becomes the input for other. It is an integrated approach to farming. "Farming system" is a complex inter-related matrix of soil, plants, animals, implements, power, labour, capital, and other inputs controlled in parts by farming families and influenced to varying degrees by political, economic, institutional and social forces that operate at many levels (Mahapatra et al, 1992). Integrated Farming (IF) is a whole farm management system, which aims to deliver more sustainable agriculture. It refers to agricultural systems that integrate livestock and crop production. Integrated farming systems has revolutionized conventional farming of livestock, aquaculture, horticulture, agro-industry and allied activities. It is sometimes called as Integrated Biosystems or Integrated Agriculture (Manjunatha, 2014). It comprises of inter-related set of enterprises with crop activity as base, will provide ways to recycle produces and "waste" from one component becomes an input for another part of the system, which reduces cost and improves soil health and production and/or income.

Why IFS is needed?

- For reducing the risks due to biotic and abiotic stresses
- High input costs
- For meeting the rising need of food, feed, fibre, fuel and fertilizer
- Nutritional requirement of family
- Increased demand of soil nutrients
- For increasing the income
- Employment
- Standard of living
- Sustainability

(http://www.rroij.com/open-access/integrated-farming-system—an-holistic-approach-a-review.pdf)

Goals of Integrated Farming Systems

- Maximization of yield of all component enterprises to provide steady and stable income.
- Rejuvenation of system's productivity and achieve agro-ecological equilibrium.

- Avoid build-up of insect-pests, diseases and weed population through natural cropping system management and keep them at low level of intensity.
- Reducing the use of chemicals (fertilizers and pesticides) to provide chemical free healthy produce and environment to the society.

Factors determining type of farming

- Physical factor (Climate, soil, topography)
- Economic factor
    - Marketing cost
    - Labour availability
    - Capital
    - Land value
- Consumer demand
    - Prevalent pest and diseases
- Social factor (type of community, easy transport, marketing facilities)
- Objective (income, production, minimizing cost, etc.)
- Environment (availability of resources and components)

(Manjunatha, 2014).

Factor deciding nature and size of enterprises

- Farm size
- Marketing facilities
- Climate
- Technologies available
- Soil type and condition
- Income level
- Credit facility
- Skill/Knowledge

(Manjunatha, 2014)

Components of Integrated Farming System

- Crop husbandry
- Livestock production
- Poultry
- Duckery
- Horticulture
- Aquaculture
- Apiculture
- Sericulture
- Mushroom cultivation
- Agro-forestry
- Biogas plants

(http://agritech.tnau.ac.in/agriculture/agri_ majorareas_ifs_ l.html)

Integrated-farming systems have different models based on different agroeco-system, like Irrigated low and uplands, Rain fed and dry land areas and Hill regions. All above components of IFS differed in different models.

Contribution of livestock to the farming system

Livestock constitute a "living bank" providing flexible financial reserves in times of emergency and serve as "insurance" against crop failure for survival. Crop and livestock is considered to be the most dominant farming system in India. However, under present scenario, the importance of integration of livestock, poultry, fishery and horticulture is likely to increase significantly. In fact, livestock plays an important role in the national economy by augmenting family income and generating gainful employment in rural areas. The importance of livestock in India goes beyond the function of food production, as it has been an important source of draught power, source of manure for crop production and fuel for domestic use.

Livestock environment interaction : Generally, farmers do not practice single livestock rearing system but incorporates different livestock (cows, buffaloes, sheep and goats, pigs and small numbers of poultry in the backyard) to meet their domestic needs along with other agricultural components, like horticulture, plantation, vegetables, sericulture and agro-forestry. In this system, animals are raised mainly on agricultural waste and the complementarities between different components are tried to exploit to its maximum level. The animal power is used for agricultural operation and the dung is used as manure and fuel. It may be possible to reach the some level of yield with proportionately less input in the integrated farming and the yield would be inherently more sustainable because of waste of one enterprise becomes the input of another leaving almost no waste to pollute the environment or to degrade the resource base.

Implication of livestock on soil fertility: Soil fertility maintenance is the combined result of the interactions among plants, animals, and their by-products, a complex but essential component of the whole farming system. Through animals plant produce is converted to manure. Dung helps to improve soil texture and to decompose litter more easily. With a traditional feeding system, and farmyard manure (FYM) preparation method, an adult large ruminant animal provides about four tones of FYM and six large ruminants are sufficient to provide required FYM for one hectare of farmland under a rice – maize – wheat system for one year.

Livestock as a source of farm power : In general, male animals are used for draught purposes usually in pairs. In land preparation, generally animals are used especially in hill areas, where mechanization is not yet available.

Livestock as a source of manure : The excreta of animals have been used as manure for crop production. The animal's manures are not only rich in major nutrients but also contain several micronutrients. The demand of livestock manure is very high for agricultural as well as horticultural crops. In general, the total output of dung (fresh weight) from cattle and buffalo per day to be about 10 kg and 12 kg, respectively giving a total of 3.6 tones and 4.3 tones of dung per animal per annum, respectively. Assuming the animals are stall fed, the annual output of N,P and K for cattle would be 12.6 kg N, 5.4 kg P and 7.2 K, and from buffalo 15 kg N, 6.5 kg P and 8.6 kg K. The availability of manure for use in agriculture and fish production can be calculated from the average dung production and nutrient value of the manure. The nutrient content of the excreta varies with species. Generally, the value of the manure, in increasing order is cattle, sheep and goat, followed by pig, chicken and ducks. Animal urine is very rich in nitrogen and potassium. The value in cattle urine has been reported to be 0.9 - 1.2 % N, a trace level of P and 0.5 - 10 % K. Urine output per kg body weight is in the range 17-45 ml/kg body weight.

Few successful IFS model developed for Uttar Pradesh

Model: AICRP-IFS Centre BHU, Varanasi

IFS model is developed at AICRP-IFS Centre BHU, Varanasi consisted crops (0.81ha), dairy animal (4 cows), (400 broilers), horticultural crops (0.06ha), fishery (0.1ha) and mushroom (0.01ha). In the very first year of the study, total farm production in terms of rice equivalent yield (REY) was 43.76 t/ha and gross and net returns as high as Rs. 6,56,481 and Rs. 2,50,465 $ha^{-1}year^{-1}$ respectively, which emphasized the IFS approach. Production of sufficient quantities of cereals (4,046 kg), pulses (744 kg), oilseeds (206kg), milk (10,222 litre), fruits (240 kg), vegetables (2,219 kg), green fodder (23,722 kg), dry fodder (8,680 kg) and mushroom (106 kg), *etc.* much more than annual demand of food and fodder of the family and also improved nutritional status because of additional food products *viz;* milk, fruits, meat, *etc.* and thereby prevented them market dependency for domestic consumption. (AICRPFS, 2013).

IFSRI, Modipuram in 2004-05

The model developed on 1.5 hectare area comprises of crops (0.72 ha), dairy (0.32 ha), horticulture (0.22 ha), fishery (0.10 ha) and miscellaneous (0.14 ha) which was used for goat, apiary, vermicompost, threshing floor and farm building, etc. This model initially was consisting of field crops including fodders, dairy with improved milch animals (Two buffaloes of murrah breed+one cow of sahiwal breed), horticulture (A multistoried fruits and vegetables unit), apiary (10 bee boxes) and pisciculture (A mix culture of fishes including rohu, katla, mrigal, nain and grass carp). This was further strengthened by establishment of a small vermicompost unit (0.01 ha) in 2006 and goat unit (15 goat animals) in 2007. The goat unit, however, was not found suitable and profitable under stall feeding and was removed from the programme in subsequent years. In addition, fruit plants (Stone fruit "Bel", jackfruit, aonla, jamun and citrus spp. Kagji Nimboo) were also planted all around the farm boundaries as wind breaks to protect the field crops and add in to income of the farm. At boundary of horticultural unit's Carisa carendis locally known as "karonda" was planted which served as live fencing and provided considerably high fruit yield (4-6q/year) as a bonus. All the farm wastes, by products and crop residues, etc. were properly recycled in to the system itself so that nothing go as waste and output of one enterprise serves as a input for other enterprise. Under crop production besides food for family consumption, provided green fodders and feed concentrates to the dairy animals and also green biomass as feed of fish and goat. Net return from different commodities are (Rs. ,000) 74.43, 87.02, 10.26, 4.94 and 4.2 from crop, animal husbandry, horticulture, fishery and apiary, respectively.

Integrated livestock – fish culture

Integrated livestock-fish culture would be more successful, if proper stocking density of fish and animals are followed. The use of animal waste to fertilize fish ponds leads to greater fish yield, as the manure provides active nutrients (NPK) for the metabolic cycle in the ponds and promotes the growth of plankton, which is the natural food for fish. Cattle, pigs, poultry and ducks can be raised on the embankments or near by the ponds so that the manure can directly be utilized for pond fertilization. There are several types of integrated fish farming systems and the most common ones are discussed below:

i) ***Cattle – Fish farming :*** Fish farming can become more production-oriented, if integrated with cattle farming. Cattle are fed with the grass grown in and around the pond banks and manure is either collected or washed directly from the cattle sheds into the ponds for fish culture.

ii) ***Pig–Fish farming :*** Small pigsties are constructed over the fish ponds, while the bigger ones are constructed on the dikes and pig manure is allowed to enter the pond directly or collected and fermented in suitable pits before applying in the ponds. Fresh pig manure is regarded as highly efficient for pond fertilization and fish can utilize directly the feed spilled by the pigs, which would otherwise go as waste. On an average, 30 to 40 pigs are sufficient to fertilize one ha pond water area.

iii) ***Goat /Sheep-cum-Fish farming :*** Intensive goat and sheep raising is increasing due to high demand for chevon and mutton. Manure from goat and sheep is also potential for integrated animal-fish farming system.

iv) ***Poultry–Fish farming :*** The poultry-fish system requires little space, low capital investment and provide quick returns. Poultry dropping are rich in highly soluble inorganic salts and have high N and P values as compared to other livestock manures. Layer or broilder chicken can be raised in houses built above the fish ponds or on the dikes. This type of integration can be practised both, in large commercial ventures and in small farms.

Besides the feed for fish is available round the year, the egg and meat produced by poultry provides an additional income to the farmers. Commercial strains for meat and egg production (dual purpose birds, like Vanaraja birds) are now available and have been proved successful. Approximately 60 kg/ha/day deep litter manure to be applied in fish culture pond and 500 – 600 poultry birds are enough to fertilize one ha of fish pond.

v) ***Duck–Fish farming :*** The duck house is usually made up of locally available materials, like bamboo, wood, etc. The fish gather protein-rich natural food from the pond ecosystem and may consume directly the feed spilled by the ducks. Ducks usually consume tadpoles, mosquitoes and dragon fly larvae, which are not consumed by fishes. Another advantage is that ducks feed on snails, which are vectors of certain fish parasites. Ducks are not only fertilize ponds nut also release nutrients from the pond soil by its dabbling activity and also enhance the availability of oxygen for fishes resulting in enhanced pond productivity.

The local ducks are not suitable for commercial raising and for that Khaki Campbell and Indian runners are recommended. Approximately, 200–300 ducks are enough to fertilize one ha of fish pond.

Number of animals required to fertilize 1 ha pond water area

S.No.	Animals/fish	Recommended numbers/ha water area
1	Cattle/buffalo	4-5
2	Goat	50-55
3	Pig	30
4	Duck/Layers	450-500
5	Composite fish culture	7000-8000

Goat based integrated farming system approach

Integration of crops, horticulture, goat rearing, dairy, fisheries, poultry, etc. a viable option to provide regular income to millions of small land holder, minimize cost of production through multiple use of resources and risk. *Goat farming is boon for millions of landless, marginal and small farmers*- studies done in Bundelkhand revealed that as a family with 15 adult females' goats can earn an annual income of Rs. 52,000 to 55,000. With introduction of good goat husbandry practices by appointing local youth to facilitate the activities as Field Guides, 35 million goat keepers in the country who are living below the poverty line, can enhance their income by four folds from Rs. 8000 to 35,000 per annum (BAIF's experience in Jharkhand, Odisha and Rajasthan).

SWOT analysis of small land holding farmers in India

Strength	Weakness	Opportunities	Threats
Sufficient Manpower	Fragmented Holdings	Loans with low interest	Weather related adversities
Hardworking nature	Poverty	Subsidies for livestock addition	Technology failure would affect economy
Mostly fulltime farming	Low literacy	Presence of more than one enterprise	
	Low risk bearing ability		

Advantages of Integrated Farming Systems

- Regular income and year round employment
- Provides food and nutritional security
  - Eco-recycling of agriculture residues/by-products/wastes
  - Better soil quality for sustainable agriculture
  - Minimization in pollution hazards
  - Improves micro climate
  - Conservation of natural resources
  - Minimizes the risk of failure in productivity

(http://www.rroij.com/open-access/integrated-farming-system—an-holistic-approach-a-review.pdf)

Limitations of IFS

- Lack of awareness about sustainable farming systems
- Unavailability of varied farming system models
- Lack of credit facilities at easy and reasonable interest rate
- Non-availability of ensured marketing facilities specially for perishable commodities
- Lack of deep freezing and storage facilities
- Lack of timely availability of inputs
- Lack of knowledge/education among farming community specially of rural youth

(http://www.rroij.com/open-access/integrated-farming-system—an-holistic-approach-a-review.pdf)

❑❑❑

Chapter 4

Perspective of Indigenous Livestock Breeds and its Importance

Deepak Sharma, Satyendra Pal Singh and Madhu Tiwari

Department of Animal Genetics & Breeding, College of Veterinary Science and Animal Husbandry, Uttar Pradesh Pandit Deen Dayal Upadhyaya Pashu Chikitsa Vigyan Vishwavidhyalaya Evam Go Anusandhan Sansthan, Mathura

Livestock sector have a crucial role in Indian economy and is an vital sub-sector of Indian Agriculture. This is the only sector in which poor can be benefitted and simultaneously contribute to the Indian economy as compared to getting benefited from growth generated in other sectors. The overall growth rate in livestock sector is stable and is around 4-5% and this has been accomplished despite the fact that stake in this category was not sizable. The progress in the category results in even reinforcement of the rural economy particularly in lessening the poverty amongst the poor and marginal peoples. The benefit of growth should be equitable, providing betterment mainly to the weaker section and landless workers and should help poorly supplied areas, like draught prone, arid and semi-arid areas .Livestock sector should generate additional employment opportunity to people in the rural areas, especially to the female population. Livestock should provide major source of income in the selected areas having potential for mixed crop-livestock farming system, and the growth in the sector should result in the improvement in the rural areas.

The contribution of livestock sector in country GDP at the current rate was 4.4% to national GDP and 26.9% in GDP from Agriculture in the year 2015-16. Among the livestock and their products, milk contributed maximum (66.7%) as a single commodity. India ranks first in the world for milk production for more than last 20 years. During the year 2015-16, country produced 155.5 million tons of milk with 337 ml per capita availability. India possesses vast variety of livestock wealth, as it maintains 11% of the total world livestock population. According to 19th livestock census, India possessed 512.05 million of livestock comprising of 190.90 million cattle, 108.70 million buffalo, 65.07 million sheep, 135.17 million goats, 10.29 million pigs and the rest being constituted by other species, such as yak, mithun, camel, horse, donkey and mule. All the breeds of indigenous livestock have a long evolutionary history and the natural selection, which essentially led to their establishment in their respective ecological niche. All of these breeds are distinguished from each other by certain morphological as well as production parameters.

The Indian livestock, irrespective of the species, is an admixture of two or more genetic variants/breeds and is generally referred to as non-descript or deshi and thus, cannot be precisely allocated to any documented breed. The numerous lesser known breeds, strains and new genetic populations of different farm animal species exist, which have not been properly studied and documented. The native farm Animal Genetic Resources possesses unique genes or combinations of genes, which are responsible for like disease resistance, stress resistance, quality animal products, feed efficiency and many more traits of economic and environmental importance. Indigenous bovines are rich in variability and excellent in desirable attributes for different environment and production systems.

Livestock Population Scenario and Dynamics

The total livestock population consisting of Cattle, Buffalo, Sheep, Goat, Pig, Horses & Ponies, Mules, Donkeys, Camels, Mithun and Yak in the country is 512.05 million numbers in 2012. The total livestock population has curtailed by about 3.33% over the animal population tally. Livestock population has shown positive growth significantly in Gujarat (15.4%), Uttar Pradesh (14.%), Assam (10.8%), Punjab (9.6%) Bihar (8.6%); Sikkim (8.96%) and Meghalaya (7.4%).

Table 1: Livestock population (2012 Livestock census)

S.No.	Species	Number (in millions)	Ranking in the world population
1.	Cattle	190.9	**Second**
2.	Buffaloes	108.7	**First**
	Total Bovine population (including Mithun and Yak)	**300**	**First**
3.	Sheep	65	**Third**

4.	Goats	135.2	**Second**
5	Pigs	10.3	-
6	Others	1.7	-
	Total livestock	**512.3**	

Table 2: Production of livestock in India, 2015-16

S.No.	Product	Quantity	Ranking in the world production
1.	MILK in million tonnes	**155.5**	FIRST
2.	MEAT million tonnes	**7.02**	NA
3.	WOOL in million kgs.	**47.9**	NA

Table 3: Livestock and Poultry Production in India

Species	Livestock Census, 2007 (no in millions)	Livestock Census, 2012 (no in millions)	Growth Rate
Cattle	199.1	190.9	-4.1
Buffalo	105.3	108.7	3.19
Sheep	71.6	65.1	-9.07
Goat	140.5	135.1	-3.82

Cattle genetic resources of India

The well-defined recognized breeds of cattle constitute around 18% of the total cattle population in the country and rest 82% of the cattle are exotic/cross-bred (22%) and non-descript type (60%).Among descript breeds, very few are maintained for milk production (Sahiwal, Gir, Tharparkar and Red Sindhi), some are dual-purpose breeds (Deoni, Hariana, Kankrej and Rathi, etc.), while the rest are draft breeds, maintained by farmers for producing bullocks. The different breeds are economically well-suited to the areas where they exist. A massive and diverse range of agro-ecological zones in India have helped to grow number of cattle populations. The cattle breeds can be classified as on the basis of its body size, horn size and utility. The cattle breeds can be classified as on the basis of its body size Vechur, Malnad Gidda, Punganur, Motu, Purnea, Kosali and Hill cattle are known as small type. The breeds Bachaur, Bargur, Binjharpuri, Dangi, Gaolao, Ghumsuri, Tho-Tho, Pullikulam, Kenkatha, Khariar, Krishna Valley, Nimari, Rathi, Siri, Umblachery, and Kherigarh are of medium size. The large size breeds include Ongole, Gir, Hariana, Deoni, Mewati, Nagori, Tharparkar, Kankrej, Malvi, Kangayam, Red Sindhi, Sahiwal, Khillar, Hallikar, Amritmahal, and Gangatiri.

The cattle breeds can be classified as on the basis of horn size Kankrej had the thickest horns. Long horns were available in Hallikar, Bargur, Khillar, Pullikulam, Kangayam, Amritmahal, Krishna Valley breeds. The short type horns breeds are Hariana, Siri, Rathi, Ongole, Bachaur, Nagori, Gaolao, Mewati, Krishna Valley, Ponwar, Binjharpuri and Gangatiri.

The description of 41 well-defined recognized breeds of cattle, their distribution & characteristics are presented in Table 4.

Table 4: Descript cattle breeds of India, its distribution and their characteristics

S. No.	Name of Breed	Breeding Tract	Utility	Characteristics	Image (Source*)
1.	Amritmahal	Hassan, (Karnataka)	Draught	Grey in colour but varies from white to almost black. Long horns; emerge from the top of the poll fairly close together in backward and upward direction.	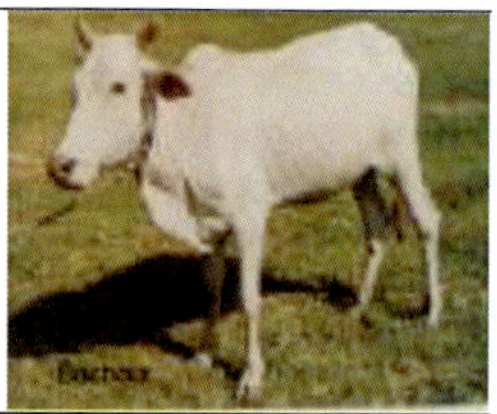
2.	Bachaur	Sitamarhi, Darbhanga, (Bihar)	Draught	Medium sized, compact animal and white or grey colour. Short and stumpy horn.	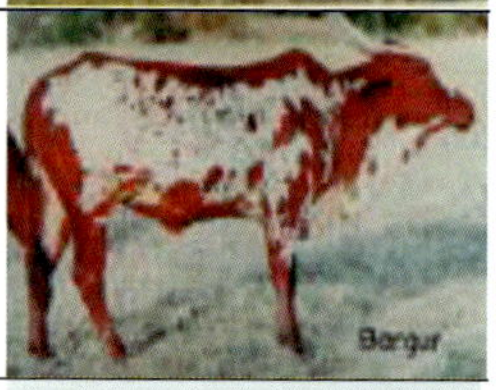
3.	Bargur	Erode (Tamilnadu)	Draught	Brown with white markings, Horns are closer at root and inclined and backward	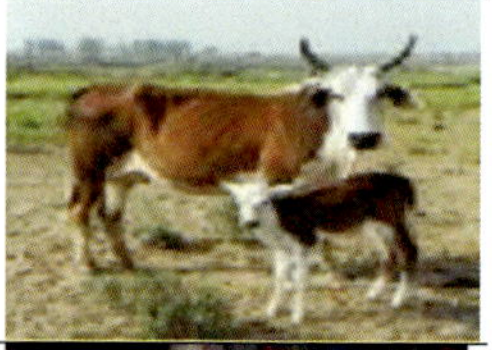
4.	Belahi	Ambla, Panchkula (Haryana)	Draught	Medium sized and reddish brown colour. Sickle shaped horn.	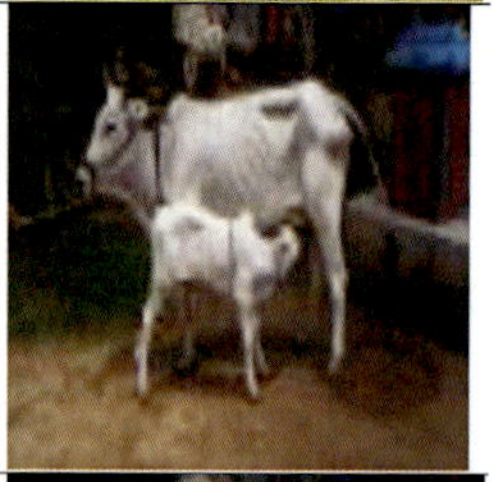
5.	Binjharpuri	Jajpur, Bhadrak (Odisha)	Dual	White color, horns curved upward and inward	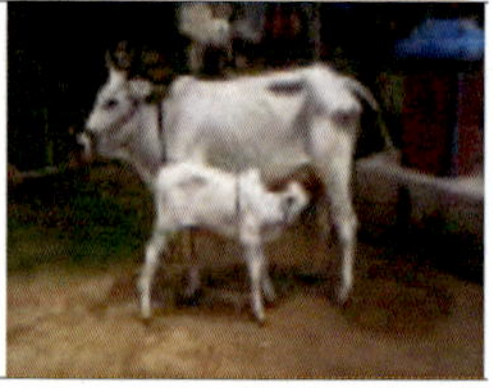

6.	Dangi	Dang (Gujarat), Nasik, Ahmadnagar (Maharashtra)	Draught	White with red and black spot unevenly over the body. Thick and short horn.	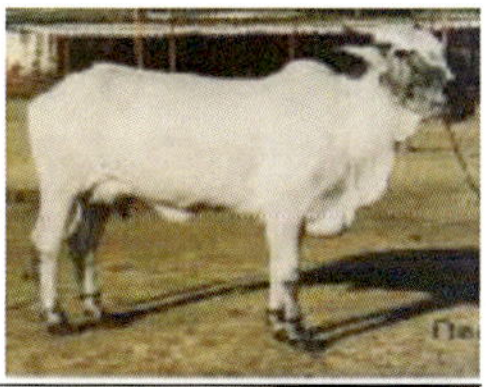
7.	Deoni	Bidar (Karnataka), Parbhani, nanded (Maharashtra)	Draught	Black and white spotted body colour, short horn with blunt ends. Bulging forehead.	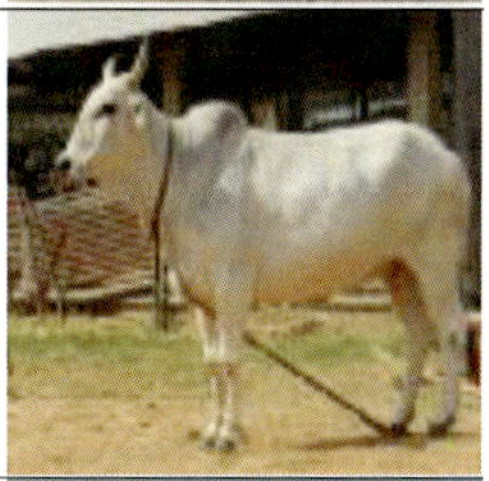
8.	Gangatiri	Varanasi, Balia (Uttar Pradesh), Bhojpur (Bihar)	Dual	Complete white, grey colour, medium sized horn, prominent forehead with groove in middle	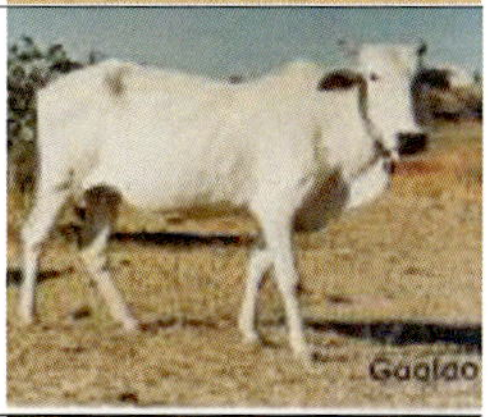
9.	Gaolao	Durg, Chindwada (MP), Wardha, Nagpur (Maharashtra)	Dual	White in colour, males are generally grey over neck, short and stumpy horn.	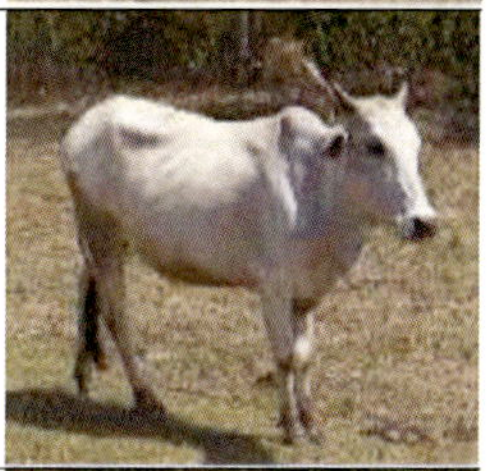
10.	Ghumusari	Ganjam (Odisha)	Draught	white sometimes grey in clolour. Horns curved upward and inward	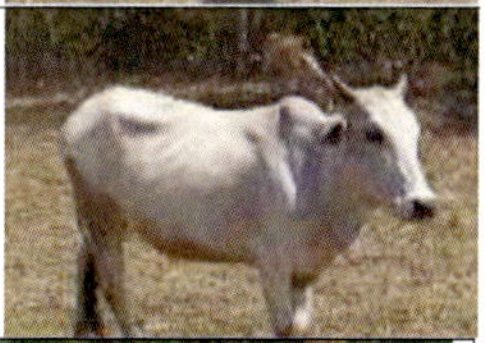
11.	Gir	Bhavnagar, Junagarh (Gujarat)	Milch	Pure red and sometimes speckled red. Horns are peculiarly curved. Starting at the base of the crown they take a sideways downward and backward curve and again incline a little upward and forward taking a spiral inward sweep, ending in a fine taper thus giving a half moon appearance. Long and pendulous ears folded like a leaf.	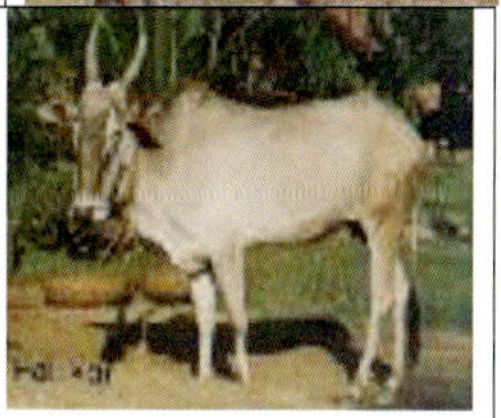

12.	Hallikar	Hassan, Mysore (Karnataka)	Draught	White to light grey, horn emerge near to each other from top of poll and are carried upward and backward, each in a straight line for nearly half their length and then with gentle and graceful sweep bend forward and slightly inward ending up with pointed tips, White markings or irregular patches round the eyes and cheeks, and neck or shoulder region are the distinctive features of this breed.	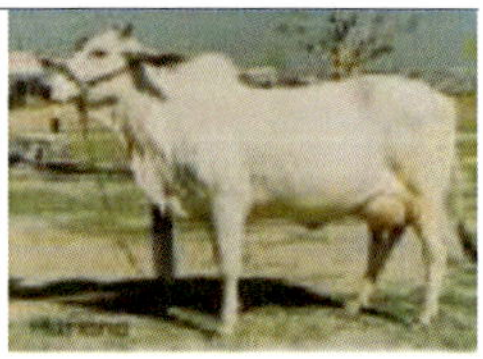
13.	Hariana	Hissar, Rohtak, Jind (Haryana)	Dual	White or light grey, small horn, bony prominence at the center of poll	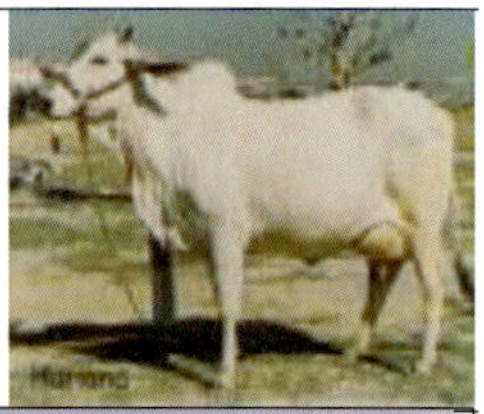
14.	Kangayam	Coimbatore (Tamil Nadu)	Draught	Grey or white in colour, Long crescent shaped horn	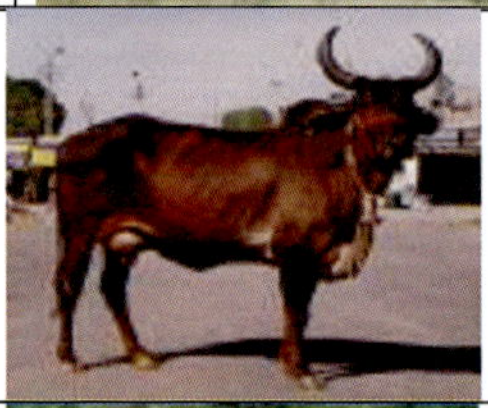
15.	Kankrej	Mahesana (Gujarat)	Dual	Silver grey in colour, lyre shaped horn, heaviest breed of cattle	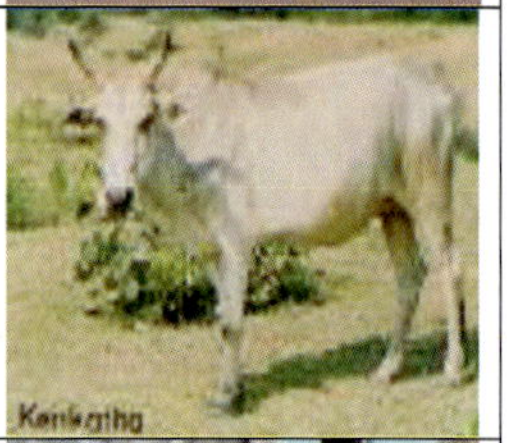
16.	Kenkatha	Banda (UP)	Draught	grey in colour, horns directed forwarded, small animal	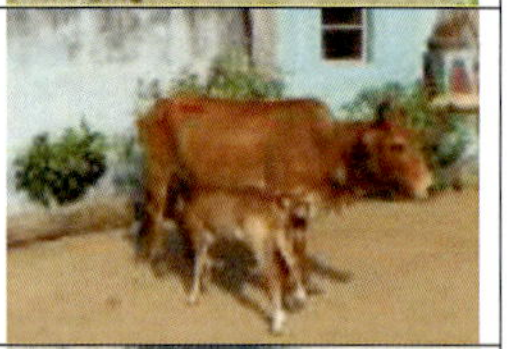
17.	Khariar	Balangir (Odisha)	Draught	Brown or grey in color, straight horn	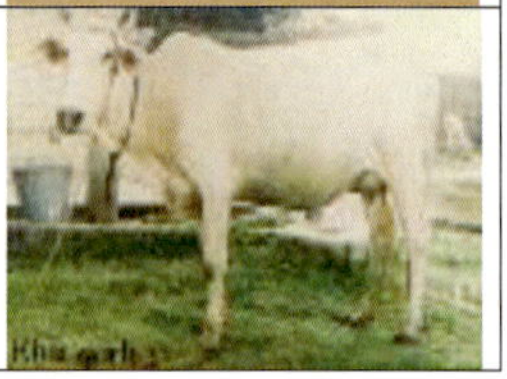

18.	Kherigarh	Kheri (Uttar Pradesh)	Draught	White coat colour, horns are upstanding, curving outward and upward.	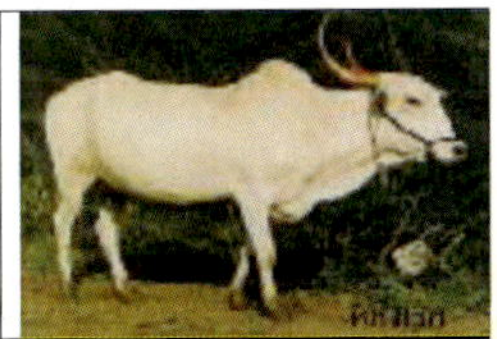
19.	Khillar	Pune (Maharashtra), Dharwad (Karnataka)	Draught	Grayish white in colour, bow shaped long horn, distinct groove in the center of forehead	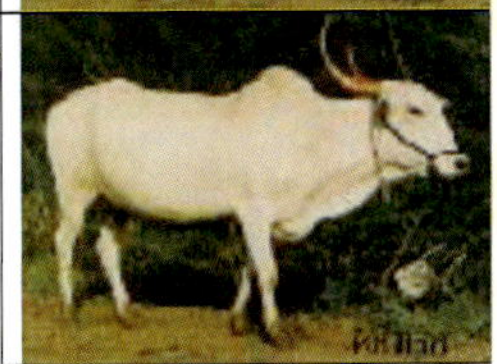
20.	Kosali	Raipur, Durg (Chhatisgarh)	Dual	Light red to whitish grey in colour, small, stumpy and straight horn	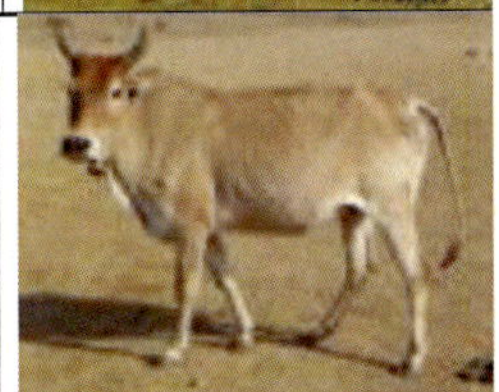
21.	Krishna Valley	Satara (Maharashtra), Raichur (Karnataka)	Draught	grey white in colour, horns small and curved, massive body	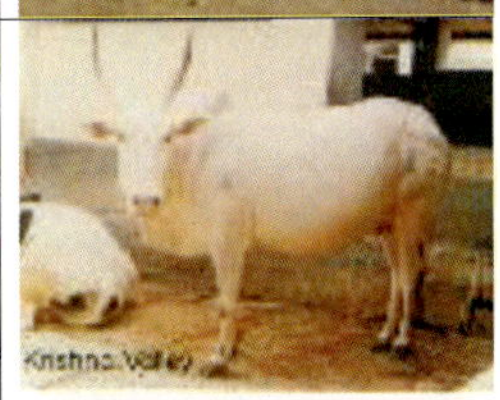
22.	Malnad Gidda	Hasan, Udupi (Karnataka)	Dual	Black in colour, small and straight horn, small compact body	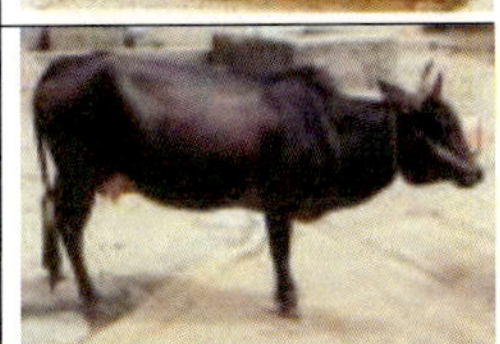
23.	Malvi	Rajgarh (Madhya Pradesh)	Draught	White and white greyish in colour, lyre shaped horn	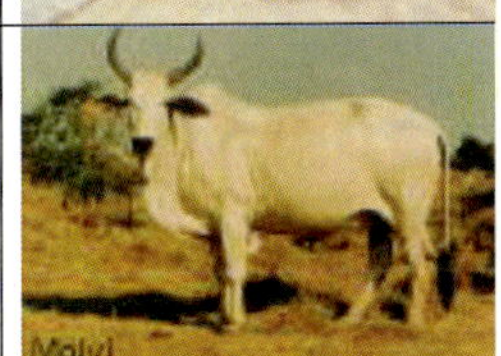
24.	Mewati	Faridabad (Haryana), Alwar, Bharatpur (Rajsthan), Kosi, Mathura (Uttar Pradesh)	Draught	White in colour, darker shade on neck, shoulder, outward, upward and inward pointed ends horn, long and narrow face	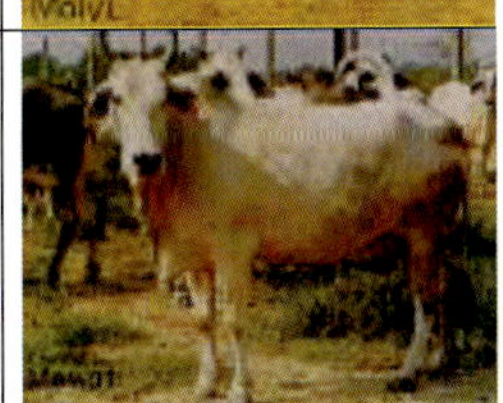
25.	Motu	Malkanagari (Odisha)	Dual	Brown sometimes grey in color, straight upward with rounded tip, small size animal	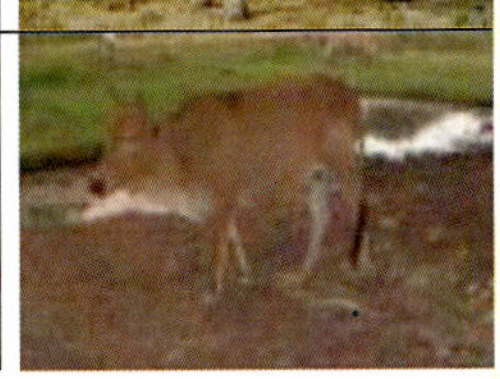

26.	Nagori	Nagaur (Rajsthan)	Draught	white or light grey in colour, hornsoutward and upward with gentle curve	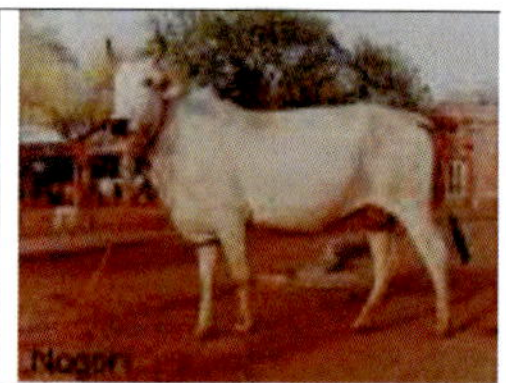
27.	Nimari	Nimar (Madhya Pradesh)	Draught	brownish red and white gives chitkabri appearance, horns emerge backward from outer angle of poll	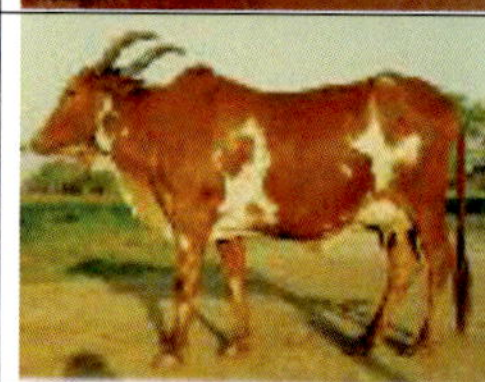
28.	Ongole	Nellore, Guntur (Andhra Pradesh)	Dual	Glossy white in colour, short and stumpy horn, majestic gait	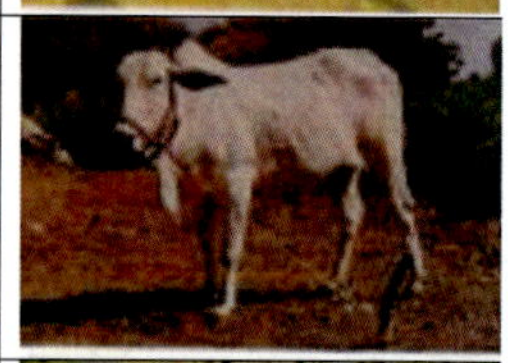
29.	Ponwar	Pilibhit (Uttar Pradesh)	Draught	brown or black with white patches, horns emerge outward, upward and then curved inward	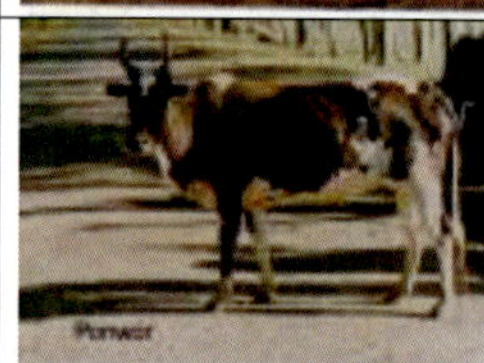
30.	Pulikulam	Madurai (Tamil Nadu)	Draught	Dark grey in male and whitish grey in female, horns outward upward and inward, small size compact body	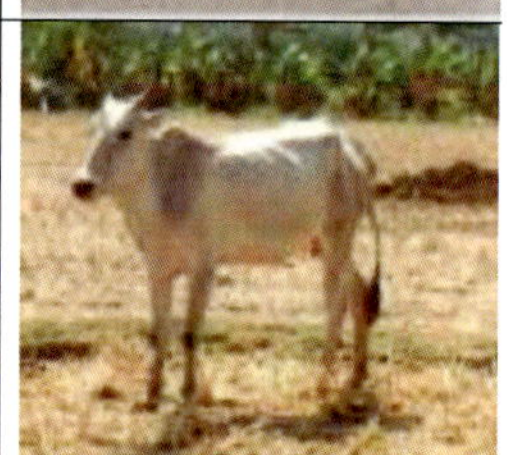
31.	Pungnur	Chitoor (Andhra Pradesh)	Dual	white, grey to light brown to dark brown in colour, crescent shaped horn	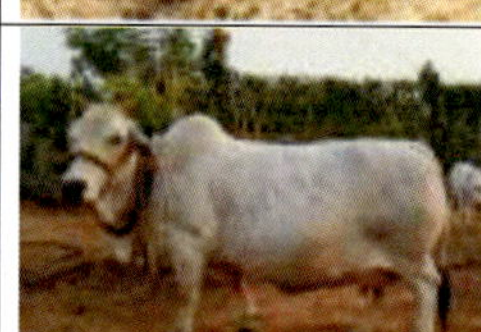
32.	Rathi	Ganganagar, Jaisalmer (Rajsthan)	Dual	Brown with white patches all over the body, short horn curving outward,	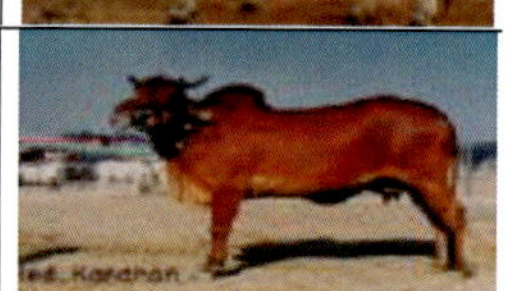
33.	Red Kandhari	Parbhani, Latur (Maharashtra)	Draught	deep dark red in colour, medium sized evenly curved horn	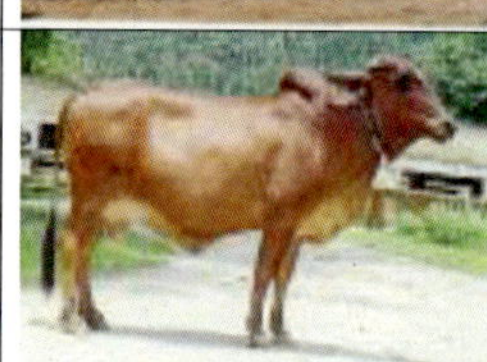

34.	Red Sindhi	Baluchistan province (Pakistan)	Milch	red colour, horns are thick at base, emerge lately curved upward	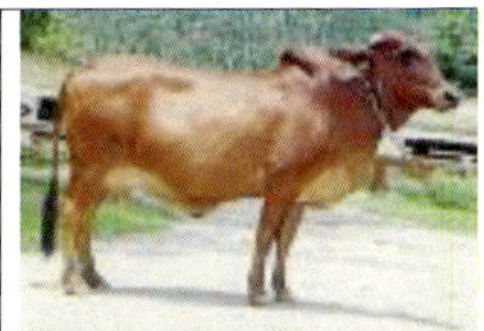
35.	Sahiwal	Ferozpur, Amritsar (Punjab)	Milch	brownish pale red in colour, short and loose horn, loose skin, pendulous naval flap	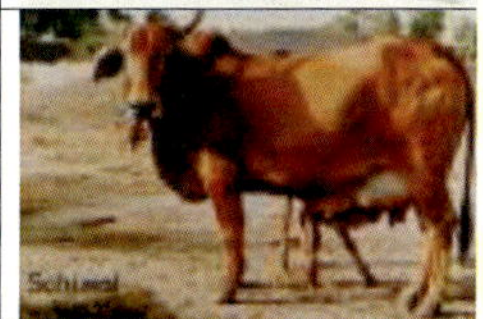
36.	Siri	Darjeeling (West Bengal), Gangtok (Sikkim)	Draught	Black or brown with white patches, medium horn curved outward, hump is covered with tuft of hair	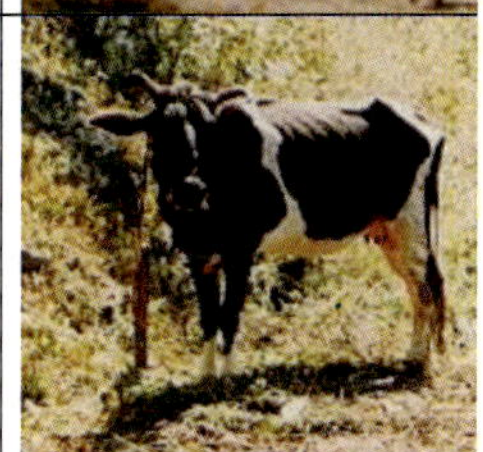
37.	Tharparkar	Kutchch (Gujarat), Jaisalmer, Jodhpur (Rajasthan)	Milch	white or light grey in colour, horns are thick and short	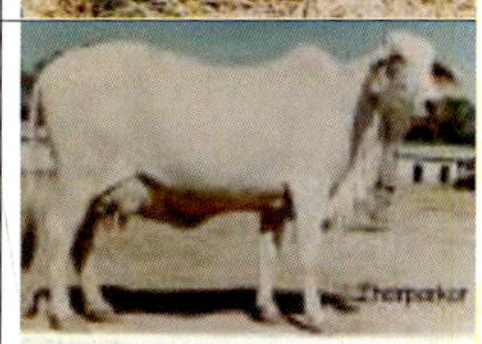
38.	Umblachery	Nagapatinam (Tamil Nadu)	Draught	grey in colour,horns are small and thick	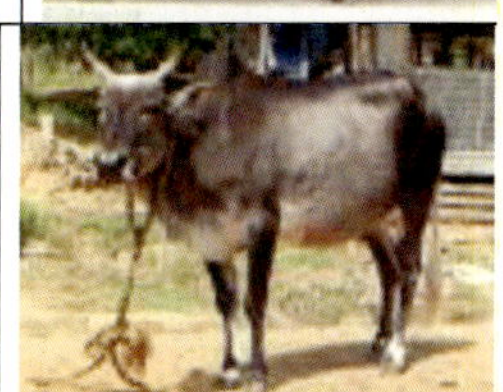
39.	Vechur	Kottyayam (Kerla)	Dual	light red and fawn colour, small and thin horn, extremely small sized compact animal	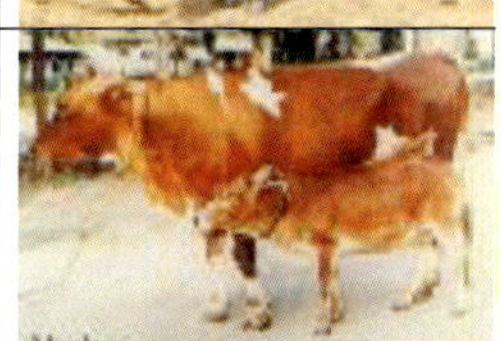
40.	Badri	Uttarakhand	Dual	Small in size having long legs and varied body colours – black, brown, red, white or grey. Hooves and muzzle are black or brown in colour.	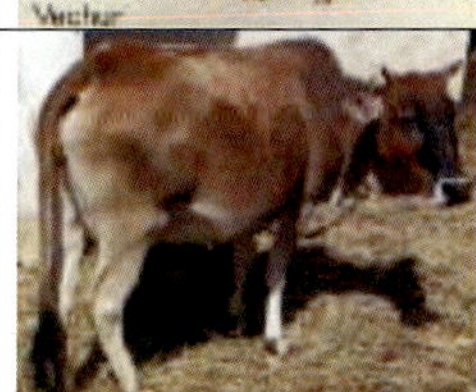
41.	Lakhimi	Assam	Dual	Small sized and have relatively short legs. Coat colour is variable mainly brown and grey.	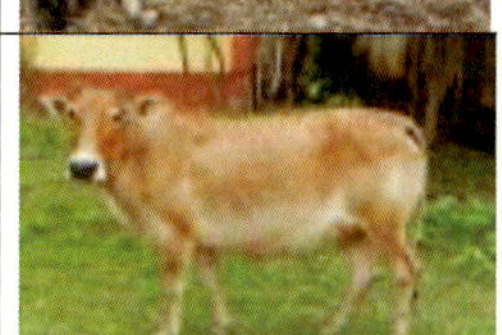

*Image Sources

1. http://14.139.252.116/agrportal/index.htm
2. Umblechery- https://en.wikipedia.org/wiki/Umblachery#/media/File:Amblacheri_02.JPG
3. Belahi- http://dairyknowledge.in/article/belahi
4. Punganur- https://goo.gl/hYRkGe'
5. Gangateeri -https://en.wikipedia.org/wiki/Gangatiri#/media/File:Gangatiri_02.JPG
6. Ghumsari- http://dairyknowledge.in/article/ghumusari

Genetic diversity of Buffalo breeds

Buffalo is a matter of pride for the country, as it is a multi-purpose animal supporting in several aspects. Buffalo provides milk, meat and draught power, in addition to several minor products. The original domesticated stock of buffaloes is believed to have been derived from the Indian wild buffalo, *Bubalus arnee.* Riverine and Swamp buffaloes were domesticated almost together (around 2000BC), former in the Indus Valley Civilization and the latter in the Yangtze Valley. Riverine and Swamp which differ in terms of chromosome number (50 vs. 48), body size (heavy vs. medium built), the main purpose (milk+ draft vs. draft+meat), behaviour and body colour.

Buffalo numbers in the country has been showing positive growth at a regular rate with minute escalation in milk production. Highest increase in the past five years was in Haryana (25.1%) followed by Uttar Pradesh (20.6%), Madhya Pradesh (13.9%), Gujarat (13.6%), Uttrakhand (12.2%), Andhra Pradesh (10%) and Rajasthan (6.6%). as out of total buffalo population around 50% are breedable female so farmers tend to rear buffalos for milk production. Indian states UP, Rajasthan, Punjab, Haryana, Gujarat and Maharashtra have maximum buffalo numbers and responsible for approximately 60% of the overall buffalo population. Most of the milch breeds of buffaloes are found in these States. In eastern area, around 10% of total buffalo population is fond having around one million swamp buffaloes, which are used for drought purposes mainly.

As per 19th livestock census, the total buffalo population in the country is 108 million, out of which 17.05% population is pure belong to registered breeds and 39.53% buffaloes are grades of purebred buffaloes. Presently the buffaloes are contributing 76.2 m MT (2016) of milk in the country, which is about 49% of total milk produced thus making it economically viable milch species. Moreover, the butterfat percentage is quite high among buffaloes with an average of 6.5% fat. According to ICAR-NBAGR, India have 13 registered buffalo breeds - Murrah, Nili-Ravi, Jaffarabadi, Mehsana, Nagpuri, Pandharpuri, Bhadawari, Surti, Toda, Banni, Chilika and Kalahandi. Murrah is acknowledged as best breed in the world and imported by many countries. Bhadawari is known for high fat in milk. India possesses a superior genetic resource of buffalo species and excellent milch breeds, like Murrah, Mehsana, Surti, Nili Ravi and Jaffarabadi are present in sufficient numbers and are spatially distributed. Murrah is the pre-dominant buffalo breed and is the breed of choice included in breeding programme of most of the Indian states, for upgrading the non-descript/local buffaloes followed by Surti, Mehsana and Jaffarabadi. Toda and Bhadawari are the two breeds that are threatened to extinction.

Buffalo breeds of India, based on their phenotype can be classified into six distinct groups as: (i) Murrah group comprising Murrah, Murrah grades and Nili-Ravi (ii) Gujarat group comprising Banni, Jaffarabadi, Surti, Mehsana and their grades (iii) Uttar Pradesh group has Bhadawari (iv) Central India group includes Nagpuri, Pandharpuri and Marathwadi breeds in Maharashtra, Kalahandi and Chilika breed in Odisha (v) South India group comprises Toda (vi) North-Eastern group includes Swamp buffaloes mainly distributed in Manipur and Assam. The description of 13 well-defined recognized breeds of buffalo, their distribution & characteristics are presented in Table 5.

Table 5: Descript buffalo breeds of India, its distribution and their characteristics

Sr. No.	Name	Home Tract	Main Use	Characteristic	Photograph
1	Banni	Kutchchh districts of Gujarat	Food-Milk	Mainly Black, sometimes Copper. Horns Curved. Medium to large, heavy with 24 to 30 cm diameter in adult animals. Horns are vertical and upward in direction with inverted double/ single coiling.	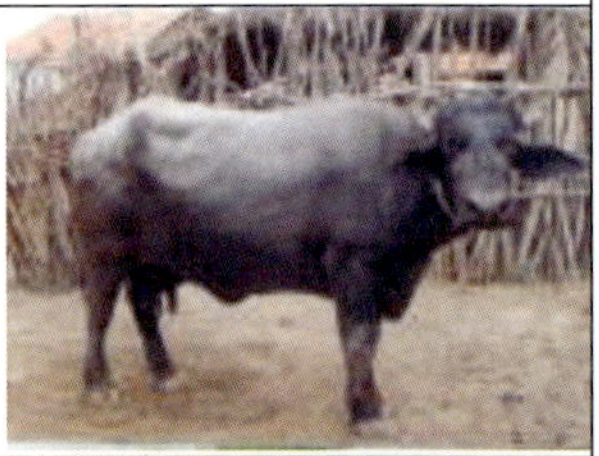
2	Bhadawari	Bhind, Morena districts of Madhya Pradesh and Agra, Etawah districts of Uttar Pradesh	Food-Milk; Work-Draught	Blackish copper to light copper. Colour of legs is usually like wheat straw. Horns are black curling slightly outward, downward before running backward parallel and close to neck and finally turning upward. Two white lines "Chevron" locally called as Kanthy are present on the lower side of the neck.	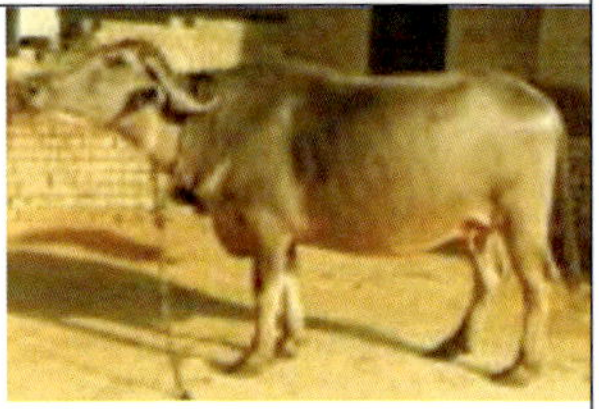
3	Chilika	Ganjam, Puri, Khurda, Cuttack districts of Odisha	Food-Milk; Work-Draught; Manure	Colour Brownish black or Black. Horn Curved Upward, inward. Medium sized with compact body, strong legs and small udder	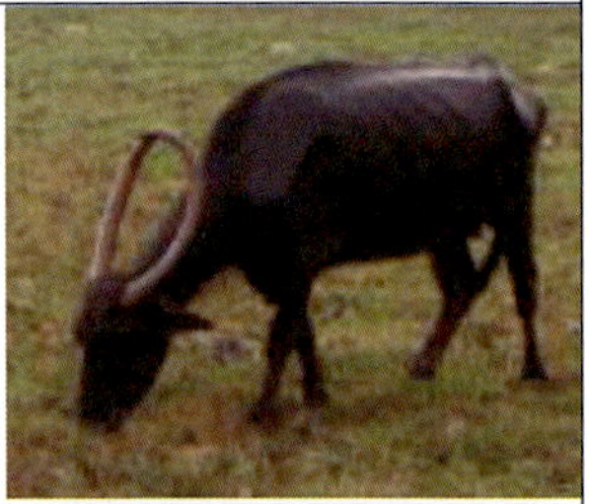
4	Jaffarabadi	Amreli, Bhav-nagar, Jamnagar, Junagadh, Rajkot, Porbandar districts of Gujrat	Food - Milk; Work - Draught and Transport	Black but some animals having white or grey tail switch are also seen. Horns exibit wide variation, but usually emerge out by compressing the head, go downward sideways, then upward and inward finally forming a ring like structure. Horn are long. Horn shape is peculiar of this breed. It makes eyes to look small - termed as study eye, especially in males.	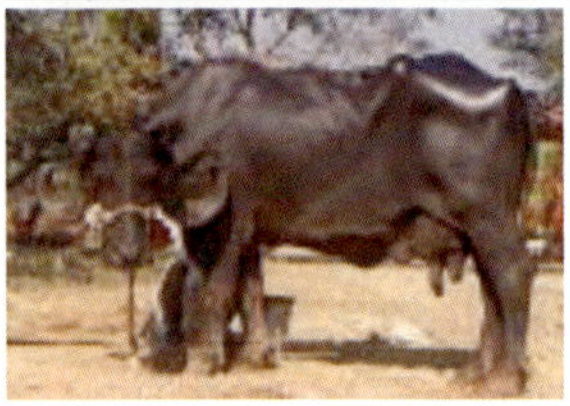

5	Kalahandi	Kalahandi distrtict and adjoining area in Rayagada district of Odisha	Milk, draught,	Coat colour is usually blackish grey, sometimes grey. Horns Horizontal going backwards, upward, and inward, Curved to make half circle appearance. About 50cm long. Muzzle, eyelids, tail and hoofs are black. Head convex, hump small, udder round and medium in size. Tail extends below hock with coarse hairs on switch	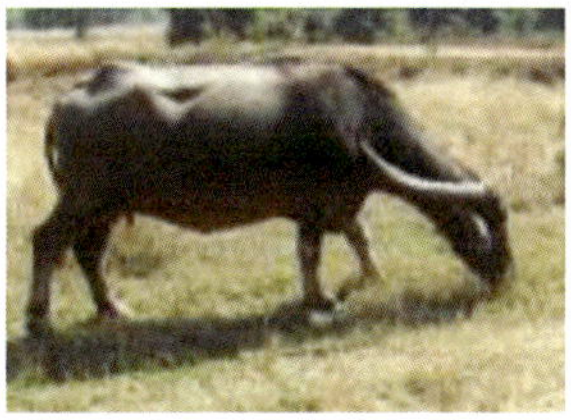
6	Marath-wadi	Parbhani, Beed, Nanded, Latur, Jalna districts of Maha-rashtra	Milk; Draught and Transport	Grayish black to jet black. Some animals have white markings on forehead and lower parts of the limbs. Horns are parallel to the neck, reaching up to shoulder but never beyond shoulder blade. Length of horns differentiates these buffaloes from Pandharpuri buffaloes. Horns reach upto shoulder unlike in Pandharpuri buffaloes where these may reach up to pin bones some time.	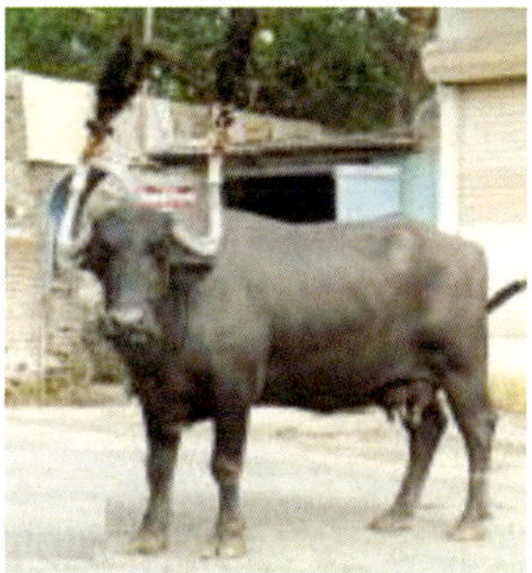
7	Mehsana	Ahmadabad, Banas Kantha, Mahesana and Sabar Kantha districts of Gujarat	Milk.	Mostly black, a few animals are black brown or brown. Horns are generally sickle shaped with the curve more upward then in the Surti breed and less curved then in the Murrah breed. They are generally bent downward and then take a curve like the horns of a ram. Eyes are very prominent, black and bright bulging from their sockets with folds of skin on upper lids.	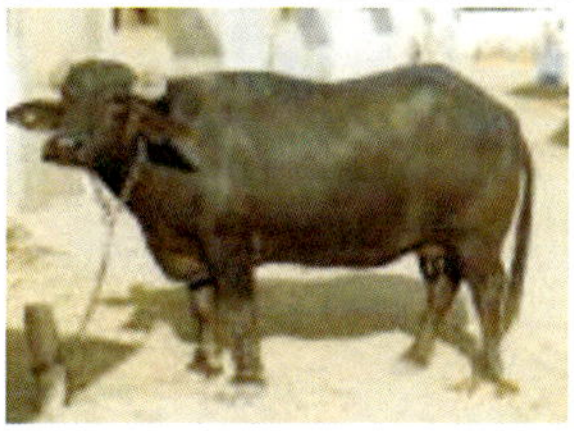
8	Murrah	Rohtak, Gurgaon, Jind and Hissar district of Haryana and Delhi	Milk and Meat; Work - Draught	Colour Jet Black. Horn Tightly curved in a spiral form, Short in size	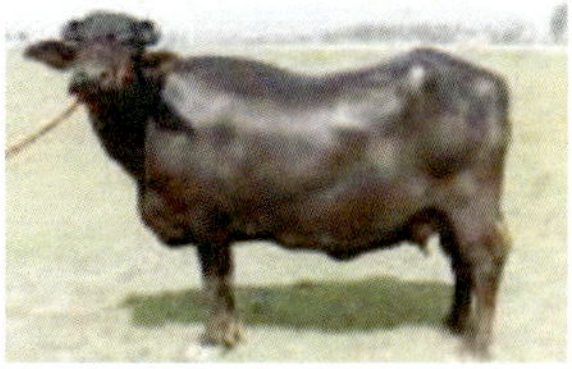

9	Nagpuri	This breed is native to the Vidarbha region of Maha-rashtra. Akola, Amravati, Yavatmal, Wardha and Nagpur Districts of Maha-rashtra	Food - Milk; Work - Draught	Black coloured animals with white patches on face, legs and tail tips. Puranthadi strain is slightly brownish. Horns are flat, curved and carried back on side of the neck nearly to shoulders like a pair of swords, horn tips pointed, upward in orientation mostly. Horns are heavier in males than in the females. Horns are long.	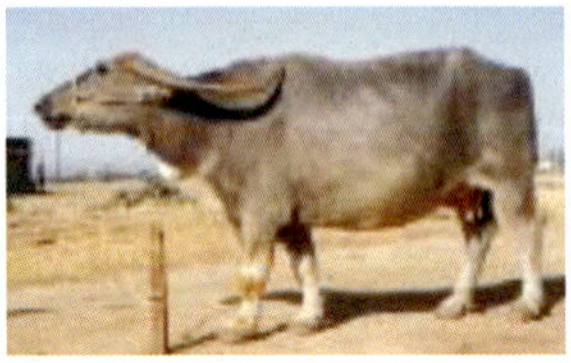
10	Nili Ravi	Nili Ravi buffaloes are found in Fazilka, Ferozepur, Zira and Makhu tehsils of Ferozepur district; and Patti and Khem-karan tehsils of Amritsar district	Food - Milk	Colour Normally black. Horns are tightly curved and circular in cross section, small in size. Usually walled eyes and white markings on forehead, face, muzzle, legs and tail. The most desired character of female is the possession of these white markings known as "Panch Kalyani".	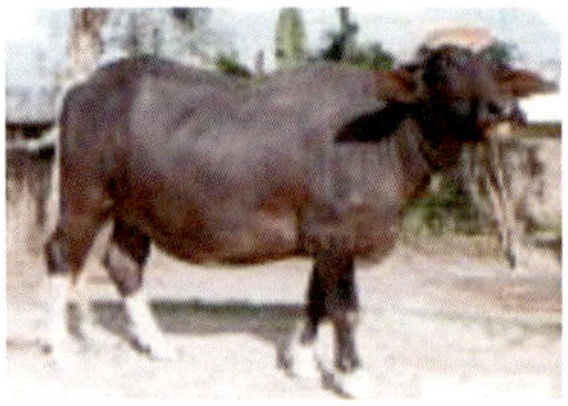
11	Pandhar-puri	Sangli, Solapur and Kolhapur districts of Maha-rashtra	Food - Milk; Work - Draught	Usually black and White markings are found on forehead, legs and tail in few animals. Horns are very long and extend beyond shoulder blade.	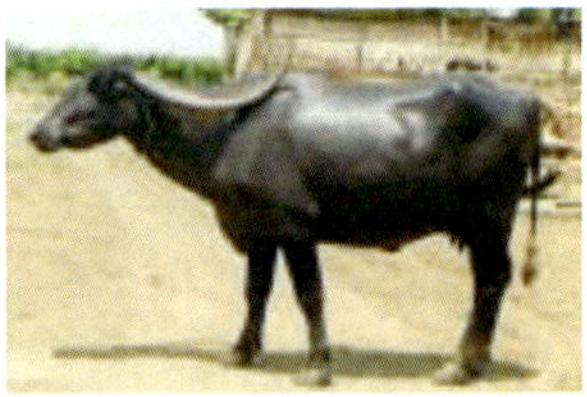
12	Surti	Vadodara, Bharuch, Kheda, Surat districts of Gujarat	Food - Milk	Coat colour varies from rusty brown through siliver- grey to black. Skin is black or brown. Medium sized animal, two white bands below the neck. Horns are flat; sickles shaped and are directed down ward and backward, and then turn upward at the tip to form a hook.	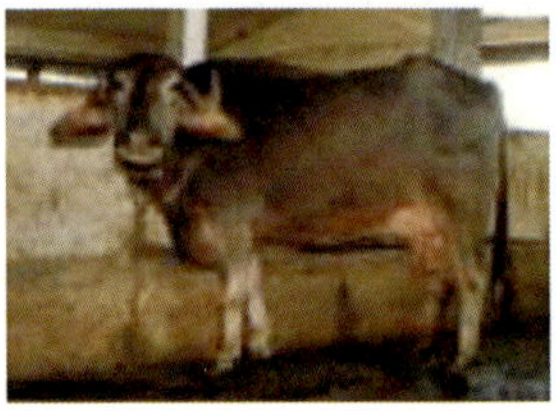

13	Toda	Nilgiri District of Tamil Nadu	Work - Draught; Socio-cultural - Religious ceremonies	In adult buffaloes the predominant coat colours are fawn and ash-grey. Horns long (62cm) and are variable in shape. They are usually set wide apart, outward, slightly downward and upward with the points being recurved inward, forming characteristically a crescent shape or semicircle. A narrow band of dense hair covering the top line from the crest of neck to the point of origin of tail, two chevron markings - one just around the jowl and the other anterior to the brisket.	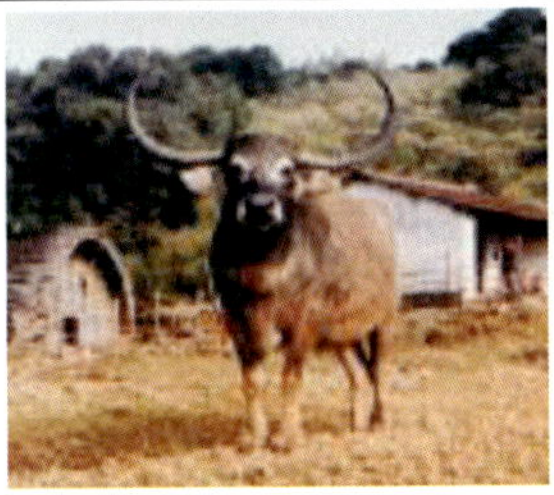

Source: http://14.139.252.116/agris/breed.aspx visited on 27/01/2018

Sheep genetic resources of India

Small ruminants play an important role in the rural economy. They are principally maintained by poor sections of rural community providing them a source of livelihood. In hilly, drought prone and desert areas, the weaker section population mainly rely on animal husbandry and sheep in particular sheep have ability to graze very close, and utilize spares vegetation on which other species of livestock may not able to sustain. Sheep farming can be started with less investments and farmers and landless labourers can generate more profit. sheep rearing have numerous hand up, such as: indigenous sheep get well along with Indian extreme environment and indigent management practices, Sheep are suitable for wool and meat, and farmer can get average of 1-2 kids per sheep per tupping, The meat rate is increasing day-by-day, Average meat recovery of 22-30 kg/ sheep and Penning leads to manurial value to land.

Sheep genetic resources of India are represented by 42 well-defined breeds and sizeable non-descript populations in various agro-ecological conditions. The defined breeds have developed owing to natural selection for adaptation to ecological conditions coupled with human intervention to meet out his requirements. The non-descript populations of sheep have developed as a result of indiscriminate breeding and intermixing of breeds. The sheep genetic resources of

India can be classified according to their distribution in northern-temperate, northwestern arid and semi-arid, southern peninsular, and eastern regions identified based on agro-ecological conditions and prevalence of sheep types over there. Most of the Indian sheep breeds are used for dual purpose, such as for mutton and carpet wool. North-western arid and semi-arid regions have some important sheep breeds, such as Chokla, Jaisalmeri, Marwari, Magra, Malpura Nali, and Sonadi. The Chokla and Nali breeds are found in Rajasthan and are suited for carpet-wool producing sheep breeds. The state of Rajasthan possessed highest sheep population as per record.

The description of 42 well-defined recognized breeds of sheep, their distribution & characteristics are presented in Table 6.

Table 6: Descript sheep breeds of India, its distribution and their characteristics

S. No.	Name of Breed	Breeding Tract	Utility	Characteristics	Image (Source*)
1	**Balangir**	Balangir, Sambalpur, Sundergarh districts of Odisha.	Meat; Fibre - Wool	White or light brown or of mixed colour. Ears are small and stumpy. Fleece is extremely coarse, hairy and open. Legs and belly are devoid of wool.	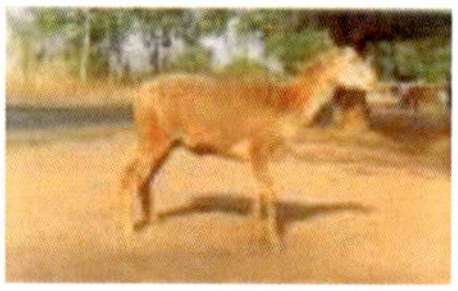
2	**Bellary**	Bellari and Davangere districts and adjoining areas of Haveri and Chitradurga districts	Meat; Fibre Wool	Coat colour comprises black and white. Most of the animals are black with patches of white all over the body including head, thorax, abdomen, belly and legs. Ears are tubular and medium in size.	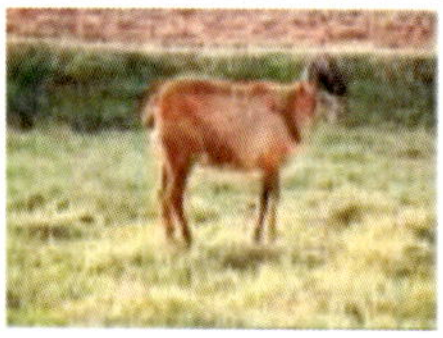
3	**Bhakarwal**	Jammu & Kashmir	Meat; Fibre - Wool	Generally white. Head is black in colour. Horns are curved backward and downwards. Ears are horizontal and directed backwards. Body coat is wooly. Head, face and legs are devoid of wool.	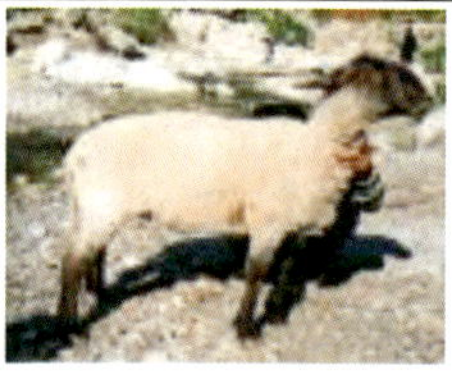
4	**Bonpala**	Sikkim	Meat; Fibre - Wool.	Fleece colour ranges from completely white to completely black and have generally mixed colour of black and white. Horns are directed slightly upward before running backward, and then twisted forward and outward. Tall, leggy, well - built animals. Nose is typically roman type.	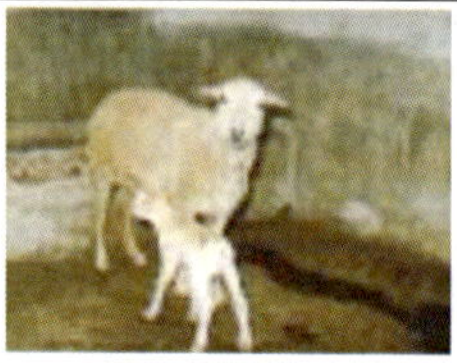

5	**Changthangi**	Leh district of Jammu & Kashmir	Fiber - Wool; Meat	Horns are long, curving backward and downward, Good fleece covers of extraordinarily long staple. Ears are drooping and medium in size.	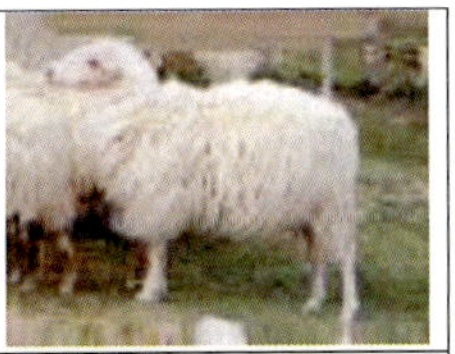
6	**Chevaadu**	Tirunelveli district of Tamilnadu	Meat, Skin, Religious and cultural use	Dorsal part of the body is light brown in colour and the ventral part, from the jaw to inguinal region, is lighter than the dorsal part of the body and these animals are called as "Arichevaadu".	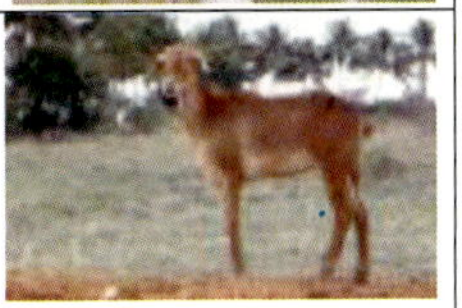
7	**Chokla**	Nagaur, Sikar, Churu district of Rajasthan	Fibre - Wool; Food - Meat	The coat colour is white. The face colour is dark brown (Raata Munda). Light to medium sized animals, face is generally devoid of wool. Ears are tubular.	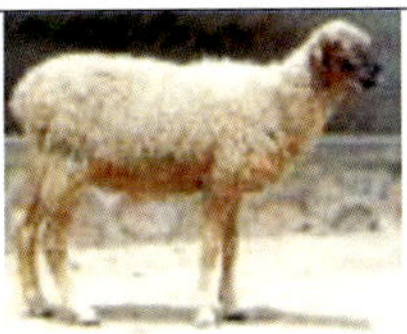
8	**Chotta-nagpuri**	Chottanagpur region of Jharkhand and adjacent districts of West Bengal	Meat; Fibre - Wool	Mostly brown in colour, some are white, black or black and brown. Ears are small and parallel to the head. Fleece is coarse, hairy and open. Females are polled.	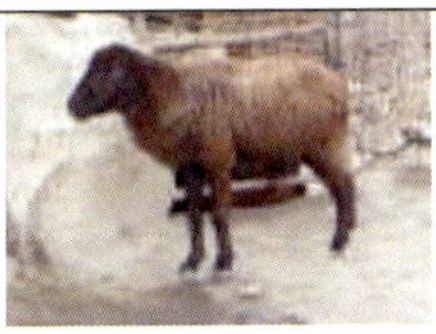
9	**Coimbatore**	Tamil Nadu, and Kerala	Meat; Fibre - Wool	Body colour is white with varying extent of black or brown on face, ears and neck also extending up to shoulder, chest and back. Ears are medium sized and horizontally placed.	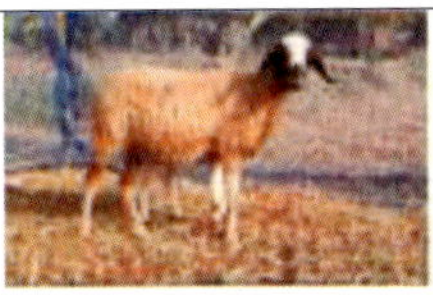
10	**Deccani**	Maharashtra A.P. and Karanataka. The soils in the breeding tract ranged from light to deep black cotton soils.	Meat; Fiber - Wool	Colour Predominantly black or black with white markings	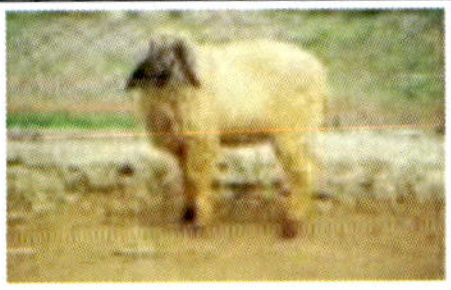
11	**Gaddi**	Himachal Pradesh	Fibre - Wool ; Meat	Colour Usually white although tan, brown and black and mixtures. The ears are small. Fleece is relatively fine and dense	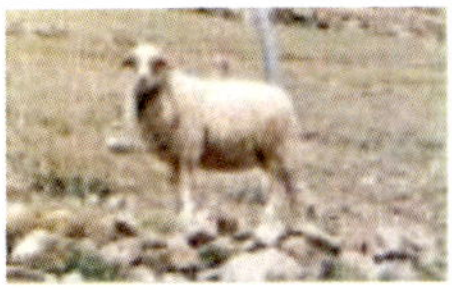

12	**Ganjam**	Odisha	Meat	Medium sized animals. Ears are medium sized and drooping (13 cm). Nose line is slightly convex. Fleece is hairy and short.	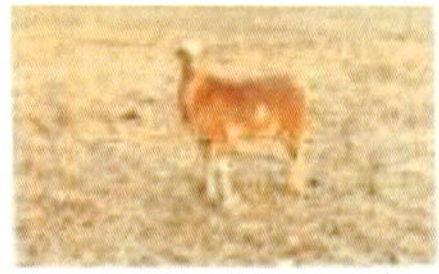
13	**Garole**	West Bengal. Breeding tract comprises of Sunderban area	Meat	Mostly grey in colour. White, Black, and Brown. Horns are Straight and little curved in the end. Small in size. Garole sheep have the ability to graze in knee-deep conditions in marshy land.	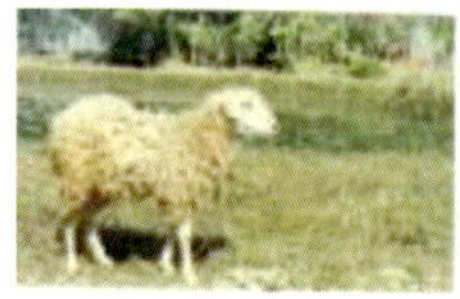
14	**Gurez**	Found in Gurej Tehsil of Baramulla district in Northern Kashmir.	Meat; Fibre - Wool	Body colour is predominantly white with brown or black colour on muzzle and around eyes. Body is mostly well covered with white fleece.	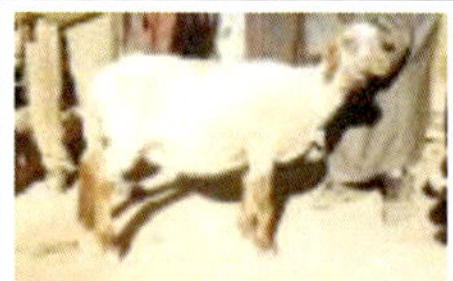
15	**Hassan**	Hassan district of Karnataka	Meat; Fibre - Wool	Colour White body with light brown or black spots. Fleece is white.	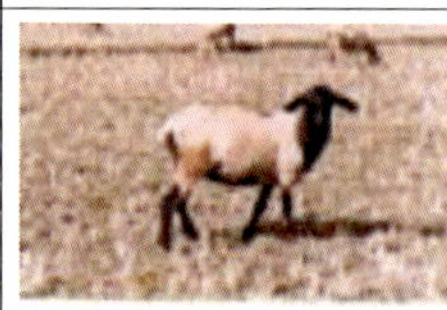
16	**Jaisalmeri**	Barmer, Bikaner, Jaisalmer, Jodhpur districts of Rajasthan	Fibre - Wool; Food - Meat	Face is black or dark brown, the colour extends up to the neck.	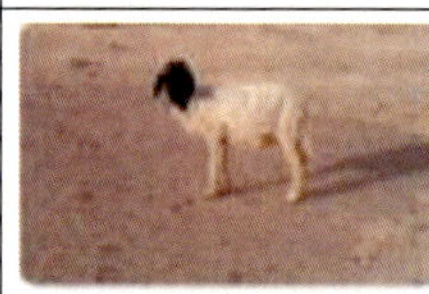
17	**Jalauni**	Madhya Pradesh and Uttar Pradesh	Meat; Fibre - Wool	White body colour with white or black face. Straight nose line. Fleece is coarse, short stapled, open and generally white in colour.	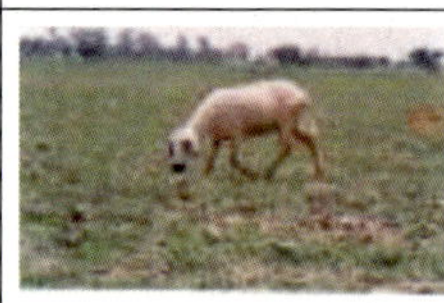
18	**Karnah**	Jammu & Kashmir	Fibre - Wool; Food - Meat	Body colour is white with a few animals having black or brown spots on face. Horns take a backward turn and then forward and upward with pointed tips.	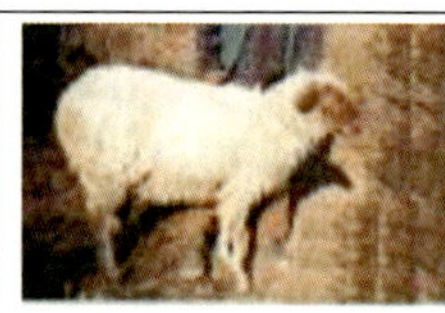
19	**Katchaikatty Black**	Madurai district of Tamil Nadu	hair, ram fighting and meat	Animals are medium in size, compact body. Face concave with depression, Tail is short and slender	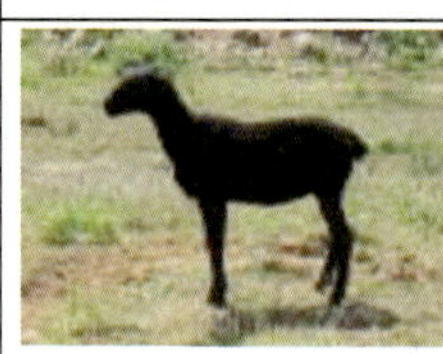

20	**Kendrapada**	Odisha	Meat	Colour Brown,	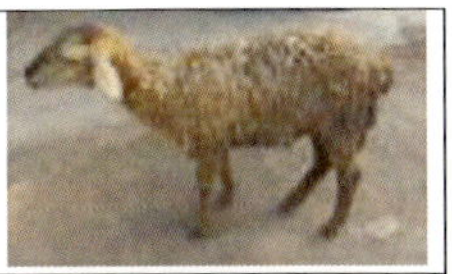
21	**Kenguri**	Karnataka.	Meat	The body coat is dark brown or coconut coloured. In most cases, there is a white spot on the forehead and sometimes on legs and other body parts also. Horns are Thick & curved with pointed tips running Backward, outward and downward.	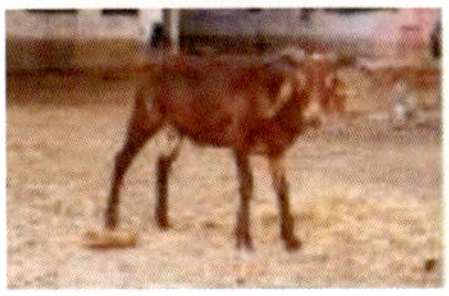
22	**Kilakarsal**	Tamil Nadu	Meat	Dark tan coat dorsally, black colour ventrally – under belly and inner side of legs. Black colour noticed above eyelids and either side of the lower jaw. Ears are leaf like, semi pendulous and medium sized.	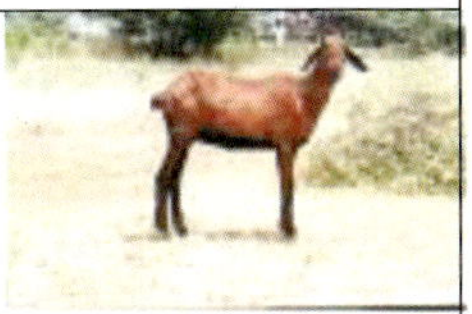
23	**Madras Red**	Tamil Nadu	Meat	Colour Red. Intensity varies from tan to dark brown. Some have white markings at the forehead, inner aspect of thigh and lower abdomen. Typical prominent Roman nose. Ears are pendulous.	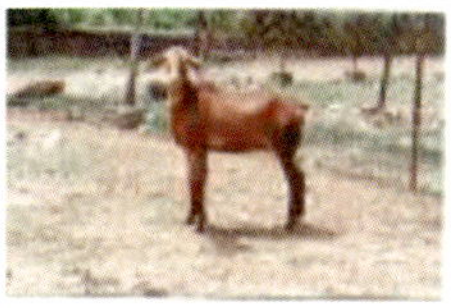
24	**Magra**	of Rajasthan	Wool; Food - Meat	Colour White. Face is white with brown patches around the eyes. Skin colour is pink. Ears are stumpy or small and tubular.	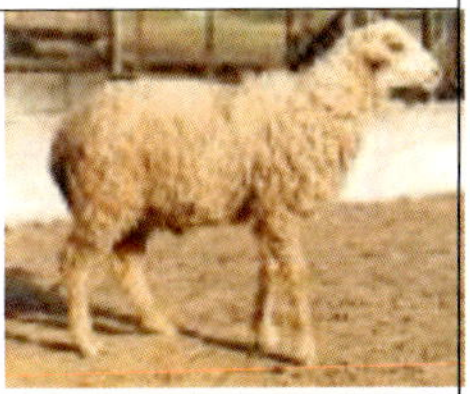
25	**Malpura**	Rajasthan	Fibre Wool; Meat	Face colour is light brown extending up to the neck. Fleece is white. Both polled. Nose is typically roman. Ears are short and tubular with a small.	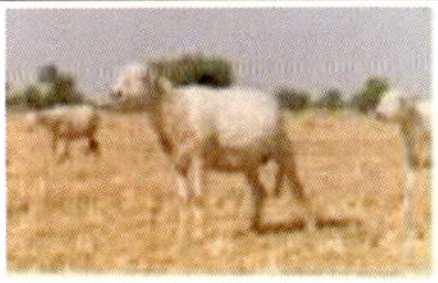
26	**Mandya**	Mysore and Bangalore rural districts	Food - Meat	The coat color is white with light brown face usually extending up to neck. Compact body with a typical reversed U- shape conformation from the rear. Roman nose.	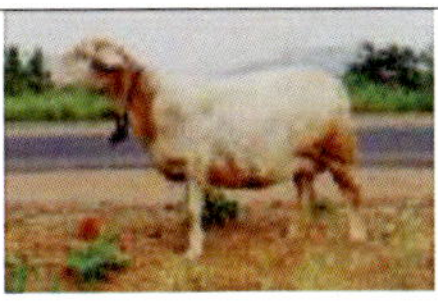

27	**Marwari**	Rajasthan	Fibre - Wool; - Meat	Face is typically black and the colour extends up to lower part of neck. Fleece is white. Ears are tubular and extremely small in size. Nose is straight, flat and tapering.	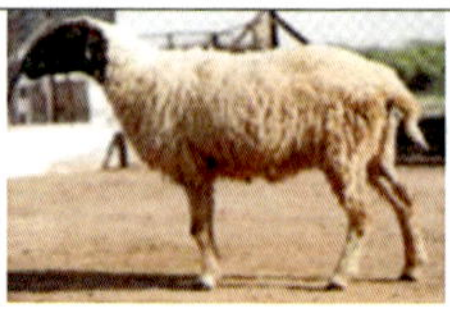
28	**Mecheri**	Salem district and Perundurai Taluk of Erode district.	Meat; Skin	Body colour is light tan with darker shade over the neck. Both polled. Animals are medium in size with leggy stature. Nose line is slightly roman. The chest is broad. Ears are of medium size.	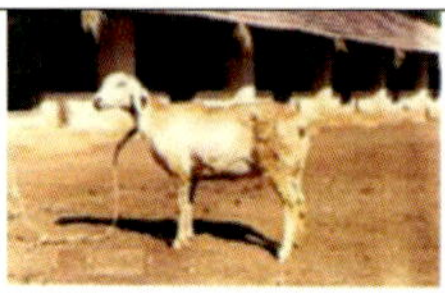
29	**Muzzafarnagri**	Uttar Pradesh and Uttarakhand	Meat; Fibre - Wool	Face and body white with occasional patches of brown or black. Both polled. Face is slightly convex. Ears are long and drooping. Fleece is white, coarse and open.	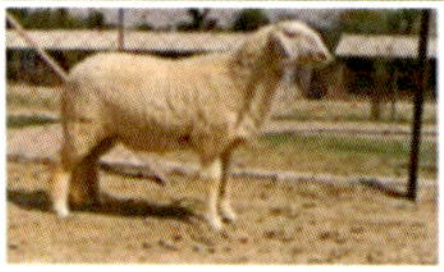
30	**Nali**	Rajasthan	Fibre - Wool; Meat	Colour White. Face is light brown which may extend to the neck. Ears are large and leafy. Fleece is white and coarse	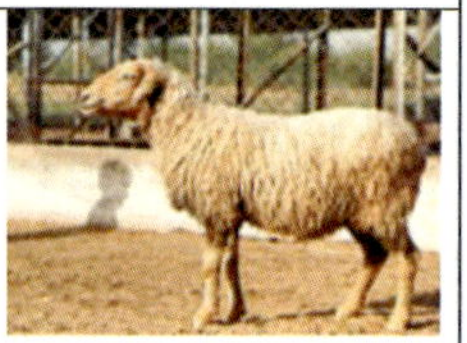
31	**Nellore**	Andhra Pradesh	Meat	Body colour Red or white with or without black colour on the ventral side. Tall animal with little hair except at brisket, withers and breech. Ears are long and drooping.	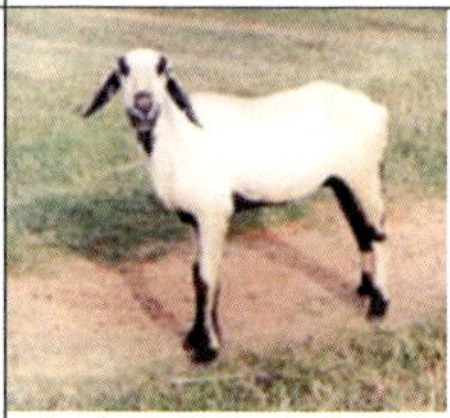
32	**Nilgiri**	Nilgiri hills of Tamil Nadu state	Meat; Fibre - Wool	The coat colour is generally white. A small horny scur is present in males. Face line is convex, giving a typical roman nose. Ears are generally pendulous.	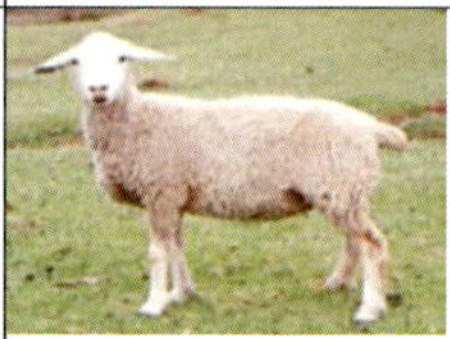
33	**Patanwadi**	Gujarat	Fibre - Wool; Meat	Face colour is light to dark brown. Fleece is white. Typically roman nose. Ears are medium to large with hairy tuft. The migratory sheep have larger body and long legs. They have coarse fleece.	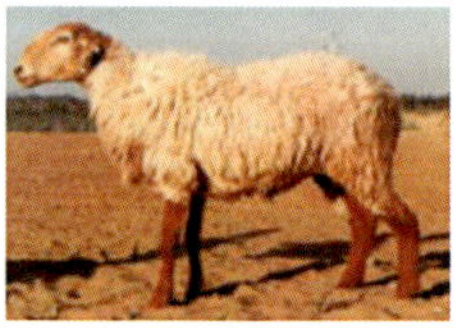

34	**Poonchi**	Poonch, Rajouri district of Jammu & Kashmir	Fibre - Wool	Predominantly white in colour, including the face, but spotted animals are also seen. Medium sized animals. Nose and forehead is flat. Ears are medium in size and drooping. Body is covered with white, medium to coarse fleece.	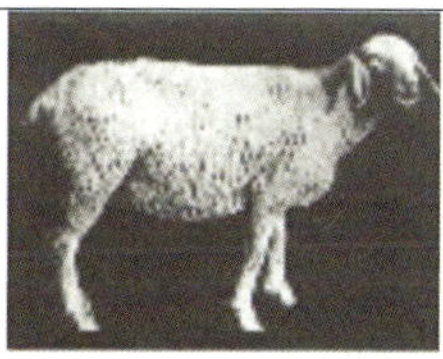
35	**Pugal**	Rajasthan	Meat; Fibre - Wool	Fleece colour varies from white to light brown. Face is black with small light brown strips on either side above the eyes. Lower jaw is typically light brown. Both polled. Ears are short and tubular. White fleece of medium carpet quality.	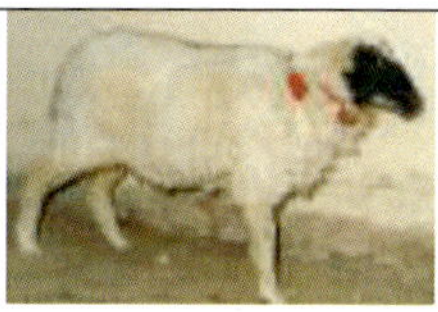
36	**Ramnad White**	Tamil Nadu	Meat	Pre-dominantly white with black colour on the ventral aspect of the body, in the region of inner canthi of eyes extending to poll, angle of mouth, lower lip, chin, throat, brisket, tips and border of the ears, and fore and hind limbs. Body is covered with short hair.	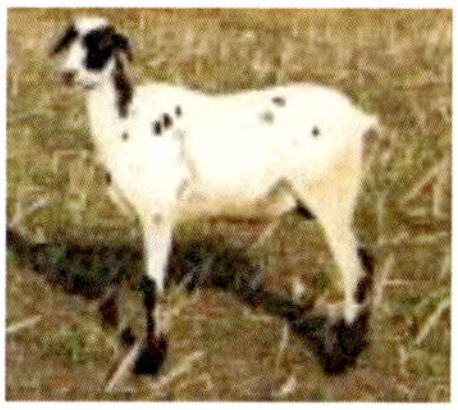
37	**Rampur Bushair**	Himachal Pradesh	Fibre - Wool; Meat; Pelt	Fleece colour is predominantly white with brown extremities including face, neck, belly and legs. Medium to large in size. Ears are flat and drooping. Roman nose. Fleece is of medium quality and dense.	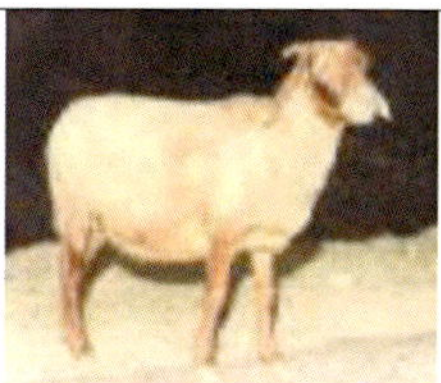
38	**Shahbadi**	Gaya, Shahbad districts of Bihar	Meat; Fibre - Wool	Fleece colour is mostly grey, sometimes with black spots. Ears are long (16.63 cm) and drooping. Fleece is extremely coarse, hairy and open. Legs and belly are devoid of wool.	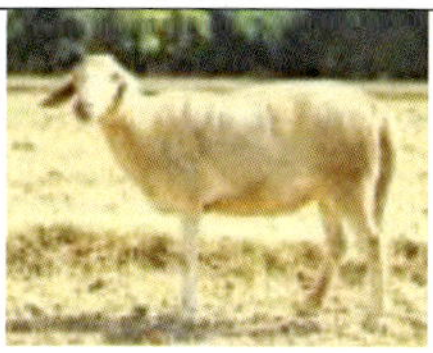

39	**Sonadi**	Rajasthan	Fibre - Wool; Meat	The face colour is light brown or white. Body is covered with white, open and coarse fleece. Ears are long (16-17cm), flat and drooping. White fleece, extremely coarse and hairy.	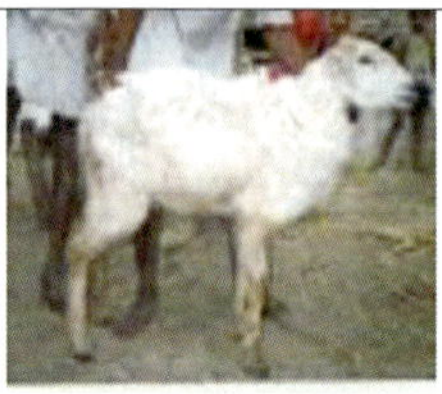
40	**Tibetan**	Northern Sikkim and Kameng district of Arunachal Pardesh.	Meat; Fibre - Wool	Mostly white with black or brown face. Brown or white spots are also observed on the body. Spiral horns running upward, downward and upward with a sharp tip. The nose line is convex. Fleece is relatively fine and dense. Brown or black wool on neck.	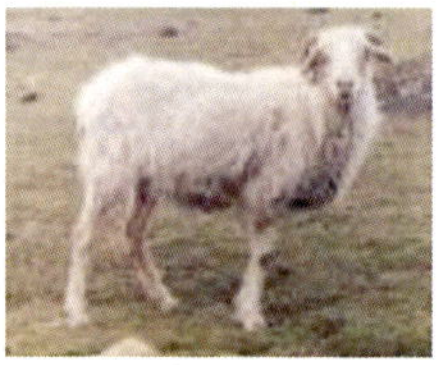
41	**Tiruchi Black**	Tamil Nadu	Meat	Body is completely black. Horns are found in males only. Small sized animals. Ears are short (9.59 cm), directed downward and forward. Fleece is extremely coarse, hairy and open.	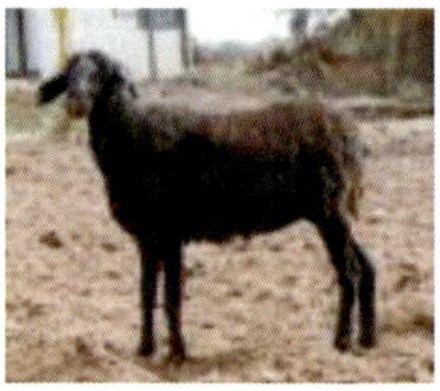
42	**Vembur**	Thoothukudi/Tuticorin districts of Tamilnadu	Meat	Body colour is white with fawn to black patches all over the body. Horns are found in males, only Tall animals. Ears are long and drooping. The body is covered with short hairs.	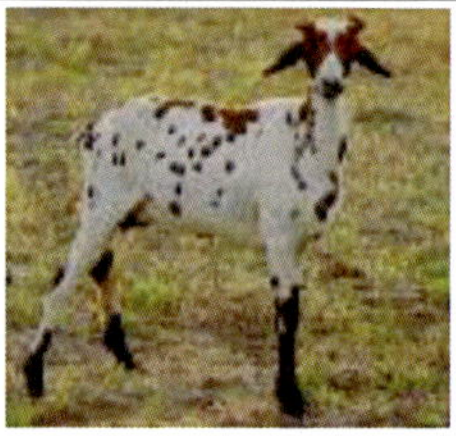

*Source: 14.139.252.116/agris/breed.aspx visited on 27/01/2018
Poonchi- http://www.sheepfarm.in/poonchi-sheep-breed-profile-information visited on 27/01/18

Goat genetic resources of India

Goat husbandry is the backbone of the economy of small and landless farmers in India. It is a guarantee against crop devastation and provides another source of livelihood to the farmers throughout the year. Goats provide dependable source of income to 40% of the rural population who are below the poverty line.The estimated population of goats of the country is 135.17 million consisting of 37.61 m males and 97.55 m females (19th Livestock census, 2012). The goat contributes about 26.40% to the total livestock population of the country and that next to the cattle (37.28%). However, goat population has been decreased by 3.82% as compared to the population (140.53 million) reported in 18th Livestock census, 2007, in spite of the fact that approximately 41% of goats are slaughtered for meat per year. Among the different states, the maximum decrease in goat population was recorded in West Bengal (-23.65%), while Assam showed 42.81% increase in goat population followed by Bihar (19.54%), Chhattisgarh (16.52%), Gujarat (6.87%) and Uttar Pradesh (5.36%). Presently, goat genetic resources of India are represented by 28 well-defined breeds. The geographical distribution of descript goats has been shown in Table 7.

Table 7: Descript goats breeds of India, its distribution and their characteristics

S. No.	Name	Home Tract	Main Use	Characteristic	Photograph
1	Attapady Black	Palakkad / Palghat districts of Kerala	Mutton	Colour Black. Horns Present in sex, Curved and oriented backwards and Small in size. Extremities are black. Tail is bunchy type.	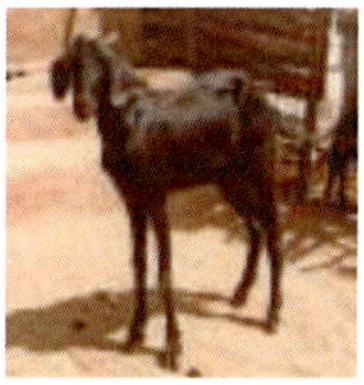
2	Barbari	Mathura, Agra and Etah, Etawah districts of U. P. and Bharatpur districts of Rajasthan.	Milk and Meat	Colour-White with tan spots, black spots in few. Horns are twisted, directed upward and outward. Large in size. Small sized animals, twisted horns. Ears - small and erect, tubular.	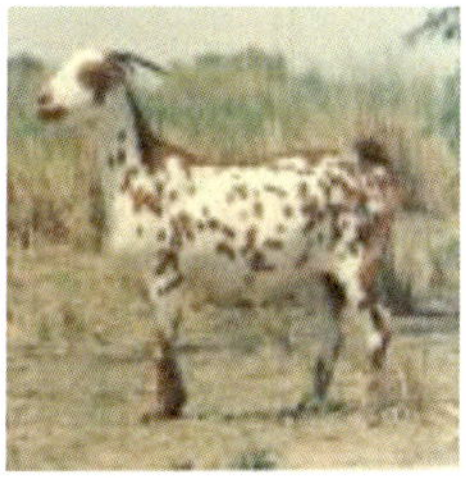
3	Beetal	Ferozpur, Amritsar and Gurdaspur districts of Punjab	Milk and Meat	Beetal goats are tall animals, having roman nose and long ears (24.8 cm).Black coat is common. Horn Small in size (about 12 cm), carried horizontally with slight twist, directed backward and upward.	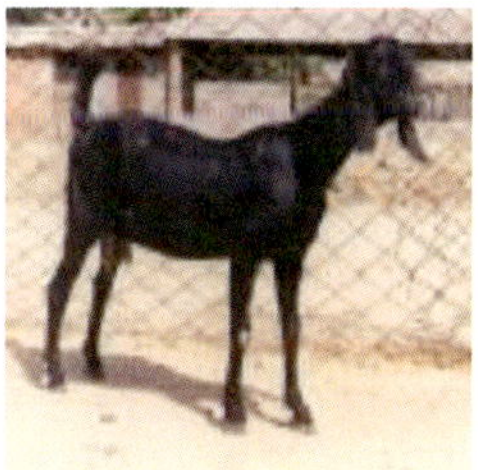

4	Berari	Amravati, Wardha, Nagpur and Akola districts of Maharashtra	Mutton	Colour, Light to dark tan. Horns Flat, small, oriented upward and backward. Black coloured ring around neck in adult male. Black hair line along with the vertebral column extending upto tail in both sexes.	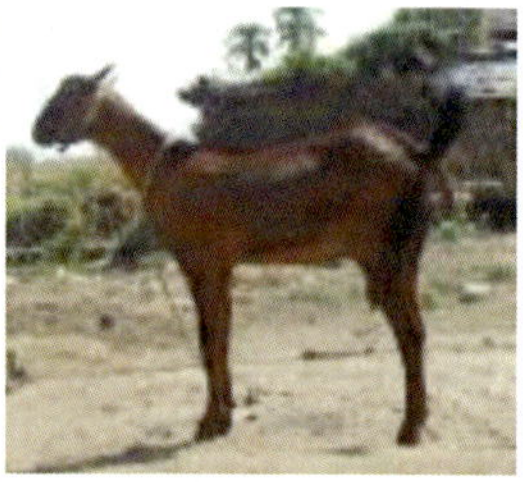
5	Black Bengal	West Bengal, Bihar, Jharkhand, Orisha, Assam and Tripura.	Meat	Colour predominantly black, brown, grey and white are also found. Small in size, directed upward and sometimes backward. Small-legged goat. Haircoat is short and lustrous. Nose line is slightly depressed.	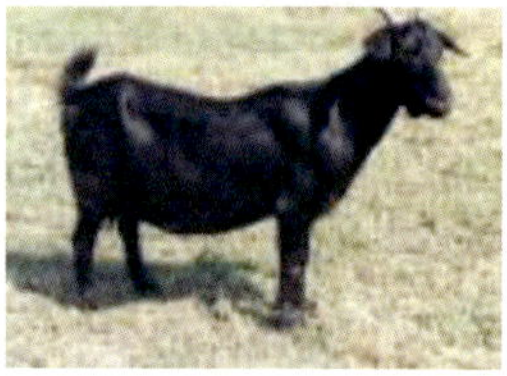
6	Changthangi	Leh and Kargil districts of Jammu &Kashmir	Fibre-Hair (Pashmina); Meat	Horn large and twisted like a corkscrew, turned outward, upward and inward to form a semi-circle. Medium sized animals and sturdily built. Ears small, erected and stumpy.	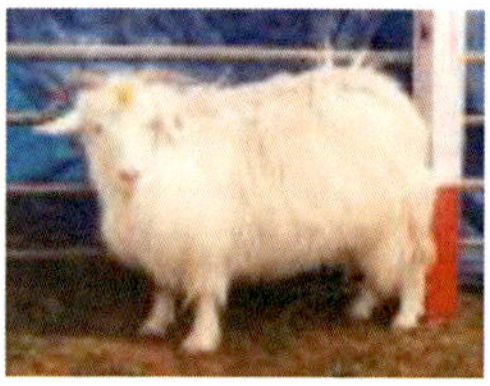
7	Chegu	Chamba, Kinnaur and Lahul&Spiti districts of Himachal Pradesh	Fibre - Hair (Pashmina); Meat.	Colour compact white, black, grey, brown. Horns are long, cork shaped, directed upward, backward and inward/outward, medium to large in size. Reddish/tan/black coloration mostly around head & neck, and abdominal areas.	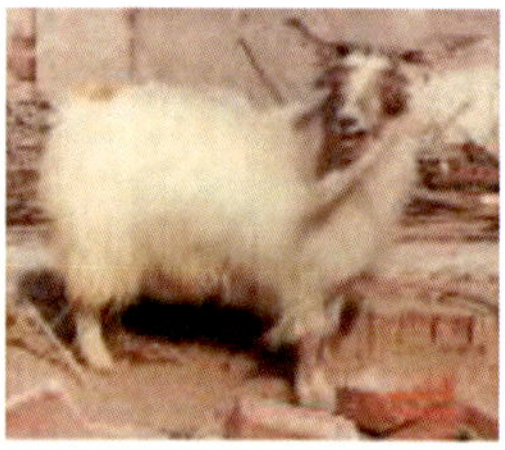
8	Gaddi	Himachal Pradesh and Jammu & Kashmir	Meat; Fibre - Hair;	White is dominant colour. Black coloured animals are also present. Horns directed upward and backward and occasionally twisted and are long in size. Ears are drooping and pointed.	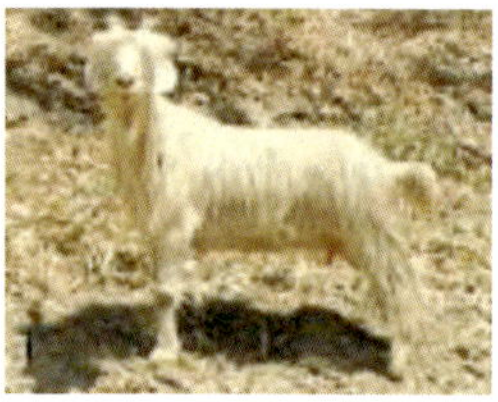

9	Ganjam	Ganjam, Rayagada, Gajapati, Khurda and Nayagarh districts of Odisha	Meat, milk	Black or Brown black. White, brown and spotted animals are also found. Horns twisted and curved. Long, parallel and pointed backward and upward. Head convex, ears are long and drooping.	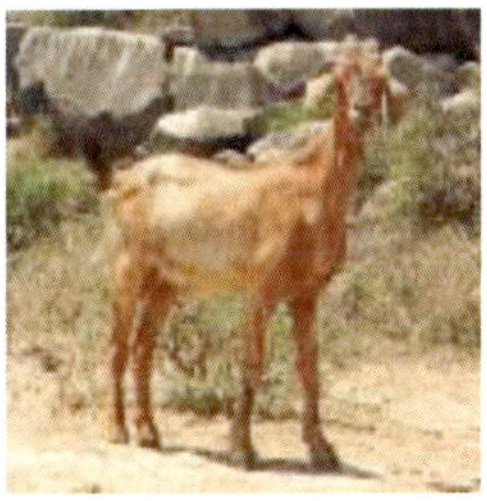
10	Gohilwadi	Amreli, Bhavnagar, Junagadh, Rajkot and Porbandar districts of Gujarat	Meat and Milk	Colour black, Horns are slightly twisted and turned upward, outward and backward. Nose line is slightly convex. Ears are tubular and drooping. Body covered with coarse long hairs.	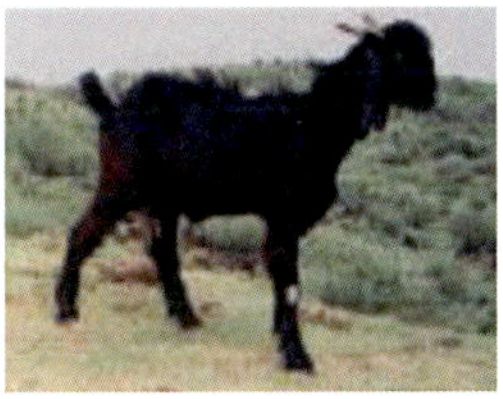
11	Jakhrana	Alwar district of Rajasthan.	Milk and Meat	Colour predominantly black, black with white spots. White ears, White face mask. Horns curved upward and backward and medium sized. Straight face line. Forehead is narrow and slightly bulging.	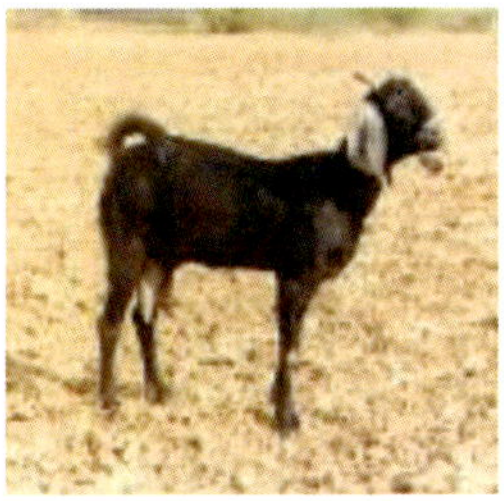
12	Jamunapari	Chakarnagar area of Etawah district of Uttar Pradesh	Food - Milk and Meat	Colour white with patches of tan mostly on head and neck. Horns small, sword shaped running backward and upward. Face is large and convex having tuft of hairs. Ears are long (about 30cm) flat and drooping.	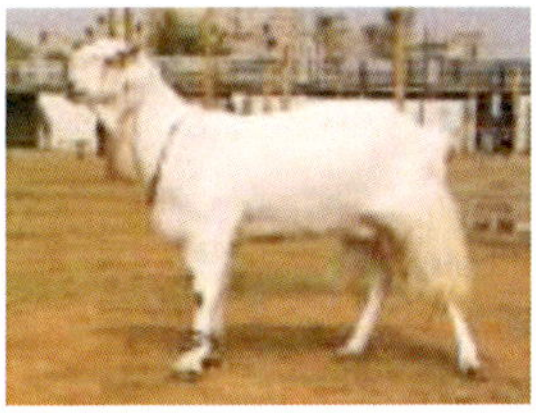
13	KanniAdu	Tamil Nadu	Meat	Colour generally Black with two white stripes on either side of the face and white colour in the underbelly and inner side of the legs. Horns directed backward and curved upward are predominantly present. White lines on the edge of ears.	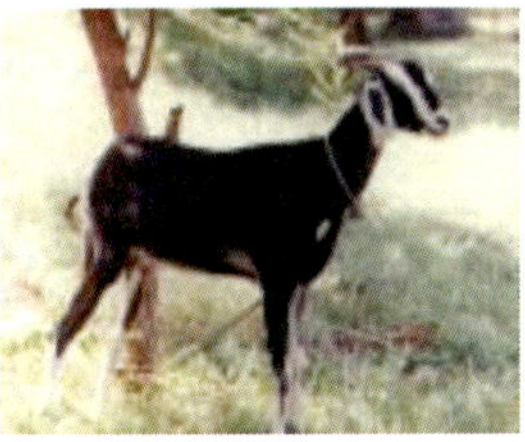

14	KodiAdu	Tamil Nadu	Meat, Skin and Manure	Colour white with splashes of black or reddish brown colour. Horns directed upward, backward and curved downward or upward and sharp at the tip. KodiAdu goats are tall, long, lean and leggy animals with compact body.	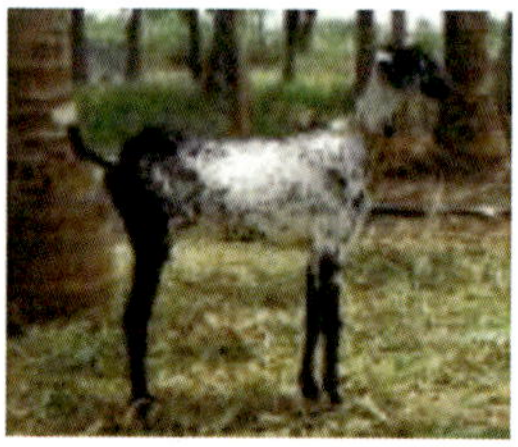
15	Konkan Kanyal	Hilly tract of Konkan coastal region. Sindhu durg district of Maharashtra	Mutton	Colour black with white marking on collar, lower jaw and ventral surface. Horns cylindrical, backward. Bilateral white strips from nostrils to ear. Legs- long, laterally black, medially white and white from knee to fetlock joint.	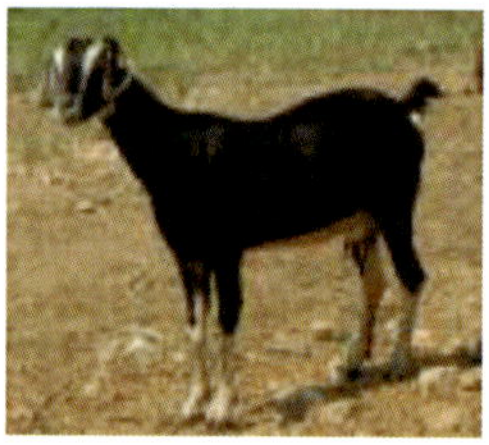
16	Kutchi	Mahesana, Kutchchh and Patan districts of Gujarat	Food - Meat and Milk	Coat is pre-dominantly black. White spots on neck, mouth and ear region. Horns are small to long, corckscrew type horns.	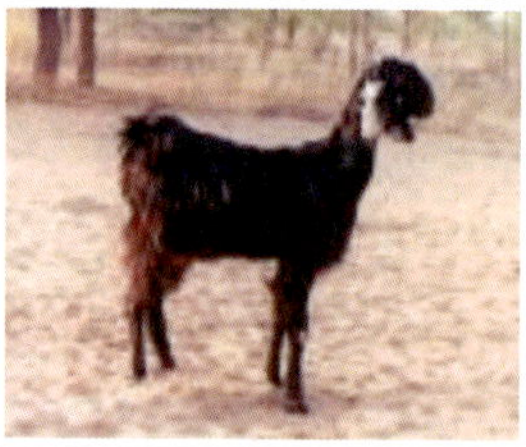
17	Malabari	Kannur/Cannanore and Calicut district of Kerala	Milk and Meat	Colour majority complete white. Some are black or brown. Horns Small in size and slightly twisted directed outward and upward. Medium sized ears, directed outward and downward reaching up to the nose.	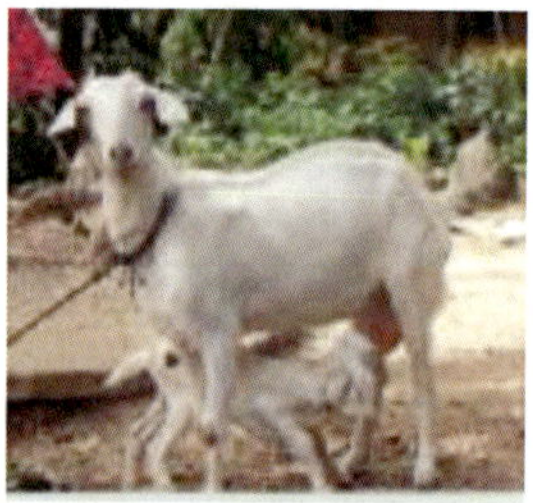
18	Marwari	Bikaner, Jaisalmer, Jodhpur, Nagaur and Pali districts of Rajasthan	Meat and Milk	Colour Black. Horns corkscrew type, directed upward and backward. Small to long in size. Long shaggy hairy coat. Pendulous ears. Thick beard in both sexes.	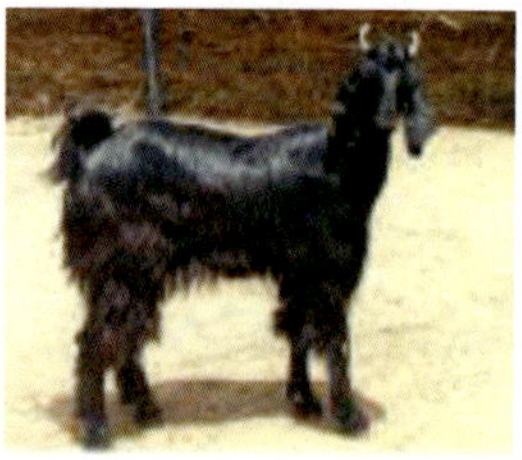

19	Mehsana	Ahmadabad Gandhi-nagar, Mahesana, and Patan district of Gujarat	Meat and Milk	Colour black with white ear base. Horns medium sized. Screw type, twisted slightly, curved upward and backward and pointed at the tips. White spots are present on the upper part of upper muzzle and look like a ring in some of the animals.	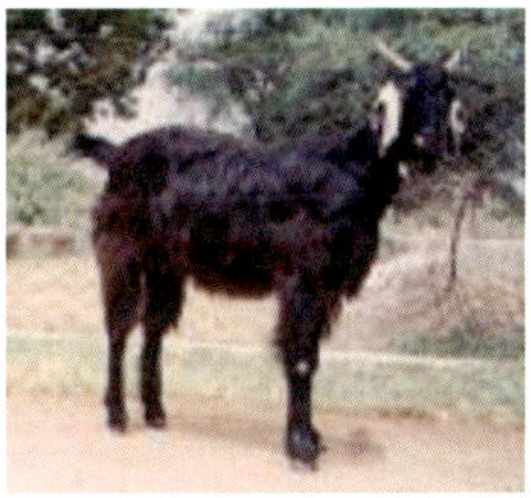
20	Osmanabadi	Ahmad-nagar, Solapur and Osmanabad districts of Maharashtra	Meat	Predominant colour is black. White colour is noticed only on ears and some spots on neck and forehead. Horns are straight/ curved and small in size running backward, upward and downward.	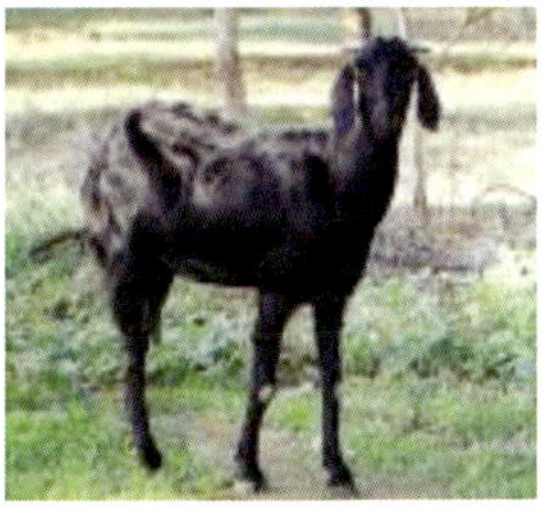
21	Pantja	Pantnagar, U.S.Nagar, Nainital (Uttara-khand) and adjoining districts of U.P	Dual (Che-von, Milk)	Fawn to brown colour, Small sized. Triangular, twisted, slightly upwards and backwards, pointed tip. White streak on either side of face. Ears are pendulous.	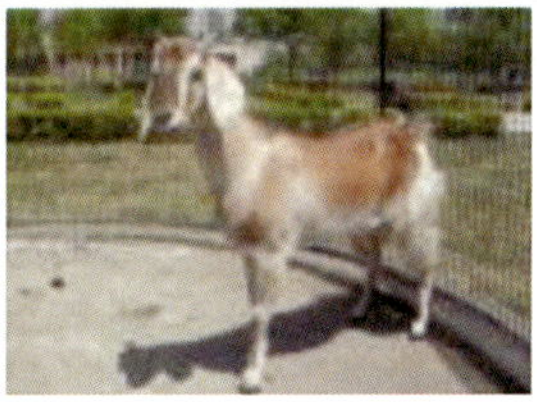
22	Salem Black	Tamil Nadu	Meat and Skin	Colour completely black with glossy hair coat. Salem Black goats are tall, long, lean and leggy animals with compact body. The ears are medium in length, leaf-like and semi-pendulous. Neck is thick, broad and well set to the thorax in males.	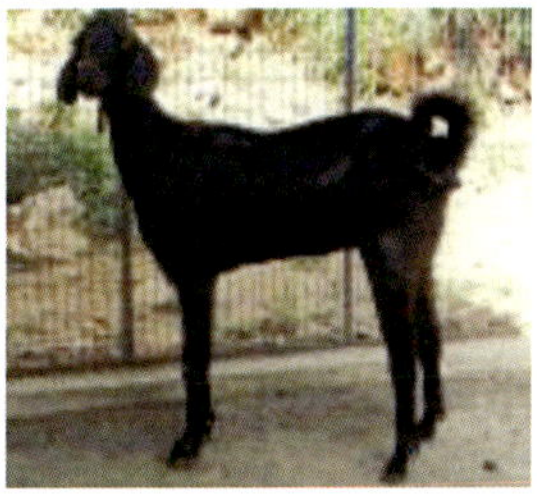
23	Sangamneri	Nashik, Ahmad-nagar and Pune districts of Maharashtra	Milk and Meat	Colour generally white. White mixed with Black and Brown are also seen. Horns are thin pointed, directed backward and upward. Hair coat is extensively coarse and short.	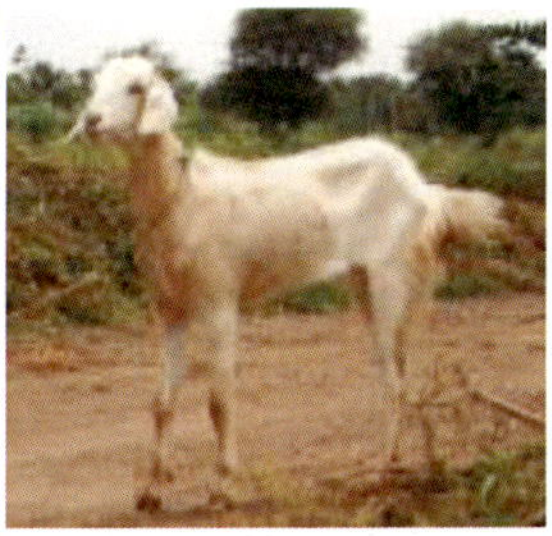

24	Sirohi	Ajmer, Bhilwara, Chittorgarh, Sirohi and Udaipur districts of central and southern Rajasthan.	Milk and Meat	Coat colour is pre-dominantly brown with light or dark brown patches. Horns are slightly twisted and curved, directed upward and backward. Flat and leaf like drooping ears.	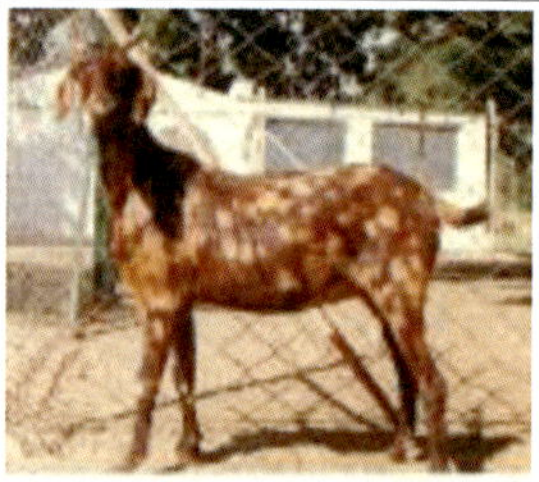
25	Sumi-Ne	Nagaland	Meat	Colour white with characteristic black markings on head, neck and legs. Ears are horizontal. Horns are pointed. Beard is present. Presence of long hair in adult animals is the most important phenotypic character. The length of the fibre, however, is more in case of male as compared to that of females	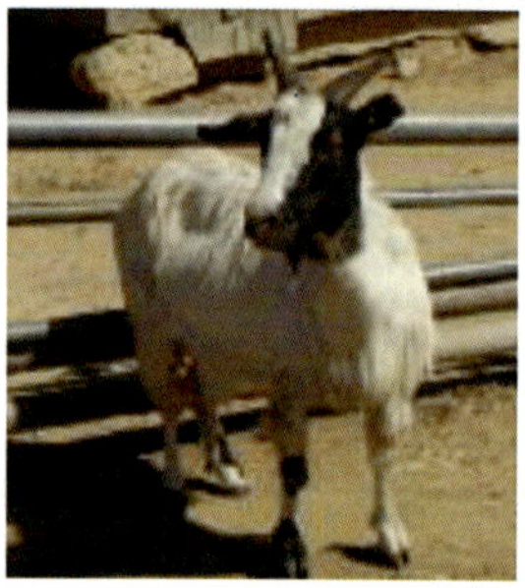
26	Surti	Gujarat	Meat and Milk	Colour white, black, tan, coffee and greyish color. Mottled animals are also found. Horns Small to medium in size, directed backward. Pendulous and medium sized ears. Well-developed udder with large conical teats.	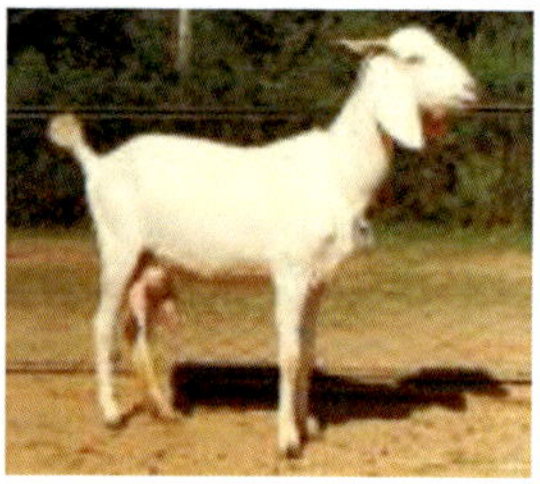

*Source: http://14.139.252.116/agris/breed.aspx visited on 27/01/2018

Importance of livestock diversity

Under the changing climatic conditions, we need to emphatically and scientifically acknowledge the superior traits of livestock breeds so that future generations can be benefitted from the invaluable genetic resources. In coming years, livestock-keeping will be continued to play an important role in the livelihoods of large numbers of small-scale farmers and pastoralists, many of them among the world's poor. Therefore, animal genetic resources will be critical for global food security and livelihoods in fulfilling the demand for energy, protein, and other critical nutrients. As per one estimate of FAO (2009), about a billion people rely directly on livestock for their livelihoods. In order to meet the country demand for animal products maintaining sufficient livestock diversity would be necessary to ensure adaptation potential in times of uncertainty and climate change.

This loss in livestock diversity has become a fundamental challenge as maintaining diversity is pre-requisite for adapting to future changes. It is expected that climate change will have direct effect on livestock productivity as well as indirectly through changes on the availability of feed and fodder. The rise in temperature due to climate change will create heat stress in livestock, less stable crop yields and lead to more frequent outbreaks of pests and diseases. Climate change will be the biggest challenge for deciding the direction of efforts of the global scientific community to preserve global food production system (Renaudeau *et al.*, 2012; Thornton *et al.*, 2009). Our Indigenous Livestock breeds have several anatomical and physiological factors that control the ability of animals to thermoregulate. Different animals have different respiration capacity, relative lung size, relationship between surface area per unit body weight, Properties of skin and hair, metabolic heat production and endocrinological profiles -these factors influence heat stress response. That uniqueness in characters is the result of evolutionary forces and their interactions over longer periods of time. The diverse livestock and poultry breeds of our country are adapted to various extremes of climatic conditions, production system and feed resources. The Indian native cattle *viz.* Sahiwal, Tharparkar, Hariana, Rathi, Gir and Nagori, *etc.* can survive in extremes of agro climatic. Kankrej an important cattle breed, is known for its adaptability to high temperature, powerful draught capacity and resistance to tick borne disease.

Similar to cattle, India is blessed with immense richness of buffalo diversity. In India, buffaloes are considered as major dairy species that contributes more than 50% of milk production in addition to draught power and meat. Buffaloes are established as an economically important species not only in India but also in many Asian and Mediterranean countries and its genetic improvement ranks high amongst agricultural research needs of these countries. India has exceptional and diversified buffalo germplasm. Murrah is known for high fat rich milk while Bhadawari have the highest milk fat. Chilka buffalo is known for adapting to brackish-water salinity conditions and similarly Banni buffalo is a unique breed adapted to drought hot-dry climate and it has nocturnal grazing ability. Likewise swamp buffalo of north-east India have excellent draft power.

Similarly India has remarkable diversity in sheep and goat. Gaddi sheep breed is adapted to temperate and low-oxygen environment. Garole sheep is known world over for its high prolificacy and adaptation to mangrove ecology. On the other hand, Chokla, Malpura, Marwari sheep and many other breeds from arid zones have adapted themselves to desert conditions. Many breeds of goat are also adapted to different ecological niche with high temperature, humidity or both, for example; Andaman goat is adapted to saline conditions, Changthangi is adapted to higher altitude temperate condition, whereas Jakhrana is well acclimatized to semi-arid condition. These diversified livestock populations provide great resource and options in meeting future challenges in changing environment, and human demands.

Conclusions

Indian animal production system comprised primarily of a mixed crop-livestock farming system. It is paramount for the security and existence of large numbers of poor and marginalized community of India. This kind of livestock husbandry system, provide income; create employment, less dependency on machines and utilization of draught power and manure. This production system expects special connotation in the relation of continued economic progress, enhancing income. It is well-established fact that India contributes significantly to world's livestock resources as documented by livestock census, 2012. Both the national economy as well as the socio-economic development of the country is supported by the livestock sector. The livestock sector is doing well in the area of animal products; now farmers are getting acquainted with value addition and are ready to export their farm produces, like dairy, wool, and other products. During the recent past, there has been a net loss of diversity because of an increased rate of disappearance of some of the traditional breeds of livestock (FAO, 2007). It is also pondered that species related to production and marketing systems with fast formalistic change show high extent of breeds that are currently at-risk and that also which have already been extinct. The indigenous farm animal breeds can be averted through their sustainable utilization. Efforts, like identifying unique biomolecules, producing high quality products with value addition could be more important as a measure of transforming the utility or making indigenous livestock more utilizable in today's context. Thus, it is imperative to have a thorough knowledge of the population structure and genetic diversity, as it can provide a far-sighted basis for the obligation of conservation. It will also help in sensible handling of native breeds as genetic resources to meet probable future demand of adaptation to ever mutable environment or production demands.

References

FAO. 2007. The State of the World's Animal Genetic Resources for Food and Agriculture, edited by Barbara Rischkowsky and Dafydd Pilling. Rome.

FAO. 2009. Status and trends report on animal genetic resources – 2008. CGRFA/WG-AnGR-5/09/Inf. 7.

FAO. 2013. In vivo conservation of Animal Genetic Resources. FAO Animal Production and Health Guidelines No. 14. Rome.

Thornton PK, Kruska RL, Henninger N, Kristjanson PM, Reid RS, Atieno F, OderoAN and Ndegwa T. (2002). Mapping poverty and livestock in the developing world. A report commissioned by the U K Department for International Development, on behalf of the Inter-Agency Group of Donors Supporting Research on Livestock Production and Health in the Developing World. Nairobi, International Livestock Research Institute.

Renaudeau D, Huc E and Noblet J. (2007).Acclimation to high ambient temperature in Large White and Caribbean Creole growing pigs. Journal of Animal Science 85: 779-790.

❑❑❑

Chapter 5

Role of Nutrients in Enhancing Livestock Productivity

Vinod Kumar, Shalini Vaswani and Avinash Kumar

Department of Animal Nutrition, College of Veterinary Science and Animal Husbandry, Uttar Pradesh Pandit Deen Dayal Upadhyaya Pashu Chikitsa Vigyan Vishwavidhyalaya Evam Go Anusandhan Sansthan, Mathura

Introduction

Livestock sector productivity depends on many factors, like genetic ability, feeding strategies, farm management and health. In developing countries, like India, it is evolving in response to rapidly increasing demand for livestock products. For higher productivity, a good dairy feeding program must consider the quantity, suitability of the feed and a time bound feeding programs. Imbalanced in feeding of dairy animals in particular leads to excess feeding of some nutrients whilst others remain deficient. To ensure high productivity, it is necessary to plan for feed resources through short and long term planning. Here are few examples of imbalance feeding in our feeding schedule and their bad effects: (1) Excessive grain feeding, (2) Oilcake (as *sani)* alone (3) Feeding of particular type of green or dry fodder in excess when in plenty (4) No supplementation of minerals supplement to compensate milk production requirement. All these feeding mismanagement leads to a number of production diseases in dairy animals. Balancing the ration of a dairy animal warrant proper knowledge of its (1) maintenance, growth and production requirements, (2) feed ingredients option available for feeding (3) Knowledge of nutrient composition (4) a sound feeding strategies for low cost. All these factors are keys to feeding a productive or transition animal for preventing production disease and higher production. In following paragraph, there is an outline of nutrient requirements of dairy animals and means to achieve a balance ration.

Role of nutrients in productivity

The nutrient requirements for animals include water, energy (TDN), protein (CP), minerals (calcium, phosphorus, magnesium potassium, sodium, and trace elements) and vitamins (especially vitamins A, D and E). The specific nutritional requirements for individual animals differ due to differences in genetic make-up, age, capacity, growth rate and desired gain or production, pregnancy, lactation, work, stresses, sickness, etc. the requirement for maintenance, growth and production of particular animal is calculated for dry matter (DM), total digestible nutrients (TDN), crude protein (CP), minerals and carotene. Requirements are met by giving available feed and fodder in a particular area to meet the requirement. The difference between nutrients in feeds fed and the actual requirements of the cattle must be made up by extra feed or supplements. The best quality feeds and pastures are reserved for the fast-growing and high-producing animals.

Energy : Energy is an important nutritional factor related to poor reproductive function in animals. The metabolic use of available energy in ruminants ranking each physiological state in order of importance are as follows: 1) basal metabolism, 2) activity, 3) growth, 4) energy reserves, 5) pregnancy, 6) lactation, 7) additional energy reserves, 8) estrous cycles and initiation of pregnancy, and 9) excess energy reserves (Ryan *et al.*, 1992). Energy content in diet of Indian animals is measured as total digestible nutrient (kg) or metabolizable energy or net energy. On an average for a crossbred animal a daily maintenance requirement of energy for lactating animal is about 30 g TDN and 107.0 Kcal ME/$W^{0.75}$kg and milk production requirement for per kg 4% FCM, energy requirement are 436 g TDN and 1082 Kcal ME. Out of which, about 45% energy is partitioned for maintenance and rest 55% for milk production (Saha *et al.*, 2013). The maintenance requirement lactating Indian cattle as TDN was 39.5 g/kg $W^{0.75}$ and for milk production and weight gain were 332 g/kg FCM and 1.78 g/g body weight gain, respectively (Paul *et al.*, 2004). In subcontinental condition, low quality fodders pre-dominates feeding regimen of dairy animals as a result, deficiency of energy in diet leads to adverse effect on health and production. Negative energy balance during early lactation in dairy cows leads to an altered metabolic state that has major effects on the production of IGF family members. Low IGF-I concentrations are associated with poor fertility. Metabolites and metabolic hormones that change in relation to negative energy balance, insulin-like growth factor-I (IGF-I) is strongly associated with the calving to conception interval and pregnancy outcome and their effect on oocyte (Leroy *et al.*, 2006), ovary (Llewellyn *et al.*, 2007), uterus (Butler, 2001) and oviduct (Fenwick *et al.*, 2008) effects embryo development, contributing to the high rates of embryonic mortality in dairy cows. In growing animals, low energy ration leads to decrease in growth rates and thus takes more time in gaining mature body weight.

Protein : A deficiency or excess of dietary protein has adverse effect in production. Over-feeding of protein has been associated with decreased pregnancy rates in female dairy cows (Blanchard *et al.*, 1990) and buffaloes (Qureshi *et al.*, 2002). The exposure to high levels of ammonia or urea may impair maturation of oocyte and subsequent fertilization or maturation of developing embryos. Overfeeding protein during the breeding season and early gestation, particularly if the rumen receives an inadequate supply of energy may be associated with decreased fertility (Dunn and Moss, 1992). This decrease in fertility may result from decreased uterine pH during the luteal phase of the estrous cycle in cattlefed high levels of degradable protein (mustard cake *sani*). Energy costs for detoxifying ammonia into urea (waste product resulting from excess protein) may aggravate an existing energy shortage resulting in reduced ovarian activity. This means that excess protein requires extra energy to remove it from the body. If cows are in a negative energy balance and are losing weight, they will lose even more weight because of the excessively high protein. Animals that lose excessive weight have a harder time re-breeding and probably won't until their weight begins to come back. Cows fed excess protein (more than 10-15% above requirements) required more services per conception and had longer calving intervals. The maintenance requirement of CP was estimated to be 6.27 g/kg $W^{0.75}$ whereas CP requirements for milk production and weight gain were 82.3 g/kg FCM and 0.44 g/g body weight gain, respectively (Paul *et al.*, 2004). For examples a cow weighing 350 kg, producing 10 liter of FCM need 1290 g CP and 6.6 kg TDN daily. Approximately dry matter intake of cow is 10 kg; diet of cow should have 10-13% protein and 65% TDN. This has to be met by feeding good quality fodders and concentrate to avoid production problems. Requirement of high yielding dairy cows i.e. Holstien cow producing 30-35 litre milk will be very high i.e. about 3.5-4.0 kg protein or ration DM containing about 16% protein.

Fat : Cows receiving high level of energy during the postpartum period had increased LH pulse frequency and decreased the period from parturition to ovulation (Perry *et al.*, 1991). Fatty acids and cholesterol are substrates for reproductive hormone synthesis (progesterone, prostaglandins). Therefore, the effects of fat may be independent to those of increased energy availability. In subcontinent animal diets usually contain 2 to 3% fat. Supplementing fat to improve reproduction was initially attempted to increase the energy density in the diet. High fat diets for cattle contain 5 to 8 % fat. Exceeding these dietary fat levels >8% impairs rumen function. For example a 400 kg body weight cow consuming 10 kg dry matter have about 300 g crude fat in their diet, thus there is scope of adding upto 500 g fat in daily diet for high yielders without any detrimental effect on rumen fermentation. Feeding high fat diets to cycling heifers and postpartum cows increased progesterone production and the lifespan of the corpus luteum (CL). Higher progesterone levels during the luteal phase generally result in improved fertility. Increasing dietary fat also results in increased follicular growth. Fat content of the diet should be increased above the typical 3% of diet DM for cows in the early postpartum period in order to meet the energy requirement. Feeding calcium salts of long chain fatty acids also improved pregnancy or conception rates (Thatcher and Staples, 2000).

Minerals : Minerals play an important role in nutrient utilization and several biochemical functions concerning production and reproduction. Minerals are very important nutrients for dairy animal production. Deficiency of minerals may leads to certain structural, physiological or immunological disorder affecting growth, production and reproductive health of animals. Minerals deficiency is an area specific problem and supplementation strategy must be revised accordingly. Requirements of minerals for reproduction and immunity are generally higher than maintenance requirement of animals. Supplementation of minerals requires correct knowledge of bioavailability, sources, requirement of animal and mineral interactions with other nutrients. (Kumar, 2015). The availability of minerals to cattle depends upon the production system, feeding practices, and environment. Macro-minerals include: calcium, phosphorus, magnesium, potassium, suphfur and salt are needed in relatively large amounts in the body. The trace minerals include: cobalt, copper, iodine, iron, manganese, selenium and zinc and are needed in very small or "trace" amounts in the body. Animals obtained minerals through the consumption of natural feeds, fodders and supplementation of inorganic salts in the ration. Mineral deficiencies and imbalances have long been held responsible for low production among cattle and buffaloes fed on crop residues in tropical agro-climatic condition. Mineral deficiencies and imbalances are often cited as causes of poor reproduction. It is clear that adequate amounts of minerals must be provided, but little is known about the effects of marginal deficiencies and imbalances. The same is true of excessive intakes of minerals, which may indeed be harmful.

Calcium (Ca) : Ca plays a very importance role in structural and physiological functions. Ratio of Ca: P between 1.5:1 and 2.5:1 for lactating cows caused no problems. Lactating cows must be provided with adequate amounts of Ca to maximize production and minimize health problems. Other function of calcium is to allow the muscle contraction. A reduction in muscle contractility affects rumen function; lower dry matter intake, thus negative energy balance. This results in increase in fat mobilization leading to fatty liver syndrome and ketosis. It has been shown that plasma calcium concentration of 5mg/ml reduces abomasal motility by 70% and the strength of the contraction by 50%. Low calcium concentrations also prevent insulin production, further exacerbating this situation (Goff, 1999). Muscle tone in the uterus will also be adversely affected with cows experiencing prolonged calving and retained placenta. Uterine involution may also be impaired giving rise to fertility problems. A major concern in the mineral feeding of dry cows relates to providing optimum levels of Ca and P in order to decrease the occurrence of milk fever. Indian lactating cows need about 0.40 to 0.60% to low yielders and ration containing 0.75 to 0.80 per cent Ca on DM basis should be provided to high producing cows.

Phosphorus (P) : It is the second most abundant mineral element in the body with 80 to 85% of P in the body being found in the teeth and bones. Essentially, P is involved in metabolic reaction and energy transfer within the body. It is required for normal milk production, growth, and efficient use of feed and by the rumen micro-organisms in the digestion of cellulose and synthesis of microbial protein. A decreased fertility rate, feed intake, milk production, decreased ovarian activity, irregular estrous cycles, increased occurrence of cystic ovaries, delayed sexual maturity and low conception rates have been reported, when phosphorus intakes are low (Cromwell, 1997). In a field study, when heifers received only 70-80% of their phosphorus requirements and serum P levels were low, fertility was impaired (3.7 services per conception). Services per conception were reduced to 1.3 after adequate P was supplemented. Increasing P supplementation from 0.4% to 0.6% of the ration had no effect on days to first estrus or services per conception. However, in some instances, responses have been reported in the field, when phosphorus supplementation was increased to 0.5% or 0.6%. Increasing the dietary concentration of P above requirement does not improve reproductive performance. Scientists have found that reproductive performance was not different on the lower but adequate concentration of phosphorus, when compared to cows fed a higher concentration (above requirements) of dietary phosphorus. Thus, increasing the concentration of dietary P above requirement (more than 0.38-0.40%) does not improve reproductive performance (Amaral-Philips, 2011).

Selenium (Se): Se is involved in normal spermatogenesis and is an essential component of a range of selenoproteins, including glutathione peroxidase, thioredoxin reductase and iodothyronine deiodinase. Se with GPx also appears to be involved as a structural protein to provide normal sperm motility. Both deficiency and excessive selenium have been demonstrated to be detrimental to normal spermatogenesis (Wiltbank *et al.*, 2007). There are two major sources of Se for animals: (1) Se naturally originating from plants, in the form of seleno-amino acids, including selenomethionine and selenocysteine; (2) inorganic Se in the form of selenate or selenite. Even if the physiological requirement for Se is low in an animal, if this is not met, the anti-oxidant system is compromised, with subsequent detrimental consequences in terms of animal health (Spears, 2000). A marginal Se deficiency in pregnant animals will lead to abortion, or calves will be weak and unable to stand or suckle. Se supplementation reduces the incidence of retained placentas, cystic ovaries, mastitis and metritis. Compromised selenium status has also been associated with poor uterine involution, and weak or silent heats. In males, Se supple mentation has been shown to increase semen quality. Symptoms of chronic Se toxicity include lameness, sore feet, deformed claws and loss of hairs from tail. In pregnant animals, Se toxicity will produce abortions, stillbirth and weak and lethargic calves as Se accumulate in the fetus at the expense of the cow (Patterson *et al.*, 2003). The dietary requirement for Se by most species is about 0.1 ppm. Revised requirement of Se for better immune response in dairy animals is 0.3 ppm (Weiss, 2002).

Zinc (Zn) : Zn is an essential component of over 200 enzyme systems of which the metabolic action include carbohydrate and protein metabolism, protein synthesis, nucleic acid metabolism, epithelial tissue integrity, cell repair and division, and vitamin A and E transport and utilization. In addition, zinc plays a major role in the immune system and certain reproductive hormones (Capuco *et al.*, 1990). Zn is known to be essential for proper sexual maturity, reproductive capacity, and more specifically, onset of estrus. Zn has a critical role in the repair and maintenance of the uterine lining following parturition, speeding return to normal reproductive function and estrus. In bulls, a Zn deficiency results in poor semen quality and reduced testicular size and libido (Daniel, 1983). Zn has also been shown to increase plasma beta carotene level, which is correlated to improvement in conception rates and embryonic development (Short and Adams, 1988). Improved Zn status also improves fertility by reducing lameness, resulting in cows more willing to show heat and improved mobility and performance of bulls. Severe Zn deficiency in cattle results in reduced growth, reduced feed intake, loss of hair, skin lesions that are most severe on the legs, neck, head and around the nostrils, excessive salivation, swollen feed with open, scaly lesions, and impaired reproduction. A deficiency of Zn in males reduces testicular development and sperm production. In females, cycling and conception rate are decreased by Zn deficiency. Severe Zn deficiency is rare, but has been observed in ruminants grazing forages. Based on Zn supplementation studies, subclinical Zn deficiency can result in impaired reproduction and decreased weight gains (Spears, 1994). The recommended dietary content of Zn for dairy cattle is typically between 18 and 73ppm depending upon the stage of lifecycle and dry matter intake. Cu, Cd, Ca and Fe reduce Zn absorption and interfere with Zn metabolism (Patterson *et al.*, 2003). Requirement of Zn in diet of dairy cows is 40 ppm (NRC, 2001).

Copper (Cu) : Cu is a necessary component of number of enzymes including superoxide dismutase, lysyl oxidase and thioloxidase (Halliwell and Gutteridge, 1999). Cu has an important role in the immune system, where its compounds are involved in reducing infections and diseases. Cu deficiency in cattle is generally due to the presence of dietary antagonists, such as suphfur, molybdenum and iron (Fe) that reduce Cu bioavailability (Spears, 2003). Dietary requirements for Cu are greatly increased by high concentrations of molybdenum and sulphur. Deficiencies of copper have also been associated with retained placenta, embryonic death and decreased conception rates. Inadequate Cu status may be related to an increased incidence of infections at calving, increased severity of infections and a higher SCC than that seen in Cu-adequate cattle. Reproductive problems that relate to Cu deficiency manifest themselves in inhibited conception rate even though estrus may be normal. Weak and silent heats have been reported. Dairy cows with higher serum Cu levels had significantly less days to first service, fewer services per conception and fewer days to open. Proper Cu supplementation of the sire is needed for production of quality semen. Feeding a total of 10 to 15 ppm Cu in the ration dry matter or supplementing with 10 ppm Cu should meet dairy cattle needs. If rations contain antagonists, such as elevated iron, sulfur, or molybdenum, replacing 35 per cent of supplemental Cu with organic Cu sources could improve Cu availability. The following mineral ratios may be helpful in maintaining Cu levels in blood: Zn: Cu 4:1, Cu: Mo 6:1 and Fe: Cu 40:1 (Hutjens, 2000).

Manganese (Mn) : Mn is a required nutrient for dairy cows; however, clinical deficiencies are extremely rare because most feedstuffs contain at least marginally adequate concentrations of Mn. Mn is an activator of enzyme systems in the metabolism of carbohydrate, fats, protein and nucleic acids. Mn appears to have a vital role in reproduction. It is necessary for cholesterol synthesis (Kappel and Zidenberg, 1999), which in turn is required for synthesis of the steroids, estrogen, progesterone and testosterone. Insufficient steroid production results in decreased circulating concentrations of these reproductive hormones resulting in abnormal sperm in males and irregular estrus cycles in females. The corpus luteum has high manganese content and may be affected by level of Mn supple mentation. Also, vaginal Mn concentration is higher in cycling than in anoestrous ruminants. A deficiency in Mn may be associated with suppression of estrus, cyclic ovaries and reduced conception rate (Patterson *et al.*, 2003). The maintenance requirement for absorbed Mn was set at 0.002 mg/kg of body weight (1.2 mg/day for an average Holstein cow), the growth requirement was set at 0.7 mg/kg of growth, pregnancy requirement was set at 0.3 mg/d, and the lactation requirement was set at 0.03 mg/kg of milk (NRC, 2001).

Iodine (I) : Iodine is important in the development of fetus and maintenance of general basal metabolic rate, as it is involved in synthesis of thyroid hormone, thyroxin, which regulates the rate of metabolism. Iodine deficiency leads to delay in puberty, suppressed or irregular estrus (Puls, 1994), failure of fertilization, early embryonic death, still birth with weak calves, abortion, increased frequency of retained placenta in females and decrease in libido and deterioration of semen quality in males (Satish Kumar, 2003). Inadequate thyroid function reduces conception rate and ovarian activity. Thus, I deficiency impairs reproduction and iodine supplementation has been recommended when necessary to insure that cows consume 15-20 mg of I each day. Recently, Excessive I intakes have been associated with various health problems including abortion and decreased resistance to infection and disease. Signs of subclinical I deficiency in breeding females include suppressed estrus, abortions, still births, increased frequency of retained placentas and extended gestation periods (Hess *et al.*, 2008). Calves born to cows that are marginally deficient in iodine are weak and may be hairless.

Cobalt (Co) : Co is needed for proper vitamin B_{12} synthesis. Maintaining adequate vitamin B_{12} status benefits both, the dam and offspring. When adequate, sufficient amounts of vitamin B_{12} cross the placenta and are present in colostrums. Milk and colostrums in particular, contain high levels of vitamin B_{12}, which is required for the conversion of propionate to glucose and for folic acid metabolism. Depletion of Co and vitamin B12 at parturition causes depressed milk production and colostrums yield and quality (Patterson *et al.*, 2003). Co deficiency is associated with an increased incidence of silent heats, a delayed onset of puberty, non-functional ovaries, and abortion. Inadequate Co levels in the diet have been correlated with increased early calf mortality. A Co deficiency ultimately results in a vitamin B_{12} deficiency. Mn, Zn, I and monensin may reduce Co deficiency. The required dietary content of Co for dairy cattle is 0.11 ppm (Miller *et al.*, 1988).

Potassium (K) : K is the third most abundant mineral element in the animal body, surpassed only by calcium and phosphorus. The K requirement for gestating and lactating sows is 0.20 per cent. Potassium requirement increases in diets with higher Na and chloride (Cl) levels. Ruminants have a higher K requirement than nonruminants. K is essential for rumen micro-organisms. The single most consistent effect of suboptimal K in the ration of ruminants is decreased feed intake. Lactating dairy cattle, particularly high producing cows, require the highest levels of dietary K. Under heat stress, their optimal level of dietary K can be as high as 1.9 per cent, but the normal National Research Council (NRC) recommendation is 1.0 per cent of dietary dry matter.

Chromium (Cr) : Cr potentiates insulin action, resulting in increased uptake of glucose and amino acids by cells in the body (Short and Adams, 1988). Dietary energy intake in early lactation does not meet energy demands for maintaining body reserves and milk yield. Low serum insulin, high serum glucagon and growth hormone (Herbein *et al.*, 1985), and high plasma NEFA concentrations (Grummer, 1993) in early lactation dairy cows indicate high catabolic activities and negative energy balance. This leads to increased gluconeogenesis and glycogenolysis in the liver and increased mobilization of protein reserves from muscle tissue. This metabolic pattern is initiated before parturition (Vazquez-Anon *et al.*, 1994). Several studies reported insulin resistance begins before parturition and continues during early lactation. Thus, during the periparturient period, insulin resistance may be an important factor in the initiation of catabolic activities (Holstenius, 1993). Cr supplementation (0.5 ppm) may enhance the action of insulin and, consequently, decrease plasma NEFA and liver tri-glyceride concentrations and improve glucose tolerance, which may result in improvement of performance and production during the periparturient period.

Salt (NaCl) : The daily salt requirements for dairy cattle are met easily by adding 1 per cent salt to a grain mix and offering additional salt free choice. Lactating cows need 2 g salt/kg milk production. Dry cows need 40g salt daily or 0.3% Na per kg DM. Salt deficiencies can affect the efficiency of digestion and indirectly the reproduction performance of cows. Sodium and chloride normally do not appear in feedstuffs in adequate amounts to meet animal requirements and should be provided free choice at all times (Elrod and Butler, 1993).

Vitamins : The vitamin requirements of dairy cows are met by a combination of rumen and tissue synthesis, natural feeds and dietary supplementation. Factory made concentrates containing supplemental vitamins greatly reduces infertility due to a vitamin deficiency. To ensure adequate vitamins intake animals must be fed with concentrates or mixed in a complete dairy cow ration (Schweigert and Zucker, 1988).

Vitamin A : It is one of the fat soluble vitamins and is known to regulate the development, cellular growth and differentiation, and tissue function. Its metabolites affect ovarian follicular growth, uterine environments and oocyte maturation. Vitamin A is required for maintaining healthy tissue in the reproductive tract. In deficient cattle, delayed sexual maturity, abortion, the birth of dead or weak calves, retained placenta and metritis have been reported (Chawala and Kaur, 2004). A deficiency of vitamin A has a direct effect on the structure and function of pituitary gland, gonads and uterus. The recommended daily supplementation for dairy cows is 35,000-45,000 units (NRC, 2001). One mg of carotene provides 400 IU vitamin A in dairy ration. Carotene is known to be in high concentrations in fresh green roughages, while grains contain relatively low amounts. Silages, especially alfalfa, contain moderate levels, while corn silage is a poor source. Dry hays, especially alfalfa, are excellent sources of carotene (Schweigert and Zucker, 1988).

Vitamin D : Vitamin D contributes to more than calcium and bone formation in cattle. The active vitamin D hormone also contributes to immune, reproductive, and mammary physiology. Multiple tissues and factors also contribute to vitamin D activity (Nelson and Merriman, 2014). A concentrates containing supplemental vitamin D in amounts sufficient should be provided to meet the cow's requirement of 10,000 IU per day.

Vitamin E : Vitamin E functions as an intra-cellular antioxidant scavenging for free reactive oxygen and lipid hydroperoxidases, and converting them to non-reactive forms, thus maintaining the integrity of membrane phospholipids against oxidative damage and peroxidation. In vitamin E and selenium deficiency condition, these free radicals accumulate and not only damage cell membranes, but also disrupt several processes linked to the synthesis of steroids, prostaglandins, sperm motility and the development of the embryo. The current NRC (2001) requirement for dairy cows is 15 IU/kg of DMI (approximately 150 and 300 IU/d for dry and lactating cows, respectively). The vitamin E (á-tocopherol) status of dairy cows is one important component of a well-functioning immune system because of its antioxidant effects on cows (Hogan *et al.*, 1993). Feeding vitamin E during dry periods until 30 days after calving resulted in 80% decrease in clinical mastitis and 60% reduction in intra-mammary infections (Weiss *et al.*, 1997). Supplementation of vitamin E at 1,500 IU daily from 60 day prepartum to 30 day postpartum to buffaloes exhibited beneficial effect on plasma á-tocopherol level and total antioxidant activity around parturition and continuation of its supplementation at 1,000 IU d-1 from 30 to 60 days of lactation improved postpartum reproductive performance of buffaloes (Panda *et al.*, 2006).

Precision nutrition : Typically precision nutrition intervention includes all nutrients required by animal to its optimum levels in ration. Balance ration include concentrate, green and dry fodder in specific ratio as per production status of animal. A good quality concentrate can be made at farm by including cereals, cereal by-product and oil-cake in 1:1:1 ratio i.e. for 100 kg about 32% cereal grain like maize, wheat, barley, bajra, jowar, etc; 32% by-product like brans, chunnies and 33% oil cakes with 2% mineral mixture and 1% salt. This mixture will provide about 200 g protein and 650-700g energy (TDN) along with minerals and vitamins. A provision of 1 kg concentrate mixture per 3 kg milk production is sufficient to take care of nutrient requirement of lactating animals. Dry animals, heifers, or breeding bull can be easily maintained after supplementation of 2 kg concentrate daily. All lactating animals requires >70% of their nutrient requirement from concentrate rest can be given by green fodder. Dry fodder should always be given as rumen filler or low maintenance fodder. No more than 15 % expenditure on ration should be on dry fodder for better nutrient availability.

In traditional feeding practices, mustard cake *sani* is done with green or dry fodder supplementation with little or no energy rich cereal grain mixture. This results in very high degradation of mustard cake in short time leading to excessive ammonia in rumen and blood. This results in loss of energy either as urea synthesis in liver or microbial protein in rumen. Both processes need energy. So, mustard cake *sani* should always be supplemented with 1-2 time cereal grain mixture or good energy source for optimum use of cake. Additional problem of excessive ammonia on reproductive health have already be discussed above. Supplementation of mineral mixture enhances optimum use of resources.

Conclusions

Nutrients have important role in hormonal, regulatory and circulatory system of the body. Supplementation of deficient nutrients in ration of dairy animal not only improves productivity but also potentiate immunity. A good choice has to be made in favour of balance feeding or supplementation feeding for higher production than traditional animal rearing on poor quality roughage with low productivity. A sound knowledge about role of resource, requirements and bioavailability of nutrients is vital in improving animal productivity. This paper highlighted role of nutrients in dairy animals.

References

Amaral-Philips, D. (2011). Phosphorus important for optimum milk production and reproduction in dairy cattle. Accessed on 08/01/2018 at http://afsdairy.ca.uky.edu/files/extension/nutrition/Phosphorus_Important_For_Optimum_Milk_Production_and_Reproduciton_in_Dairy_Cattle.pdf.

Blanchard, T., Ferguson, J., Love, L., Takeda, T., Henderson, B., Hasler, J., Chalupa, W. (1990). Effect of dietary crude protein type on fertilization and embryo quality in dairy cattle. Am. J. Vet. Res. 51: 905-908.

Butler, W.R. (2001). Nutritional effects on resumption of ovarian cyclicity and conception rate in *postpartum* dairy cows. *British Society for Animal Science Occasional Publication* **26**: 133–145.

Capuco, A.V., Wood, D.L., Bright, S.A., Miller, R.H. and Britman, J. (1990). Regeneration of teat canal keratin in lactating dairy cows. J. Dairy Sci., 73: 1051-1057.

Chawala, R. and Kaur, H. (2004): "Plasma antioxidant vitamin status of periparturient cows supplemented with a tocopherol and ß-carotene. Anim. Feed. Sci. Tech. 114: 279-285.

Cromwell, G.L. (1997). *Handbook of copper compounds and applications*. Pp: 177-202.

Daniel, R.C.W. (1983). Motility of the rumen and abomasums during hypocalcemia, Canadian J. Comp. Med. Vet. Sci., 47: 267-280.

Dunn, T.G. and Moss, G.E (1992). Effects of nutrient deficiencies and excesses on reproductive efficiency of livestock, J. Anim. Sci., 70: 1580-1593.

Elrod, C.C. and Butler, W.R. (1993). Reduction of fertility and alteration of uterine pH in heifers fed excess ruminally degradable protein. J. Anim. Sci., 71: 694-701.

Elrod, C.C., van Amburgh, M. and Butler, W.R. (1993). Alterations of pH in response to increased dietary protein in cattle are unique to the uterus. J. Anim. Sci., 71: 702-706.

Fenwick, M.A., Fitzpatrick, R., Kenny, D.A., Diskin, M.G., Patton, J., Murphy, J.J., Wathes, D.C. (2008). Interrelationships between negative energy balance (NEB) and IGF regulation in liver of lactating dairy cows. Domest. Anim. Endocrinol. 34: 31–44.

Goff, JP, Dry cow nutrition and metabolic disease in parturient cows. In: *proceeding western canadian dairy seminar red deer*.

Grummer, R.R. (1993). Etiology of lipid-related metabolic disorders in periparturient dairy cows. J. Dairy Sci. 76: 3882–3896.

Halliwell, B. and Gutteridge, J.M.C. (1999). In: Free Radicals in Biology and Medicine, third ed. Oxford University Press, New York, USA.

Herbein, J.H., Aiello, R.J., Eckler, L.I., Pearson, R.E. and Akers, R.M. (1985). Glucagon, insulin, growth hormone, and glucose concentrations in plasma of lactating dairy cows. J. Dairy Sci. 68: 320–325.

Hess, B.W., Moss, G.E. and Rule, D.C. (2008). A decade of developments in the area of fat supplementation research with beef cattle and sheep. J. Anim. Sci., 86: 188-204.

Hogan J.S., Weiss W.P., Smith K.L. (1993): Role of vitamin E and selenium in host defense against mastitis. J. Dairy Sci., 76: 2795-2803.

Holstenius, P. (1993). Hormonal regulation related to the development of fatty liver and ketosis. Acta Vet. Scand. 89(S): 55–60.

Hutjens, M.F., 2000. Feeding management of the 40 000 pound dairy herds. J. Dairy Sci., Vol. 83, Suppl 1, Abstr 108, p26.

Kumar, V. (2015). Effect of Minerals on Dairy Animal Reproduction - A review. Intl. J Liv Res. 5(6): 1-10.

Kappel, L.C. and Zidenberg, S. (1999). *Manganese: Present Knowledge in nutrition*, In: Brown ML (Ed.), International Life Sciences Institute Nutrition Foundation, Washington, **1999.** pp 308.

Leroy, J.L., Vanholder, T., Opsomer, G., Van Soom, A. and de Kruif, A. (2006). The *in vitro* development of bovine oocytes after maturation in glucose and beta-hydroxybutyrate concentrations associated with negative energy balance in dairy cows. Reproduction in Domestic Animals. 41: 119–123.

Llewellyn, S., Fitzpatrick, R., Kenny, D.A., Murphy, J.J., Scaramuzzi, R.J. and Wathes, D.C. (2007). Effect of negative energy balance on the insulin-like growth factor system in pre-recruitment ovarian follicles of postpartum dairy cows. Reproduction. 133: 627–639.

Miller, J.K., N. Ramsey and F.C. Madsen, 1988. The ruminant animal. D.C. Church. Ed. Pp. 342-400. Prentice Hall, Englewood cliffs, N.J.

Nelson, C.D. and Merriman, K.E. (2014). Vitamin D metabolism in dairy cattle and implications for dietary requirements. Accessed on 23/04/2015 at http://dairy.ifas.ufl.edu/rns/2014/nelson.pdf.

NRC-National Research Council, (2001). Nutrient requirements of dairy cattle, seventh revised ed., National Academic Press, Washington, DC, USA.

Panda, N., Kaur, H. and Mohanty, T.K. (2006). Reproductive performance of dairy buffaloes supplemented with varying levels of vitamin E. Asian-Aust. J. Anim. Sci., 9(1): 19-25.

Patterson, H.H., Adams, D.C., Klopfenstein, T.J., Clark, R.T. and Teichert, B. (2003). Supplementation to meet metabolizable protein requirements of primiparous beef heifers: II. Pregnancy and Economics. J. Anim. Sci., 81: 503-570.

Paul, S.S., Mandal, A.B., Mandal, G.P., Kannan, A. and Pathak, N.N. (2004). Deriving nutrient requirements of lactating Indian cattle under tropical condition using performance and intake data emanated from feeding trials conducted in different research institutes. Asian-Aust. J. Anim. Sci., 17: 769-776.

Perry, R.C., Corah, L.R., Cochran, R.C., Beal, W.E., Stevenson, J.S., Minton, J.E., Simms, D.D. and Brrethour, J.R. (1991). Influence of dietary energy on follicular development, serum gonadotropins, and first postpartum ovulation in suckled beef cows. J. Anim. Sci., 69: 3762-3773.

Puls, R., 1994. Mineral level in animal health. Diagnotic data. 2nd ed. Sherpa International, Clearbrook, BC, Canada.

Qureshi, M.S., Habib, G., Samad, H.A., Siddiqui, M.M., Ahmad, N. and Syed. M. (2002). Reproduction-nutrition relationship in dairy buffaloes. I. Effect of intake of protein, energy and blood metabolites levels. Asian-Aust. J. Anim. Sci., 15(3): 330-339.

Ropstad, E. and Refsdal, A.O. (1987). Herd reproductive performance related to urea concentration in bulk milk. Acta. Vet. Scnd., 28: 55-63.

Roseler, D.K., Ferguson, J.D., Sniffen, C.J. and Herrema, J. (1993). Dietary protein degradability effects on plasma and milk urea, nitrogen and milk non-protein nitrogen in Holstein cows. J. Dairy Sci., 76: 525-534.

Ryan, D.P., Spoon, R.A. and Williams, G.L. (1992). Ovarian follicular characteristics, embryo recovery, and embryo viability in heifers fed high-fat diets and treated with follicle stimulating hormone, J. Anim. Sci., 70: 3505.

Saha, D., Gupta, R.S. and Baghel, R.P.S. (2013). Energy requirements of lactating crossbred cattle (*Bos indicus*). Inter. J. Adv. Biol. Res., 3(4): 527-529.

Sathish Kumar (2003). Management of infertility due to mineral deficiency in dairy animals. In: Proceedings of ICAR summer school on "Advance diagnostic techniques and therapeutic approaches to metabolic and deficiency diseases in dairy animals". Held at IVRI, Izatnagar, UP (15th July to 4th Aug.). pp. 128-137.

Schweigert, F.J. and Zucker, H. (1988). Concentration of vitamin A, beta-carotene and vitamin E in individual bovine follicles of different quality. J. Reprod. Fertil., 82: 575-579.

Short, R.E. and Adams, D.C. (1988). Nutritional and hormonal inter-relationships in beef cattle reproduction. Can. J. Anim. Sci. 68: 29-39.

Spears, J.W. (1994). Minerals in forages. In: G. C. Fahey, Jr. (Ed.) Forge Quality, Evaluation, and Utilization. p 281. American Society of Agronomy, Inc., Madison, WI.

Spears, J.W. (2000). Micronutrients and immune function in cattle. In: Proceedings of the Nutrition Society, 59: 587–594.

Spears, J.W. (2003). Trace mineral bioavailability in ruminants. J. Nutr. 133: 1506S–1509S.

Thatcher, W.W. and Staples, C.R. (2000). Effects of dietary fat supplementation on reproduction in lactating dairy cows. In: Advances in Dairy Technology, 12: 213-232.

Vazquez-Anon, M., Bertics, S.J., Luck, M. and Grummer, R.R. (1994). Peripartum liver triglyceride and plasma metabolites. J. Dairy Sci. 77: 1521–1528.

Weiss, W.P. (2002). Relationship of mineral and vitamin supplementation with mastitis and milk quality. In: National Mastitis Council Annual Meeting Proceedings. Pp 38-44.

Weiss, W.P., Hogan, J.S., Todhunter, D.A. and Smith, K.L. (1997). Effect of vitamin E supplementation in diets with a low concentration of selenium on mammary gland health of dairy cows. J. Dairy Sci. 80: 1728-1737.

Wiltbank, M.C., Weigel, K.A. and Caraviello, D.Z. (2007). Recent studies on nutritional factors affecting reproductive efficiency in U.S. dairy herds, *Western Dairy Management Conference.*

❑❑❑

Chapter 6

Manufacturing Cost Effective Homemade Feeding Materials of Livestock

Muneendra Kumar, Shalini Vaswani and Avinash Kumar

Department of Animal Nutrition, College of Veterinary Science and Animal Husbandry, Uttar Pradesh Pandit Deen Dayal Upadhyaya Pashu Chikitsa Vigyan Vishwavidhyalaya Evam Go Anusandhan Sansthan, Mathura

Introduction

Homemade rations for dairy cattle can be a solution to the problem of cost and quality. Although commercially produced feeds offer a potential option of optimizing feed availability in order to meet the daily requirements of the dairy cow, they are usually costly and some have issues with quality. This has tended to discourage farmers. In formulating a ration for dairy cows to achieve high levels of milk production, one should aim at providing a diet that contains all nutrients required by farm animals. Energy, proteins and minerals are the three essential feed ingredients that are required by the animal for growth, maintenance and for production in terms of milk and/or pregnancy. These are generally recognized first in feed rationing. Other ingredients include vitamins. These should be availed in the required levels for normal functioning of the dairy cow and support milk production. Ideally, the farmer should provide the cow with home grown feeds to meet its maintenance requirements and any additional nutrients for production should be obtained from concentrates. Due to the high costs of bought feeds, the farmer should as much as possible strive to make use of home grown feeds. Well-prepared hay, maize meal, grasses, legumes and crop byproducts, such as sunflower heads with seed, maize stover/cobs can be used in formulating balanced rations on the farm thereby reducing the cost of feeding.

Factors to be consider while formulating homemade ration

1. The ration should be highly digestible and well balanced in terms of energy, protein, minerals and vitamins.
2. The ration being formulated has to be palatable enough to stimulate intake by the animal. Feed refused by the animal is worthless.
3. The ingredients composing the ration should be good and sound and a variety of such feeds should be used to formulate the ration for better balance of nutrients as well as palatability.
4. The ration should be fairly laxative and bulky to stimulate the walls of digestive track for maximum secretion and action of digestive juices.
5. The feed ingredients used in ration formulation should be easily available and cost effective. The least-cost ration should ensure that all requirements of the animal are met and the desired objectives are achieved.
6. Practical diet formulation must be sufficiently flexible to accommodate price and feedstuff available, while retaining the necessary nutritive balance and adequacy.
7. Ration must be properly prepared. Hard grains, like maize, barley, sorghum, etc. should must be grounded before feeding.
8. Ration must contain all limiting amino acids in balanced amount. Animal protein supplements are rich source for lysine and methionine. Among vegetable protein sources, soyabean meal is a rich source for lysine.
9. If feed contains antibacterial compound, the withdrawal period of that compound must be kept in mind.
10. The ration should be formulated and fed according to the requirement of the animals. Feeding less or in excess, both are detrimental to health.
11. In order to avoid digestive disorders, the feeding should be done at regular intervals.
12. Always avoid sudden change in the diet, as it upsets whole stomach resulting in digestive disturbances and reduction in productive performance.

13. Some feed ingredients may also contain toxic substances, which may be detrimental to the animal, when given in excessive amounts. The inclusion of these feed ingredients should, therefore, be limited or eliminated from the formulation.

14. For better digestibility the animals should get at libitum, the clean and fresh supply of drinking water.

Significance of ration balancing

The formulation of ration for various categories of livestock depends upon the nutrient requirements for a particular animal or group of animals and the feeds and fodders available for the purpose. The nutrient requirements are largely based on the size of the animal and its physiological state. Livestock feeds can be grouped into two major categories i.e. roughages and concentrates on the basic of bulkiness and chemical composition.

Roughages are bulky feeds containing more than 18% crude fibre (CF) and less than 60% total digestible nutrients (TDN). Roughages are subdivided into two major groups i.e. dry roughages (having more than 80% dry matter) and succulent (having more than 80% moisture). The dry roughages are hays (leguminous and non-leguminous), straw (wheat straw, paddy straw, barley straw, etc.) and stovers (bajra, Jowar, maize, etc.). Except good quality leguminous and non-leguminous hays, remaining are non-maintenance type roughages. Succulent roughages include mainly cultivated leguminous and non-leguminous fodders. The most commonly used kharif leguminous fodders are cowpea and guar and non-leguminous ones are jowar, maize and sudan grass. The leguminous and non-leguminous fodders of rabi season are lucerne, berseem, pea and oat and barley respectively. In addition, pasture, tree leaves silages and root crops are also grouped under this head.

Feed or feed mixtures containing less than 18% CF and over 60% TDN are classed as concentrates. They are rich in either energy or protein and accordingly are called as energy concentrates (when crude protein is less than 18%) or protein concentrates (when crude protein value exceeds 18%). Various energy concentrates are grain and seeds (maize, barley, sorghum, etc.), milling by-products (brans and chunis), roots (tapioca tubers turnip, potatoes) and molasses. Protein supplements, on the other hand may be further categorized according to the source of origin (a) animal protein supplements (meat meal, blood meal, fish meal, feather meal, etc.) and (b) plant protein supplements (oilseed cakes and meals i.e. groundnut cake, sesame cake, mustard cake, linseed oil meal, etc.). Animal origin protein supplements except dried whole and skimmed milk, contain more than 47% crude protein (CP), whereas those of plant origin, contain less than 47% CP except soybean oil meal (contains 49% CP). In addition, a third group of feedstuffs include mineral and vitamin supplements and additives which when added to the total feed mixture improve the performance of the total feed.

Types of rations

A balanced ration is one that furnishes nutrients in such proportions and amounts that will properly nourish a given animal for 24 hours. In addition, the required nutrients must be contained in the amount of DM, the animal is able to consume (DMI) in the 24 hr period.

1. Maintenance ration

The ration which just enables the animal at rest to carry on the essential processes of life, such as breathing, circulation of blood, etc. without either gain or loss of body weight is known as maintenance ration. It is dependant upon live weight of animal and also on the level of production. At higher level of production even at the same body weight, the maintenance requirement is increased.

2. Production ration

It is the additional allowance of ration for milk product over and above the maintenance requirement. An additional amount of 1 kg concentrate mixture is required for each 2.5to 3.0 kg milk produced. Production also includes growth, fattening work, etc. The additional allowance will depend upon rate of growth, fattening and type of work being done.

3. Gestation ration

It is the feed allowance which should be given to pregnant animal from fifth-sixth month of pregnancy onwards for proper growth of the foetus and to keep the mother fit for optimum milk production upon calving. An additional amount of 1.25/ 1.75 kg of concentrate mixture has been recommended for cows/ buffaloes, respectively.

Computation of ration for livestock

Ration formulation should be done in three steps i.e. 1) to calculate the probable dry matter intake (DMI) of the animal, 2) to calculate the nutrient requirement of the animal and 3) to arrive at the amount of available feeds that must be fed to fulfill the animal's nutrient requirement within its expected DMI. DM requirement varies with live weight and status/rate of the animal production. DM consumption in various Species of livestock is as follows:

S. No.	Species	DM requirement (% of live body weight)
1.	Cattle	1.5-2.5%
2.	Buffalo	2.0-3.0%
3.	Sheep	2.5-3.5%
4.	Goat (meat type)	3.0-4.0%
5.	Goat (lactating)	4.0-6.0%

To provide the required bulk in the diet, the DM allowance for cattle and buffalo should be divided as follows: One-third of the total DM requirements should be supplied from concentrate mixture and remaining two-third of the total DM from roughage portion. In roughage portion, incorporate two-third of DM from dry roughage or three-fourth DM, if sufficient legume is available. Rest, one-third DM should be from green roughage (If leguminous fodder is available, then this may be reduced to one-fourth of total roughage quota.

Thumb rule for formulation of concentrate mixture

Generally, as per thumb rule, the concentrate mixture can be prepared by mixing one-third of each of cereals, oil cakes and cereal or pulse by-products. Broadly according to this method, the concentrate mixture may also be prepared as per the following flexible formula:

S. No.	Ingredient	Parts (kg/100kg)
1.	Cereals/millets	20-60
2.	Oilcakes	20-35
3.	Cereal by-products (wheat bran, rice bran, rice polish, etc.)	10-35
4.	By-products (molasses, chuni)	5-20

The above concentrate mixture will contain 15% digestible crude protein (DCP) and 70% TDN. It should be fortified with 1-2% mineral mixture, 1% common salt, and 10-15 g vitamin A and D supplement/ 100 kg, when the animals are not receiving green.

Preparing least cost homemade concentrates

Homemade rations for dairy cattle can be a solution to the problem of cost and quality. Although commercially produced feeds offers a potential option of optimizing feed availability in order to meet the daily requirements of the dairy cow, they are usually costly and some have issues with quality. This has tended to discourage farmers. Ideally the farmer should provide the cow with home grown feeds to meet its maintenance requirements and any additional nutrients for production should be obtained from concentrates. Once you identify the most cost effective feed materials which can satisfy the nutrient requirements of the dairy cow, the next step is to combine the feeds in such ratios as to minimize costs and optimize the nutrient composition of the resulting diet. There are several methods of determining the quantities to mix. These include, Pearson square method, used when the number of feed types is two or at most four. It becomes cumbersome, when the number of feed ingredients is higher. The Pearson square has been widely used in ration formulation process. However, its major disadvantage is that one can only balance for one nutrient at a time. It, therefore, has limited application where farmers have to formulate diets balanced for protein, energy, vitamins and minerals and also being low-cost. Simultaneous equation method is appropriate, when mixing more than two ingredients to formulate the feed. Computer programs (least-cost feed formulation) used for complex mixing, where several ingredients are involved. Least-cost formulation is a mathematical solution based on linear programming. This practice is widely used within the commercial feed industry using commercially available software programmes. Least-cost formulation of diets optimizes the combination of feed ingredients that supplies the required levels of nutrients at least cost.

In order to balance a ration and to feed a lactating cow properly, it is important to know the factors that affect the nutrient requirement of the cow. The most important factors are: 1) body weight, 2) milk production, 3) composition of milk (percentage of fat), 4) stage of lactations of the cow and, 5) number of lactations. Profitability of livestock production depends on keeping costs to a minimum without sacrificing production and quality. Feed represent a large proportion of the variable cost of livestock production (60% of production cost). Various efforts has been tried to reducc cost of feed without affecting performance of animals. Incorporation of homemade and non-conventional feed resources (NCFR) can be one of the alternatives to reduce feed costs. The term NCFR has been frequently used to describe sources, such as oil palm by-products, single-cell proteins and feed materials derived from agro-industrial by-products of plant and animal origin, poor-quality cellulosic roughages from farm residues and other agroindustrial by-products, such as slaughter-house by-products and those from the processing of sugar, cereal grains, citrus fruits and vegetables from the processing of food for human consumption.

Why homemade concentrates?

Generally, a cow will eat from 2.5 to 3 % of its body weight in feed daily. For top performance, about 70 to 80 % of this feed should be a concentrate mix and the remainder good quality roughage. On good pasture, concentrate mix can be reduced 50 to 70 %, but more concentrates produce faster gains. There are many commercial concentrate mixes available. Some are high in protein for use during the first part of the feeding period. Others are high in energy for use during the last part of the feeding period. You can also make your own concentrate mixes, if the ingredients are available:

1. Concentrate use can be even higher than 1:1 concentrate to milk yield.
2. Feed costs are about 70% of total operating costs for animals, so decreasing equals significant income.
3. Concentrate supplementation for lactating cows has been proved as successful by many small holder farmers.
4. The use of local feed resources to reduce production cost should be more a primary concern for dairy farmers.
5. Most of farmers use homemade concentrates, plus by-products and commercial concentrates homemade concentrates comprised of local feed resources decrease feed cost of production, by adding value to the own production.

Conclusions

The use of two or three cheaply available farm feed materials to formulate a ration is by far the most cost effective way to increase production and profits within a dairy farm. Currently, there are feed formulators who use computer programs and complex matrices to arrive at precise quantities of various feedstuff required to make a diet of desired protein, energy and mineral levels. These can help the farmers to use the various feed materials within the farm to make a ration for their animals. The feedstuff so used to compound a ration should be mixed homogeneously to have a uniform diet. In the absence of a mechanical mixer, the farmer should first measure the required amounts, then mix a small amount and adding small quantities at a time all the while mixing thoroughly. Have the diet in the optimum texture so that the animal eats with ease.

□□□

Chapter 7

Risk Management Strategies in Dairy Sector

Sanjeev Kumar Singh, Amit Singh and Rashmi
Department of Veterinary & Animal Husbandry Extension, College of Veterinary Science and Animal Husbandry, Uttar Pradesh Pandit Deen Dayal Upadhyaya Pashu Chikitsa Vigyan Vishwavidhyalaya Evam Go Anusandhan Sansthan, Mathura

Agriculture is the backbone of the Indian economy and this sector accounts for 15 per cent of the National GDP as well as roughly 11 per cent of its exports. Half of the Indian population still relies on agriculture as the major important source of income. India ranks second in total farm output on a global level and are also a major source of raw material for a large number of domestic industries. The dairy sector is one of the major livelihood activities in rural India with an estimated production of 165 million tonnes and approximately 17 per cent of global milk production and this production is expected to reach 200 million tonnes by 2020-21.

Today, dairy is an important and growing livestock sub-sector of India's rural economy and is a livelihood option for a large number of households engaged in milk production and trade in rural India. It is a powerful avenue for generating additional income for rural households and this business passes on from generation to generation. Excessive milk production pushed rural households to perform business activities, but it is comparatively risky, since the main product (milk) is quick perishable in nature and is also confronted with several risk factors, i.e., limited and poor infrastructural facilities in villages, limited availability of pastures, availability of clean water, increasingly high cost of feed and medicine, low productivity of dairy animals, seasonal variations and irregular supply of FMD & HS vaccines, low/ non-availability of credit, high cost of production, lack of information, poor market intelligence, high transportation cost, timely delivery of products, grading, packaging, quality control, market infrastructure, agro-processing plants, marketing credit, proper pricing, standardization of weights and measures and poor access to market information.

India can be a market leader in the dairy sector, if its markets function properly. In this context, the biggest challenge before Indian Dairy industry is the inefficiency of its supply chain. The traditional system of diary marketing is dominated by the commission agents and traders who are the major price setters and most of the times farmers have to depend on them for credit also. Small and landless farmers lack marketing power and have very low share in the final consumer price. Since the dairy product is marketed through the commission agents, there is no incentive for its quality, since markets are poorly designed with non-existence of grading and sorting facilities.

The supply chain needs to be strengthened for a long term-relation between retailers and farmers for procurement and providing extension services regarding use of low-cost inputs, production technology, prices, pre-cooling, grading, sorting, packaging and on-spot quality sorting. Besides this, there is a strong need of government interventions in removing infrastructural constraints, like setting up of distribution centres, cold chain management, roads to the markets, etc.

It is necessary to ensure quality and quantity of the dairy product to the milk collection centres for smooth functioning of supply chain, since a single gateway to the regulated markets would save time and improve efficiency. To emerge as a major producer of dairy products, India needs some critical inputs, especially of supply chain management and collaboration among various stakeholders along with efficient vertical and horizontal integrations. Vertical integration of farmers through co-operatives, contract farming and retail chains would facilitate better delivery of output, reduce market risk, provide better infrastructure, attract more public investment, acquire better extension services, and would create awareness regarding prevailing and new technologies. Its multiplier effect would help in increasing income, output and employment.

The main objective is to detect the potential risks pertaining in varying degrees in the dairy-food supply chain. Risk and uncertainty, though used interchangeably in various studies, are not one and the same. In case of risk the probability is known, it is not known for the uncertainty, but both incur losses to the supply. Risk management is a proactive approach rather than reactive approach. The risk management process starts with identification of the risks and ends with the risk mitigation through the risk response development. Risk mitigation, avoidance, transferring, sharing and retaining are the various responses to deal with the risks in the dairy sector.

There are basically two types of risk at the farm level. They are agricultural risk and non-agricultural risk, such as production risk (weather, parasitic infestations and diseases), price risk (lack of demand) and input risk (shortage of inputs or when their prices vary). There are certain risks which are common to all are called as systematic (covariate) risks and risks specifically related to a particular farmer are termed as idiosyncratic risks. Risk management and mitigation can be done at the farmer level or at the community level as a whole. This can be done either with the help of self-insurances or risk pooling and mutual insurance at the community level – they have added to their work as a method of risk management strategy.

In every sphere of our life, we have to confront and manage risks. The idea of risk and risk management is not a modern manoeuvre. In order to increase efficiency, every business organization is forced to manage their supply chain effectively. The concept of supply chain risk management is rapidly developing with high rate in the contemporary business world. Supply chain members have to face and manage a number of risks in their increasingly competitive environment. Therefore, risk management could be a more effective approach to deal with several risks associated with business by identifying possible losses. Supply chain risk management is a mechanism, which aims at mitigating the negative impact of disturbance and tries to manage certain risks within supply chain. It is a process of identification of risks and mitigation of them through outcome development. The dairy supply chain comprises of dairy farms, storage and processing facilities, wholesale distributors, and retailers. As it involves many stakeholders, risks may arise from any component within its supply chain. The main risk associated with Indian Dairy may arise from economic sources (land scarcity, financial unavailability, technology disruption, improper feeding, etc.), social sources (political unrest, policy barrier, contamination, etc.) and environmental sources (natural disaster, diseases).

The main issue in this article is to present a comprehensive idea regarding the main factors and variables of different risk issues associated with the dairy sector. Hence, it is necessary to study several risk issues at storage, processing and distribution level in Indian dairy industry, since risks occurs due to hazard or associated with low financial capabilities, technological shortage, or may be socially responsible (political, unethical behaviour of employees, lack of government support, etc.), whereas some of the risks may be due to natural calamities (flood, storm, etc.) and some risks affects the processing activities (can be stated as input risk) and several number of risks arise due to poor infrastructural facilities at distribution level. The risks related to dairy sector is enumerated as per below:

Financial Risk

A number of financial risks have direct influence on the activities of all levels (storage, processing and distribution). These risks arise from different financial occurrences that often hinder the growth and development of dairy and subsequently affect the actions of supply chain. Some of the financial risks are inadequate loan facilities, complex loan procedures, high interest rate, inadequate finance and lack of insurance coverage.

Technological Risk

Certain risks arise from technological shortage, i.e., by which their production and opera-tional activities are hampered and slowed down. Technological shortage includes inadequate chilling system, shortage of cold room, absence of mechanized milking, feed mixture, improved processing facilities and so on.

Human Resource Risk

Human resource risks may further be subdivided into several types, viz., labour disputes, illiteracy, inefficiency of worker, shortage of skilled staff and frequent staff switching, since this business requires an efficient and experienced human resource on regular basis.

Absence of Fixed Government Policy

Lack of fixed policy of government in respect to feed management, breed management, loan disbursement, central distribution of milk, poor and non-transparent administrative and judicial system, bureaucratic complexities, political interference and muscleman ship, etc. places direct impact on storing, processing and distributing functions of dairy production and significantly affecting the smooth running of dairy industry in the country.

Political Risk

The political risks includes hartal (stopping of normal life by politicians or due to various protests), strike and much more political instability hampers the continuity of dairy production cycle.

Mismanagement and Unethical Behavior of Employees

Mismanagement and unethical behavior of employees along with corruption (mixing water with milk), damage of farm assets, spoilage of milk through improper handling and theft were consisted. Due to the mismanagement of staff, production costs get increased.

Natural Risk

Natural risks include natural uncertainties, i.e., flood, storm, drought, too much humidity, heavy rainfall, pollution and unhygienic environment, and quick perishable nature of milk, etc. affect the supply chain network of the dairy industry.

Hazard Risk

Hazard risks includes machine damage of cold storage (storage), cattle diseases, fire at farm shed, staff injury (processing), accident of transport vehicle (distribution), etc. which hampers the supply chain.

Input Risk

Input risk occurs due to the disruptions to the supply of input, which includes inadequate supply of quality feed, scarcity of feed, lack of upgrade vaccination and veterinary services are the most important input risks. Due to the input risk, production is hampered and production quantity is also fluctuated.

Poor Infrastructural Facilities

Poor infrastructural facilities not only hinder the growth and development of industry but also hamper the smooth distribution of product, i.e., in case of shortage of land, farm cannot be expanded. Similarly, poor conditioned roads and highways make delay and spoilage in moving the product from rural to urban areas.

Unethical Behaviour of Middlemen

Middlemen are present at every stage of the supply chain specifically they are very active at distribution level and livestock owners get rid of their various unethical practices, like added price, adulteration and deprivation.

Risk Mitigation Strategies

Numerous risk mitigation strategies have been explored in order to mitigate the risks associated with dairy supply chain. When probed deeper about supply chain, which includes insurance coverage, human resource management, government support, financial management, back-up capacity, off-farm income and investment, business policy and practice, etc.

Technological Development

The most important risk mitigation strategy in dairy supply chain risk management is technological development, which includes adoption of improved technology, like mechanized milking, mechanized feed mixing, improved processing facilities and cold storage, etc.

Insurance Management

Insurance coverage against livestock loss help to overcome different types of risks occurred from accidents, diseases, natural uncertainties and hazard risks.

Human Resource Management

Human resource management consists of hiring skilled staff, managing them by providing motivational and incentive facilities, training arrangements for them and building up of monitoring team. Skilled and efficient staffs are needed for reducing risks regarding mismanagement, temperature maintenance and different hazard risks, like machine damage, staff injury, etc. are indispensably required to mitigate risks.

Government Support

Government support for implementation of a fixed policy for dairy sector, removal political uncertainties, strengthen the regular supply of vaccine, reducing cost of feed, leasing abandoned land for the dairy farmers and supporting to develop technology and infrastructure is highly required to mitigate risk.

Feed Management

Feed management is another mitigation strategy for dairy risk management and it should focus on identification of certified feed suppliers in order to get regular supply of good quality feed.

Disease Management

As a part of mitigation strategy, one should focus on the disease management by arranging regular, upgraded and improved vaccination of the dairy animals. Any disease in livestock hinder business activities. Sometimes, it is such cataclysmic that the business even close down.

Transport Management

Due to quick perishable nature of milk, quick distribution is a necessity. Transportation and distribution need to be done in insulated vehicles to avoid excessive temperature increases. For quick and timely distribution, managing adequate transportation is must.

References

1. Mishra and Shekhar, 2011, Impact of Risks and Uncertainties on Supply Chain: A Dairy Industry Perspective, Journal of Management Research, ISSN 1941-899X, 2011, Vol. 3, No. 2.
2. Gorton, M., Dumitrashko, M., & White, J. (2006). Overcoming supply chain failure in the agri-food sector: A case study from Moldova. *Food Policy,* 31: 90–103.
3. IFCN. (2008). *IFCN dairy report: For a better understanding of milk production world-wide.* Kiel, Germany: Author. Retrieved 7 April, 2009, from www.ifcndairy.org
4. Ramaswami, B., Ravi, S., & Chopra, S. D. (2004). *State of the Indian farmer: Risk management* (Vol. 22). New Delhi: Academic Foundation.
5. Vanany, I., Zailani, S. & Pujawan, N. (2009). Supply chain risk management: Literature review and future research. *International Journal of Information Systems and Supply Chain Management,* 2(1): 16-33.

6. Gray, C. F., & Larson, E. W. (2008). *Project management: The managerial process* (3rd ed.). New Delhi: Tata McGraw-Hill.
7. Kumar, Praduman and Surabhi Mittal (2003) Crop diversification in India: Analysis by state and farm size group. Agricultural Situation in India. Special Number, August. Directorate of Economics and Statistics, Ministry of Agriculture, Government of India, pp. 273-280.
8. Surabhi Mittal, 2007, Strengthening Backward and Forward Linkages in Horticulture: Some Successful Initiatives, Agricultural Economics Research Review, Vol. 20 (Conference Issue) 2007 pp. 457-469.
9. Birthal, P.S., P.K. Joshi and Ashok Gulati (2007) Vertical coordination in high-value food commodities: Implications for smallholders, Chapter in the book Agricultural Diversification and Smallholders in South Asia, edited by P.K. Joshi, Ashok Gulati and Ralph Cummings Jr., Academic Foundation. pp. 405-440.
10. Tasnuba Nasir 1, Mohammed Quaddus1, Mohamamd Shamsuddoha2*, 2014, Dairy Supply Chain Risk Management in Bangladesh: Field studies of Factors and Variables, Jurnal Teknik Industri, Vol. 16, No. 2, Desember 2014, 127-138.
11. Thun, J.H., and Hoenig, D., An Empirical Analysis of Supply Chain Risk Management in the German Automotive Industry, *International Journal of Production Economics*, 131, 2011, pp. 242-249.
12. Mishra, P.K., and Shekhar, B.R., Impact of Risks and Uncertainties on Supply Chain: A Dairy Industry Perspective, *Journal of Management Research*, 3(2:E11), 2011, pp. 1-18.
13. Food and Agriculture Organization of the United Nations, Rome, 2017, Innovative risk management strategies in rural and agriculture finance : The Asian Experience.

□□□

Chapter 8

Selection and Breeding Strategies of Livestock to Enhance Livestock Productivity

Satyendra Pal Singh, Madhu Tiwari and Deepak Sharma
Department of Animal Genetics & Breeding, College of Veterinary Science and Animal Husbandry, Uttar Pradesh Pandit Deen Dayal Upadhyaya Pashu Chikitsa Vigyan Vishwavidhyalaya Evam Go Anusandhan Sansthan, Mathura

Livestock is an integral part of India's agricultural economy and supporting livelihood of more than two-third of the rural population. Livestock sector provides employment generation, asset creation, coping mechanism against crop failure and social and financial security. According to 19th livestock census, India possessed 512.05 million livestock population (Livestock census; GOI, 2012). India is one of the mega diversity country of the world with its rich & diverse genetic resources. Presently, India has 169 registered breed, which include 41 for cattle, 13 for buffalo, 28 for goat, 42 for sheep, 7 for horse and ponies, 9 for camel, 7 for pig, 1 for donkey and 1 for yak (NBAGR, 2017). These diverse genetic groups are reared in small herd size of 2-3 animals mainly by small, marginal and landless farmers belonging to different socio-economic level under different ecologies (Acharya and Bhat, 1984). In India, livestock production systems are mostly based on traditional knowledge, low cost agricultural residues and agro-byproducts leading to lower productivity. Climate change and global warming may have serious implications to the livestock sector. These may be manifested in the form of heat stress, loss of animal habitat, especially in coastal areas, scarcity of quality feed and fodder, and changes in epidemiological pattern of vector borne diseases, etc., ultimately leading to reduction in production and economic losses. The livestock sector is handicapped due to inadequate marketing and processing infrastructure and value addition. Therefore, this sector faces many challenges, like comparatively lower productivity, susceptibility of cross-bred cattle to various exotic animal diseases, shortage of feed and fodder and adverse impact on account of climate change that are needed to be addressed to sustain the growth in the sector. So, there is an urgent need to have a national policy with support of the state governments, to prevent the rapid erosion of genetic resources, ensure faster growth of the livestock sector, increased productivity and creation of employment opportunities in rural areas, leading to poverty reduction and to improve socio-economic status of a vast majority of our livestock producers.

Livestock farming system in India

In India, the livestock farming system are generally based on traditional, socio-economic consideration and available feed resources. These systems are traditionally based on the low cost agro by-products as nutritional inputs to animal for producing high quality food. It can be classified into 3 categories:-

1. ***Extensive animal production system (low input and low output):*** This system exists where quality feed and fodder resources are not available in sufficient quantity. The farmers have inadequate resource and infra-structure facilities. Marketing facilities for sale of milk and milk products are poor.
2. ***Semi-intensive animal production system (low input and high output) :*** It involves little external inputs such a feed, medicines or breeding stock. Most animal depends on locally available feed recourses, such as crop residue, they are relatively well-adapted to climate/ surrounding, heat & humidity and their genetic and reproductive abilities makes them self-sustainable animal system.
3. ***Intensive animal production system (high input and high output):*** It is mostly adopted by resource rich farmers in milk shed areas around peri-urban and industrial towns.

Genotype-environment interactions

Milk production is a factor of genotype-environment interactions. It is important to balance selection for both production (e.g., milk yield and composition) and functional (e.g., fertility, disease resistance, feed intake and body weight) traits. The external environmental stimuli (physical, chemical, climatic and biological) to which animals respond interact with their genotypes to determine level of expression.

Developing countries in the tropics often rely on exotic germplasm for breeding purposes. They, however, have climatic conditions, production systems and markets that are different from those where animals were evaluated. Consequently, the genotype-environment interactions can cause reduced efficiency of their genetic improvement programmes. In low input systems, the best alternative to circumvent the consequences of genotype by environment interactions is to select for adaptive traits.

Diversity losses in animal genetic resources

In developing countries, the major threats to genetic diversity losses are the extensive use of artificial selection, intensification of agriculture, indiscriminate cross breeding of local breeds with less adaptable exotic germplasm. In addition, introduction of highly productive breeds and demographic pressure are also contributing to the loss of valuable traits or decrease in population of local breeds. The intensive efforts is being made to introduce superior germplasm to overcome the low production of the local/ scrub/ deshi breeds, without any consideration to the local ecological and socio-economic situation, no serious organized effort in maintaining the purity of the breeds, inter-mating among breeds located in each others' vicinity resulting in dilution of breed characteristics, changes in cropping pattern and increased mechanization of agriculture with neglect of indigenous draught breeds of cattle.

Breeding policies/strategies

The appropriate strategy for any breeding programme would, therefore, be to set suitable selection goals that match the production system rather than ambitious performance objectives that cannot be reached under the prevailing environment. Area-specific approach utilizing the existing resources and taking into account the prevailing constraints appears to be the only reasonable sustainable solution. It is essential that the India should develop strategic planning so that available resources in different agro-ecological zones of the country can be exploited judiciously and utilized sustainably for further enhancing the milk production. Therefore, agro-climatic region and animal production system based breeding strategies is required with a focus on large scale implementation of improved animal genetics and breeding innovations (Sharma *et al.*, 2011). The National livestock policy would facilitate better inter-state co-ordination in regulating the export and import of livestock and livestock products, feed and food safety, biosecurity and conservation of indigenous breeds, which are essential for development of livestock sector (National livestock policy, 2013). Main breeding strategies adopted for cattle and buffalo in our country is summarized in Table 1.

Table 1: Breeding strategies for cattle and buffalo as recommended by Government of India.

S.No.	Type of animal	Breeding Strategy	Purpose
1.	Indigenous dairy breeds of cattle and buffalo	Selective breeding	Milk production
2.	Indigenous draught breeds of cattle and buffalo	Selective breeding	Draught power
3.	Indigenous dual purpose breeds of cattle	Selective breeding	Milk production and draught Power
4.	Non-descript cattle	Grading up with improved indigenous cattle breed	Milk production and draught Power
		Cross-breeding with exotic dairy breed followed by selective breeding	Milk production
5.	Non-descript buffalo	Grading up	Milk production and draught Power

1. Breeding strategies for cattle and buffalo

i) Genetic improvement of non-descript cattle by crossbreeding

Cross-breeding of non-descript and low producing cattle with high yielding exotic breeds suitable for respective agro-climatic conditions, will be encouraged in selected areas having adequate facility for feed and fodder and marketing facilities, etc. The cross-breeding of non-descript zebu cows with semen of exotic dairy cattle breeds has resulted in enhancing milk production by 5 to 8 times to that of non-descript cows, reducing age at first calving and shortening calving intervals in first generation crossbred progenies. It is a rapid and effective approach to genetically improve the non-descript zebu cattle particularly in urban, peri-urban and industrial towns where good marketing facilities for milk and milk products and adequate quantity of quality feed and green fodder resources exist. Holstein Friesian cattle have been recommended as the breed of choice in the irrigated plains and Jersey cattle as breed of choice in hilly terrain and coastal areas for cross-breeding. The optimum level of exotic inheritance in crossbred cattle should range between 50 and 75% (Gahlot, 2001).

The cross-breeding in dairy cattle has relatively shown good results mainly under semi-intensive and intensive animal production systems. Under semi-intensive animal production system, it is advisable to restrict exotic inheritance between 50 and 62.5% through *inter-se mating* in crossbred cattle. Therefore, the F_1 crossbred females under semi-intensive production system should be bred with genetically superior progeny-tested crossbred males having exotic inheritance between 50 and 75%. Under intensive production system, higher levels of exotic inheritance between 62.5 and 75% can be sustained. The F_1 females in the field should be bred with genetically superior progeny-tested males of exotic breeds having high progeny test index to produce progeny with 75% exotic inheritance. Further, the progeny tested crossbred males having exotic inheritance between 50 and 75% produced through *inter-se mating* can be used to sustain the exotic level between 62.5 and 75% (Mehla *et al.*, 2000). The traits as milk yield, fat % and protein % should be used as criteria for selection of crossbred bulls as well as import of frozen semen of exotic bulls. A well laid down breeding policy, along with availability of elite bulls in sufficient number, infrastructure on AI and animal health inputs, delivery of services, programme monitoring and regulatory mechanisms, is required to sustain the improved productivity of crossbreds and check the decline in performance in subsequent generations (Mathur, 2000).

ii) Genetic improvement of non-descript cattle by grading up

Upgradation of non-descript and low producing cattle with defined indigenous breeds in resource deficient areas and the breeding tracts of defined indigenous breeds, like Sahiwal, Tharparkar, Red Sindhi, Gir, Deoni, Hariana, Ongole, Kankrej, etc. should be encouraged. The non-descript cattle can be genetically improved by grading up using high genetic merit pedigreed and preferably progeny tested proven bulls of well known indigenous cattle breeds as per availability in the breeding tract (Mishra *et al.*, 2010). This system has failed to make any impact in improving the productivity of local non-descript cattle and fulfill their long term objective of transformation of non-descript cattle to the improved purebred breeds due to non-availability of adequate number of high genetic merit pedigreed or progeny tested bulls of indigenous breed, low production levels of indigenous breeds, irregular and short term basis breeding plan, which could not wean away the farmers/breeders from using scrub bulls for breeding their herds (Rout and Khatri, 2001).

Therefore, for successful implementation of grading up programme of non-descript cattle with improved indigenous breeds, the adequate number of superior breeding bulls of different indigenous breeds need to be out-sourced for production of quality frozen semen and artificial insemination (AI) infrastructure networking should be strengthened. The bulls for this purpose initially should be produced from superior dams identified from organized farms and farmer herds. These bulls should subsequently be genetically evaluated by large scale progeny testing programme through networking of organized farms and village herds. Proper monitoring of grading up programme of non-descript cattle on regular and long term basis can improve the milk yield by 500 to 800 kg in the first generation. By use of zebu bulls of high transmitting ability for grading up subsequently in initial generations, milk yield can be improved to the extent of 5 to 10 % per annum. In a period of 5-6 generations of continuous grading up, the non-descript stock will also be transformed into well-defined purebreds (Tomar, 2004).

iii) Genetic improvement of indigenous cattle breeds by selective breeding

Selective breeding of defined indigenous breeds of cattle having high milk yield, and those with excellent draft abilities, can be promoted to improve their production and reproduction potential. This will help their proliferation, conservation and genetic upgradation. The superior animals with high producing ability belonging to well-defined indigenous dairy and dual-purpose cattle breeds are maintained under intensive production system at organized farms and under semi-intensive management system at farmers' herds. Efforts need to be made to import semen of these breeds, if necessary, to avoid/reduce inbreeding. Intrusions of crossbreeding in their defined breeding tracts will be avoided.

Till now, various selective breeding schemes for genetic improvement of indigenous cattle and buffalo breeds have been undertaken generally on single and small size herds in isolation manner. These programmes could not contribute towards identification and selection of adequate number of genetically superior proven bulls in accurate and intense manner, which resulted in insignificant amount of genetic progress over the years in most of the herds of indigenous cattle breeds due to small size, absence of rigorous selection of males and females, poor replacement rate and more involuntary culling of cows on the basis of traits other than low milk production, unplanned breeding programme and poor monitoring (Gaur *et al.*, 2001). Therefore, it is suggested that the breed specific networking of organized farms and farmer's/breeder's herds should be developed to form a large associated test mate population for undertaking large scale progeny testing of breeding bulls. The closed herds could also be opened through two-way flow of superior germplasm from the breeding tract to nucleus herds and *vice-versa*. Thus, the adoption of open nucleus breeding technique will enhance genetic gain not only on organized herds, but also in the farmer's herds (Madalena *et al.*, 2001).

The areas of the country where the indigenous cattle breeds need to be improved by selective breeding are: Gujarat state for Gir and Kankrej; Rajasthan state for Rathi, Nagori and Tharparkar; Haryana, parts of Punjab, Western U.P. and Rajasthan for Hariana, Maharashtra and parts of Karnataka for Hallikar, Amritmahal and Deoni; Tamil Nadu for Kangayam and Andhra Pradesh for Ongole. By selective breeding, it is expected that genetic improvement can be achieved ranging from 1 to 1.5% per annum in organized herds and 8-10% per annum in farmer's herds in initial generations. Such breed improvement programme must form co-ordinating bodies for monitoring the germplasm production, performance recording, evaluation and selection of young bulls and testing their genetic merit through networking both at organized herds including progressive gaushalas maintaining indigenous breeds as well as farmer's herds under field conditions.

iv) Genetic improvement of indigenous buffalo breeds by selective breeding

The genetic improvement of buffalo herds maintained under intensive production system at organized farms and under semi-intensive management system in farmer's herds can be brought through selective breeding within breeds by networking approach of progeny-testing of bulls associating multiple organized herds as well as farmer's herds under field conditions. In certain pockets of states, like Gujarat, Rajasthan and Karnataka, Surti is recommended to be the breed of choice; Murrah is generally the breed of choice in the states of Punjab, Haryana and Western U.P besides few pockets in Punjab, where Nili Ravi has sizable population and it also needs to be improved through selective breeding. It is expected that genetic improvement of 1 to 1.5% per annum in milk production will be achieved at organized farms by selective breeding, through networking of multi-herds of a particular breed and 8-10% per annum in farmers' herds through introducing germplasm of high yielding buffalo bulls.

v) Genetic improvement of non-descript buffaloes by grading up

The genetic improvement of local non-descript buffaloes maintained under extensive system can be increased rapidly through mating with superior sires of improved breeds, like Murrah, Surti and Mehsana. Surti is recommended for Karnataka, Kerala, parts of Gujarat and Rajasthan, Nili Ravi for few pockets of Punjab, Murrah for Haryana, parts of western Uttar Pradesh and Punjab. Murrah is recommended for grading up in other parts of the country, where sufficient feed and fodder resources are available. It may be explored to collect semen from 50 % graded breed bull and then distribution for field insemination in the places with inadequate management and feed/fodder resources for sustaining the improvement achieved in the first generation of grading up programme.

2. **Breeding strategies for Sheep and Goat :** This aim to improve growth, body weight, reproductive efficiency, meat and wool quality and quantity, and to reduce mortality. An area specific approach should be adopted to improve quality and quantity of coarse wool and fine wool. Main focus should be to produce and distribute good quality rams/bucks of quality indigenous breeds, which can thrive in different agro-climatic conditions. Cross-breeding with high yielding exotic and other native breeds of goats also be considered.

3. **Breeding strategies for Pig :** This can focus on improving growth, prolificacy, quality and quantity of meat produced, survivability and utilization of low cost locally available feed and

managemental conditions. While efforts will continue to conserve some of the meritorious indigenous breeds of pigs in their defined local tracts, cross-breeding with high yielding, disease resistant exotic breeds be encouraged, with maximum 50% level of exotic germplasm in cross-breeding.

4. **Breeding strategies for Yak and Mithun :** It need to be supported in high altitude agro climatic regions for preservation and further development through selection, and where necessary, through cross-breeding with exotic germplasm.

5. **Breeding strategies for Equines :** Breeding of horses, mules, and donkeys be promoted to produce high quality stock for draft power and sports purposes. Selective breeding of indigenous breeds and cross-breeding can be considered.

6. **Breeding of Camels :** It aims at improving their desert specific draft power, milk production, disease resistance and sports traits. Breeding of Double hump camel in high altitude areas would be supported with import of semen to minimize otherwise high chances of inbreeding.

Molecular and assisted reproductive technologies for genetic improvement

Livestock genetic improvement programmes are based upon the technologies developed in the areas of quantitative genetics and reproductive biology. These include methodologies for selection of females based upon their expected producing ability and young males based on their expected predicted difference using pedigree information, physical attributes and subsequently evaluating sires on the basis of their progeny performance, etc. These coupled with AI and Embryo Transfer Technology (ETT) for further improving the intensity and accuracy of selection could be utilized for improvement of cattle herds maintained on organized farms and under field conditions (Gibson, 2005). Since large proportion of genetic gain is resulted through proper selection of superior breeding bulls, elite cows or she buffaloes for nominated mating may be chosen from organized herds and from farmers' herds through developing proper performance recording system under field conditions (Joshi and Kathiravan, 2010).

The advanced reproductive techniques, such as multiple ovulation and embryo transfer (MOET) and embryo manipulation (splitting, sexing and cloning, etc.) offer possibilities for faster multiplication of superior germplasm from highly selected elite donors and may facilitate to achieve the target producing large number of superior bull calves/ bulls and their adequate number of quality semen doses. Emerging developments in the area of molecular genetics has also opened the new possibility of identifying and using DNA level variation and major genes for genetic improvement of livestock. The molecular marker systems in animals (RFLP and microsatellites), genome maps, methods of detecting marker-QTL linkages and marker-assisted selection the new tools used in breeding programme for enhancing the rate of genetic progress. Marker assisted selection (MAS) can be effective on the traits, which are expressed late in the life of the animal, or that are controlled by a few pairs of alleles, such as longevity, fertility, resistance to certain diseases or defects of simple inheritance. This could be of great use in those traits in which the procedures of conventional selection have limitations in achieving efficiency or the results have not been satisfactory. The use of molecular techniques involves new opportunities and new challenges for building and using more predictive and efficient statistical models for livestock improvement. Therefore, integration of molecular markers with conventional breeding involving pedigree and phenotypic information evaluation is expected as future breeding tool for selection of animals (Vijh *et al.*, 2008).

Conclusions

In livestock, molecular characterization of genes of interest (Milk quality and quantity traits, fertility, draft, disease resistance, adaptive traits) and MAS as new breeding tools need to be explored for identifying superior animals and commercial exploitation of genetic potential of indigenous breeds. Centre and state level breeding services organizations should be established for overall monitoring and implementation of breeding programmes. Infrastructure facilities, such as establishment of AI centers, animal health centers, milk procurement and extension centers fully equipped with trained man power could be provided. *In-situ* and *ex-situ* conservation programmes should be integrated with breed improvement and development programmes. Breed nucleus herds/bull mother farms, young bull rearing centers, semen collection and cryo-storage banks should be established. A complete database should be established to carry out activities on animal identification and performance recording linked progeny testing programme for selection of large number of high genetic merit bulls. Open nucleus breeding system (ONBS) with or without MOET and other advanced reproductive techniques i.e. embryo splitting, embryo/sperm sexing and cloning, etc., could be adopted for faster multiplication of superior germplasm.

References

1. Acharya, R.M. and Bhat, P.N. (1984). Livestock and poultry genetic resources in India, IVRI, Research Bulletin No. 1, Indian Veterinary Research Institute, Izatnagar, India.
2. Gahlot, A.K. (2001). Status, challenges and opportunities of indigenous cattle development. Accessed from www.akgahlot.com.
3. Gaur, G.K., Tripathi, V.N., Mukherjee, S. and Choudhary, V.K. (2001). Efficiency of sire evaluation procedures in Frieswal cattle. *Indian Journal of Veterinary Research.* 10(2): 1-6.
4. Gibson, J.P. (2005). Strategies for utilizing molecular markers data for livestock genetic improvement in the developing world. In: Symposium on Marker assisted selection in animals.
5. Joshi, B.K. and Kathiravan, P. (2010). Buffalo genetic resources of India: present status on conservation and utilization. In Proceedings of International Buffalo Conference, New Delhi: 92-98.
6. Livestock census (2012). 19th livestock census-2012, BAHS-basic animal husbandry statistics, All India report, ministry of agriculture, department of animal husbandary and dairying and fisheries, Krishi Bhawan, New Delhi.
7. Madalena, F.E., Agyemang, K., Cardellino, R.C. and Jain, G.L. (2002). Genetic improvement in medium to low input system of animal production. In 7th World Congress on genetics applied to livestock production. August 19-23, 2002. France.
8. Mathur, B.N. (2000). Current Problems and Challenges Confronting the Dairy Industry in India. *Asian-Australian Journal of Animal Science.* 13(7): 447-452.
9. Mehla, R.K., Dhali, A., Singh, M., Singh, D., Sehgal, J.P., Singh, C., Verma, G.S., Gupta, A.K. and Yadav, B.R. (2000). Breeding policy for sustainable crossbred dairy cattle production system in India. *Asian-Australian Journal of Animal Science.* 13(7): 239.

10. Mishra, A.K., Rao, C.A.R. and Shankar, K.R. (2010). Analysis of potentials and problems of dairy production in rainfed agro-ecosystem of India. *Indian Journal of Animal Sciences* 80(11): 1126–33.

11. NBAGR (2017). website www.nbagr.res.in, Animal genetic resources of India (AGRI-IS) http://210.212.93.85/agris/breed.aspx

12. Raut, K.C. and Khatri, R.S. (2001). Some aspects of livestock development in India – a critical appraisal. *Journal of Indian Society of Agricultural Statistics*. 54(1): 52-61.

13. Sharma, A., Tyagi, S., Singh, U. and Mandal, D.K. (2011). Vision 2030. Project Directorate on Cattle. Meerut, Uttar Pradesh.

14. Sodhi, M., Mukesh, M., Ahlawat, S.P.S., Sobti, R.C., Gehlot, G.C., Mehta, S.C., *et al.* (2008). Genetic diversity and structure of two prominent Zebu cattle breeds adapted to the arid region of India inferred from microsatellite polymorphism. *Biochemical Genetics*. 46: 124–36.

15. Tomar, S.S. (2004). Text book of Animal Breeding. Kalyani Publishers, New Delhi, 300-01.

16. Vijh, R.K., Tantia, M.S., Mishra, B. and Bharani Kumar, S.T. (2008). Genetic relationship and diversity analysis of Indian water buffalo. *Journal of Animal Science*. 86: 1495-1502.

17. National livestock policy (2013). Government of India, Ministry of Agriculture Department of Animal Husbandry, Dairying & Fisheries.

Chapter 9

Promotion of Value Addition Techniques in Dairy Sector

Vikas Pathak and S.K.Bharati

Department of Livestock Products Technology, College of Veterinary Science and Animal Husbandry, Uttar Pradesh Pandit Deen Dayal Upadhyaya Pashu Chikitsa Vigyan Vishwavidhyalaya Evam Go Anusandhan Sansthan, Mathura

Introduction

Dairying in India is more comprehensive compared to crop production in the sense that it involves a majority of the vulnerable segments of the society for livelihoods. India now has indisputably the world's biggest dairy industry—in terms of milk production; last year India produced close to 146.31 million tons (NDDB, 2017) of milk, 50% more than the US and three times to China. approximately, India also produces the biggest directory or encyclopedia of any world dairy industry. The dairy sector in the it has shown remarkable development in the past decade and India has now become one of the largest producers of milk and value-added milk products in the world (APEDA, 2017). The milk revolution ("Operation Flood"), started by National Dairy Development Board (NDDB) in 1970, transformed India from being milk deficient to the largest milk producer surpassing USA in 1988. The program was led by Mr. Verghese Kurien, known as the Father of White Revolution in India.

The Indian Dairy industry is at the cusp of another revolution, moving towards increased contribution from various milk products. India, in its journey to become a full-fledged dairy industry, is assertively transitioning from just loose/ pouch milk to value-added products market and from unorganized/local to more of an organized and branded market. These two structural twains of shift from unorganized to organized market and from liquid milk/powder to value-added dairy products will provide long-term growth visibility to the organized dairy sector. The value incremented products though will requireblowout in the initial phase, will improve the margins and return on investments over long run for the entrepreneurs and companies in this sector. The demand for value-added products will be obsessed by changes in macro-economic factors like raise in urbanization, nuclear families, working women and improved per capita spending.

What is "Value-added"?

According to the U.S. Department of Agriculture (USDA) Office of Rural Business Development, "value-added" is defined as "The incremental value that is realized by the producer from an agricultural commodity or the product as the result of an: Change in its physical state of product, differentiated production or marketing, product segregation and economic benefit realized from the production of farm- or ranch-based renewable energy.

Adding value to raw milk can be undertaken on an individual farm or a group of farms, using a larger, and often more reliable, supply of the raw product. Developing such cottage industries have several requirements that need to be considered.

Revolution Phase of Value Addition in Milk

As world's largest milk producer, the Indian dairy sector can play a key role in food processing segment. This sector is slowly transforming from traditional to advanced form where more technological back up is being used to fulfill the rising market demand. During the last five to ten years, India has seen dramatic shift towards consumption of value-added products, such as cheese, yoghurt, UHT (ultra-heat treatment) milk, flavoured milk, and whey, etc. besides other milk products including a variety of sweet meats. In the food processing industry, the dairy sector has depicted high value addition (35%), whereas in the case of total agriculture, it is only 2 per cent. Milk processing in India is around 35 per cent, of which the organized dairy industry account for only 13 per cent of the milk produced, the remaining 22 per cent is processed in the unorganized sector (GoI, 2010). The organized dairy sector uses 80 per cent of the liquid milk for pasteurization and the rest for butter, cheese, and milk powder. The organized dairy sector has registered capacity to process around 65 per cent of the country's rural marketable surplus and about one-third of national milk production.

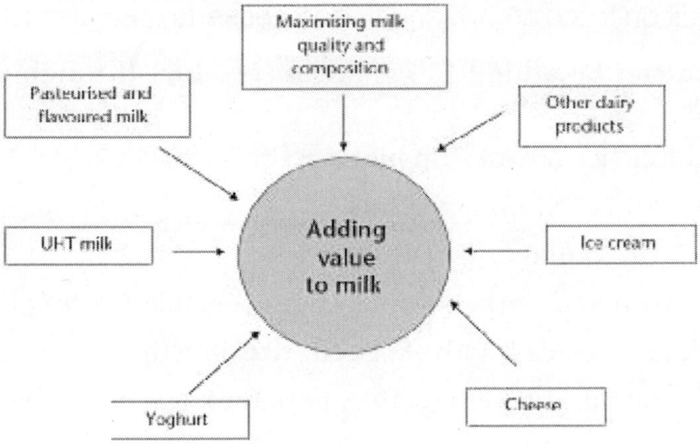

Figure 1: The diversity of dairy products that can add value to raw milk

Technology that can add value to the herd's milk by processing and marketing products can be headed as: Farm-bottled milk, cheeses, yogurt, butter, ice cream, conversion to organic, organic production of value-added products.

Bottled milk

Bottled milk is regaining the popularity and appeal it once had. Some people like the feeling of knowing the farm and conditions under which the milk they are purchasing was produced. On-farm bottling requires only the equipment necessary for the bottling, if selling raw milk. Glass or plastic containers can be used, with glass offering the appeal of environmental friendliness and nostalgia.

Advances and value addition to ice cream and frozen desserts

Ice cream is a highly delicious, very nutritious, wholesome food product that appeals to everyone. Advancement in science and technology has also lined way to innovative methods in providing more varieties, in more appealing shapes and forms with higher energy efficacy and with more precision through automatic controls. People have become reasonably health conscious and hence, the consumers have become very choosy in what they consume. Industry has already launched 'Sugar-free', 'low-calorie/dietetic', 'lactose-free' and even 'cholesterol-free' ice creams. Specific extruded ice creams mimicking shape of cartoon characters and having 'fun' aspect has been targeted specifically for the children for them to enjoy.

Value-addition to ice cream and frozen desserts

Value can be added to ice cream product through use of the following:

- Synbiotic ice cream - Prebiotic + Probiotics
- Non-fish based omega-3 fats
- Calcium/Iodine enriched ice creams
- Ice cream and Sorbets containing vegetable juices/plant sterols
- Milk fat replaced with flaxseed, rice starch, oat derivative
- New flavourings–Tea, coffee, tomatoes, spices, herbs
- Tofutti and other soy-based ice creams

Value can be added to ice cream products through use of specialty ingredients too. For instance, the SNF content of ice cream can be increased without any proneness of product to 'sandiness' owing to reduced lactose content in specialty milk powder. A single ingredient added may contribute to colour, flavour and sweetness to ice cream i.e. use of malt in ice cream.

Value addition in traditional Indian dairy products

From years, traditional dairy products remained backbone of traditional milk marketing system in India. The value added to milk through processing, product manufacturing and marketing by Indian halwais is nearly two times the price paid to the milk producers, while the western dairy products manufactured by Indian organized sector add about 50% value to milk. Fluid milk accounts for the largest product category accounting for approximately 60% of total dairy market. Ghee, paneer and khoa are the three other largest product categories. The operating margin of traditional dairy products is higher, mainly due to lower raw material cost. The raw material costs as percentage of sales prices of dahi, rasagolla, gulabjamun, peda, paneer, etc. are much lower than those of butter and milk powder (Aneja et al., 2002, FAO, 1990). Already, products like dahi, paneer, shrikhand, few khoa and chhana based sweets, lassi, chhas, etc. are sold by national and regional players. The product profile of organized dairies indicates relatively higher success in the marketing of peda (in southern India), shrikhand (in western India), dahi (across the country) and paneer (northern and western India). Other products, which show high seasonal sales, include buttermilk, curds and lassi.

Manufacture of value-added dairy products using membrane processing technologies

Membrane technology has greater applications in dairy and food industry. It is being utilized both, in traditional dairy processing and for new and innovative applications, like production of value-added dairy products. It is used for the processing of milk as well as whey, for the fractionation of dynamic dairy ingredients, etc. The key membrane technologies are the pressure driven membrane processes viz., Microfiltration (MF), Ultrafiltration (UF), Nanofiltration (NF) and Reverse osmosis (RO). UF and MF technologies are the primary membrane separation technologies used by the dairy industry for the fractionation of milk constituents (Pouliot, 2008). UF has been used successfully to concentrate dairy proteins in both, whey and milk proteins from the much smaller compounds, such as lactose, vitamins and minerals. MF traditionally has been used in the dairy industry for bacteria removal, defatting of whey and micellar casein enrichment for cheese making. Some value added ingredients developed using the membrane technology are Milk Protein Isolates, Milk Protein Concentrates (MPC), Milk derived whey protein, α-lactalbumin, β-lactoglobulin, Milk mineral concentrate, Caseins products, Lactoferrin, Phospholipids, Gangliosides, High protein powder, etc.

Recent advances in value added fermented milks

Fermented milk products are believed to have originated in the Middle East region as a means of extending the shelf life of milk, and over time they have permeated around the world. According to the definition given in the general standards of identity for fermented milks published by the International Dairy Federation, fermented milks are prepared from milk and/or milk products (e.g., any one or combinations of whole, partially or fully skimmed, concentrated or powdered milk, buttermilk powder, concentrated or powdered whey, milk protein (such as whey proteins, whey protein concentrates, soluble milk proteins, edible casein and caseinates), cream, butter or milk fat (all of which have been manufactured from raw materials that have been at least pasteurized) by the action of specific microorganisms, which results in a reduction of the pH and coagulation. Some of the proposed health benefits of consumption of fermented dairy products are: aids in relieving symptoms of lactose intolerance; protection against gastro-intestinal infection; anticarcinogenic effects; improving immunity; reducing cholesterol levels; treating constipation;

antihypertensive activity and antiallergenic qualities. In the present scenario, India accounts for less than 1.0 % of the total world's market under fermented milks segment. Currently, most of the fermented milk products available are predominantly dahi (Indian yogurt) and a few beverages such as flavored milk, fermented and unfermented milk and butter milk. But, the market has expanded beyond these most common fermented milk products and the new entrants are juices, smoothies, cereal, nutrition bars and infant/toddler formula.

Cheese a value added dairy product

Cheese is probably the most popular and well- known value-added dairy product. Hundreds of cheese varieties are produced, ranging from soft cheeses (mozzarella, ricotta, etc.) to hard cheeses (cheddar, colby, swiss, etc.). Cheese is considered an important food item with high nutritional value and is available in great diversity of flavors, texture, tastes, varieties and shapes. Around 2000 individual varieties of cheeses are being produced in the world, classified on the basis of their form, manufacturing, ripening and chemical composition. Cheese is more compact with longer shelf life as compared to any other dairy product, hence contributing to its worth and value for portability, long life and high content of fat, protein and minerals. Cheese manufacturing is one of the classical examples of milk preservation. It is formed by coagulation of the protein 'Casein' which is mainly present in milk obtained primarily from cows, buffalo and very little from goats and sheep. Fat content present in milk along with protein are found in various proportions. During cheese production, the milk is usually acidified, and coagulated by adding the enzyme after which, solids are separated and pressed into final form of cheese.

Value added organic dairy products

Organic products represent the produce which may not immediately be considered as value-added dairy products however, if the milk or cow has a certain attribute or is being raised in a specified manner that increases its product value, then only these can qualify as value-added. The growing demand for organic dairy products is driven primarily by consumers' belief in the higher quality and safety of these products, and their awareness of the positive environmental, animal welfare, and ethical impacts of organic agricultural practices. Many are concerned about the use of antibiotics and genetically engineered Growth Hormone that is injected into an estimated 30 per cent of lactating cows in conventional dairies. These are some of the reasons why consumers choose organic dairy products despite higher prices. Organic milk comes from cows that are not given any hormones, antibiotics, or pesticides. They have access to open pastures and are fed 100-per cent organic feeds grown in fields that are chemical-free for at least 3 years. Organic milk must be handled separately from conventional milk and never intermixed. Organic milk and milk products must be processed, either on-farm or off-farm, in a certified organic plant.

Prospect of value added dairy sector

India's dairy market presents lucrative and impactful opportunities. During the last 15 years, Milk Cooperatives have converted about 20% of milk procured into traditional and value-added products that offer about 20% higher revenue. This share of value-added products is estimated to increase to 30% by 2021-22. The Department of Animal Husbandry, Dairying & Fisheries (DAHDF) has initiated a number of schemes with the objective of doubling the dairy farmers' income in line with the resolution of the government to double the farmers' income by 2022. The government has undertaken three important projects for dairy development-National Dairy Plan Phase I (NDP I), National Programme for Dairy Development (NPDD) and Dairy Entrepreneurship Development Scheme. Dairy Entrepreneurship Development Scheme is being implemented by NABARD (National Agricultural and Rural Development Bank) in association with the state governments through nationalized banks at the district level. Dairy Processing & Infrastructure Development Fund (DIDF) is an ambitious scheme, which was launched in 2017-18 with an aim to double the income of the milk farmers and to further the efforts of the White Revolution. This scheme is being implemented by the NDBB through the state government through co-operative milk organizations/milk federations of the concerned state.

The aim of the scheme is doubling of dairy farmers' income which is not possible without creating additional milk processing infrastructure. This plan envisages assigning a higher priority to the judicious use of available resources through the adoption of modern technologies, which will ultimately help all the stakeholders involved including the milk producers.

Conclusions

The key to the success of value-added products is to market a supreme quality product that is reasonably priced and obtainable in a convenient location for the consumer to purchase. The contemporary consumer expects the food that they eat to be healthy and capable of preventing illness. The expanding business prospects provided by these products and their accompanying value-addition call for focused efforts towards continuous innovation and renovation of these product technologies. It is necessary to adopt new technology and practice improved system of dairy management to add value to the business of dairy industry. For development of technology, considerable R&D work has been carried out by various research institutes. Thus, value addition techniques generate so many opportunities for the dairy sector to empower the recent dairy product world.

□□□

Chapter 10

Sustainable Economic Model for Enhancing Farmers Income Through Dairy Farming

Rajneesh Sirohi, Yajuvendra Singh and D.N.Singh

Department of Livestock Production Management, College of Veterinary Science and Animal Husbandry, Uttar Pradesh Pandit Deen Dayal Upadhyaya Pashu Chikitsa Vigyan Vishwavidhyalaya Evam Go Anusandhan Sansthan, Mathura

India is the largest milk producing country in the world, producing 15o million metric tonnes of milk. India is also the world's largest and fastest growing market for milk and milk products. About 85 per cent of farmers in the country belong to the small and marginal category. While, on an average, livestock contributes about 12 per cent of farmers' income in India, the same for small and marginal farmers and landless Iabourers is 36 per cent. Furthermore, while farmers' income is growing at 3.5 per cent annually, income from livestock is growing at about 14.5 per cent. Therefore, in order to double income of farmers, it is important to focus on the dairy sector for these categories of farmers. Dairy sector has the advantage of the presence of expertise, variety of products, large market and infrastructure. unlike crops, there is no price volatility in case of milk.

Therefore, there is a need to mobilize more people to the dairy sector. Co-operatives have played a vital role in the development of the dairy sector. Milk co-operatives need to be spread throughout the country with value addition by private sector and multinationals. Dairy farming can be made more glamorous and profitable through commercialization. Financing by commercial banks can be encouraged. Market is not a problem for the dairy sector, while India itself has a large market, neighbouring countries have milk deficit. All that the farmers need is access to professional inputs, finances, and markets.

Co-operative society is an organization of group of people with collective responsibilities and thoughts for the development of needy, especially under-privileged. "A co-operative is an autonomous association of persons united voluntarily to meet their common economic, social and cultural needs and aspirations through a jointly-owned and democratically-controlled enterprise." It is based on the values of the development of agriculture, forestry, banking, credit, agro-processing, storage, marketing, dairy, fishing and housing and its network covers 85 per cent of rural households. It occupies a key position in agricultural development with support in resource and input use, harvesting of water resources, marketing channels, storage facilities, distribution channels, value addition, market information and a regular monitoring network system. Co-operatives are also engaged in economic activities, like disbursement of credit, distribution of agricultural inputs (seeds, fertilizers, and agrochemicals), etc. Co-operatives have inherent advantages in tackling the problems of poverty alleviation, food security and employment generation. It is considered to have immense potential to deliver goods and services in areas where both, the public and private sector have failed. By and large, co-operatives (except a few large ones) are "local institutions", addressing "local needs", employing "local talent", and led by "local leaders". A situation is emerging wherein there is a possibility of people migrating back to rural areas, as the co-operatives exhibit vast potential for generating self-employment opportunities at grassroots. Dairy co-operative is a success story in India. To prevent the exploitation of marginal milk producers by the private dairy, farmers in Gujarat formed the "Kaira District Co-operative Milk Producers' Union Ltd." in Anand. Under this Union, co-operatives were formed at every village to collect surplus quantities of milk from small producers and a modern dairy was established to process the milk locally. The products were sold under the brand name Amul since 1955. The success of this dairy soon spread across the neighbouring districts of Gujarat. To support these Dairy Federations and to expand the activities, the Gujarat Co-operative Milk Marketing Federation, an apex marketing body was set up in 1973.

Presently, 170 Milk Producers' Co-operative Unions and 15 State Co-operative Milk Marketing Federations are involved in milk processing. However, many of these dairy federations could not function successfully, in the true spirit of a people's movement, barring a few states. Nevertheless, the dairy co-operatives account for the major share of processed liquid milk marketed in the country. During 2004-05, there were 12.95 million members of dairy co-operatives who sold milk and milk products worth Rs.3320 crore. Dairy Co-operatives have been instrumental in transforming the rural economy on the lines of co-operative sugar factories.

For sustaining profit from a dairy farm require a scientific management syatem. An efficient management of cattle will be incomplete without a well-planned and adequate housing of cattle. Improper planning in the arrangement of animal housing may result in additional labour charges and thus, curtail the profit of the owner. During erection of a house for dairy cattle, care should be taken to provide comfortable accommodation for an individual cattle. No less important is the: (1) proper sanitation, (2) durability, (3) arrangements for the production of clean milk under convenient and economic conditions, etc.

The points which should be considered before the erection of dairy buildings are as follows:

1. **Topography and Drainage :** A dairy building should be at a higher elevation than the surrounding ground to offer a good stope for rainfall and drainage for the wastes of the dairy to avoid stagnation within. A levelled area requires less site preparation and thus lesser coat of building. Low lands and depressions and proximity to places of bad odour should be avoided.
2. **Soil type :** Fertile soil should be spared for cultivation. Foundation soil as far as possible should not be too dehydrated or desiccated. Such a soil is susceptible to considerable swelling during rainy season and exhibit numerous cracks and fissures.
3. **Exposure to the sun and protection from wind :** A dairy building should be located to a maximum exposure to the sun in the north and minimum exposure to the sun in the south and protection from prevailing strong wind currents whether hot or cold. Buildings should be placed so that direct sunlight can reach the platforms, gutters and mangers in the cattle shed. As far as possible, the long axis of the dairy barns should be set in the north-south direction to have the maximum benefit of the sun.

4. **Accessibility :** Easy accessibility to the buildings is always desirable. Situation of a cattle shed by the side of the main road preferably at a distance of about 100 meters should be aimed at.
5. **Durability and attractiveness :** It is always attractive when the buildings open up to a scenic view and add to the grandeur of the scenery. Along with this, durability of the structure is obviously an important criterion in building a dairy.
6. **Water supply :** Abundant supply of fresh, clean and soft water should be available at a cheap rate.
7. **Surroundings :** Areas infested with wild animals and dacoits should be avoided. Narrow gates, high manger curbs, loose hinges, protruding nails, smooth finished floor in the areas, where the cows move and other such hazards should be eliminated.
8. **Labour :** Honest, economic and regular supply of labour be available.
9. **Marketing :** Dairy buildings should only be in those areas from where the owner can sell his products profitably and regularly. He should be in a position to satisfy the needs of the farm within no time and at a reasonable price.
10. **Electricity :** Electricity is the most important sanitary method of lighting a dairy. Since a modern dairy always handles electric equipments which are also economical, it is desirable to have an adequate supply of electricity.
11. **Facilities, labour, food :** Cattle yards should be so constructed and situated in relation to feed storages, hay stacks, silo and manure pits as to effect the most efficient utilization of labour. Sufficient space per cow and well arranged feeding mangers and resting areas contribute not only to greater milk yield of cows and make the work of the operator easier, but also minimizes feed expenses. The relative position of the feed stores should be quite adjacent to the cattle barn. Noteworthy features of feed stores are given:
    a) Feed storages should be located at hand near the centre of the cow barn.
    b) Milk-house should be located almost at the centre of the barn.
    c) Centre cross-alley should be well designed with reference to feed storage, the stall area and the milk house.

Types of Housing

The most widely prevalent practice in this country is to tie the cows with rope on a ***Katcha*** floor except some organized dairy farms belonging to government, co-operatives or military, where proper housing facilities exist. It is quite easy to understand that unless cattle are provided with good housing facilities, the animals will move too far in or out of the standing space, defecating all round and even causing trampling and wasting of feed by stepping into the mangers. The animals will be exposed to extreme weather conditions all leading to bad health and lower production.

Dairy cattle may be successfully housed under a wide variety of conditions, ranging from close confinement to little restrictions except at milking time. However, two types of dairy barns are in general use at the present time :

1. The loose housing barn in combination with some type of milking barn or parlour.
2. The conventional dairy barn.

Loose housing system

Loose housing may be defined as a system, where animals are kept loose except milking and at the time of treatment. The system is most economical. Some features of loose housing system are as follows:

1. Cost of construction is significantly lower than conventional type.
2. It is possible to make further expansion without much changes.
3. Facilitate easy detection of animals in heat.
4. Animals feel free and therefore, proves more profitable with even minimum grazing.
5. Animals get optimum exercise which is extremely important for better health and production.
6. Overall better management can be rendered.

The floor and manger space requirement of dairy cows are given in Table.

Other Provisions

The animal sheds should have proper facilities for milking barns, calf pens, calving pens and arrangement for store rooms, etc. In each shed, there should be arrangement for feeding, manger, drinking area and loafing area. The shed may be cemented or brick paved, but in any case it should be easy to clean. The floor should be rough, so that animals will not slip. The drains in the shed should be shallow and preferably covered with removable tiles. The drain should have a gradient of 1" for every 10′ length. The roof may be of corrugated cement sheet, asbestos or brick and rafters. Cement concrete roofing are too expensive.

Inside the open unpaved area, it is always desirable to plant some good shady trees for excellent protection against direct cold winds in winter and to keep cool in summer.

Floor space per animal (Sq. feet)

Types of Animals	Covered Area	Open area	Manger length per animal (inches)
Cows	20-30	80-100	20-24
Buffaloes	25-35	80-100	24-30
Young stock	15-20	50-60	15-20
Pregnant Cows	100-120	180-200	24-30
Bulls Pen	120-140	200-250	24-30

Cattle Shed : The entire shed should be surrounded by a boundary wall of 5′ height from three sides and manger, etc. The feeding area should be provided with 2 to 2 1/2 feet of manger space per cow. All along the manger, there shall be 10" wide water trough to provide clean, even, available drinking water. The water trough, thus, constructed will also minimize the loss of fodders during feeding. Near the manger, under the roofed house 5′ wide floor should be paved with bricks having a little slope. Beyond that, there should be open unpaved area (40′ x 35′) surrounded by 5′ walls with one gate. A plan for such a house along with the plan for calves shed and their sections are shown in Fig. 13.1. It is preferable that animals face north, when they are eating fodder under the shade. During cold wind in winter the animals will automatically lie down to have the protection from the walls.

Shed for calves : On one side of the main cattle shed, there shall be fully covered shed.

Care of the cow and calf during and after parturition

Success in dairying depends largely on the proper care and efficient management of the herd. All dairy operations must be planned with due regard to the comfort of the animals. Care of pregnant cows during and after calving, therefore, should receive the personal attention of the dairy farmer; otherwise he is likely to make many costly mistakes. Few hints are given here for his guidance:

A. Caring for the cow

1. Usually a dairy cow will carry her calf a period of 282 days (gestation period). However, they may range from 270 to 290 days after conception. If breeding records have been kept, which every farmer should do, the date can be calculated to within one to ten days. Knowing expected date of calving is a "must" for taking all future care of the pregnant cows.
2. In handling advanced pregnant cows, care should be taken to prevent them from being injured by slipping on stable floors or by crowding through doorways, or by mounting cows or bulls that are in heat. Separate the pregnant cows from rest and allow them to live in a little isolated way.
3. Symptoms that an animal is about to calve include swelling of the udder, swelling of the vulva and dropping away ligaments around the tall head. At this stage, she should be housed in calving pen. Birth usually takes place in one or two hours. The room should be clear, well-ventilated, well-bedded and finally, disinfected. Alternatively a small well-grassed pasture free from trash or manure and close to the farmstead (to get some observation) make a good calving place except during monsoon and cold months.
4. The majority of domesticated animals require little or no assistance in the actual act of parturition, provided they are in a reasonable healthy and vigorous state. At the same time, it is advisable that someone shall be at hand to give any help, if some emergency arises. At the first sign of calving, the front feet of the calf should appear first, then the nose. Any abnormality in presentation requires immediate attention by a veterinarian. Remember that if the labour prolongs for more than 4 hours, abnormal presentation is probable (dystokia), immediately provide veterinary aid.

5. After parturition the exterior of the genitalia, the flanks and tail should be washed with warm clear water containing some crystals of potassium permanganate or Neem leaves boiled in water. This will give a good antiseptic wash.
6. Keep the cow warm to prevent her from chill and it is desirable to give her warm water or warm Gur sarbat to drink just after parturition.
7. It is normal for the udder to become large and swollen just before calving. Controversy exists as to whether or not the udder should be milked out before calving. Special precautions should be exercised to see that old nails, loose glass pieces, etc., do not cut and injure the swollen udder. Milk the co-partially to avoid milk fever after parturition.
8. The placenta will normally leave the cow within 2-4 hours. If it is not expelled between 8-12 hours, administer Ergot mixture. Beyond 12 hours, apply manual help by a veterinarian.
9. There are always dangers that high producing cows will develop milk fever and mastitis. The dairyman should remain alert for any symptoms of the diseases. To avoid milk fever, it is best not to draw all the milk from the udder for a day or two after calving. To avoid mastitis, regular tests should be made by a veterinarian.
10. Feed the cow at first only bran mash moistened with lukewarm water to provide laxative effect. Some green grass may also be given. After 2 days mixture of oats, bran and linseed mash can be used to replace the bran mash. If the cow is in good condition at the time of calving, the amount of feed during these two days does not matter. The amount of concentrates should then be gradually increased with the aim of reaching full dosages in two weeks.

B. Caring for the Newborn Calf

1. Immediately after the calf is born, make sure that all mucus is removed from the nose and mouth. If the calf does not start to breathe, artificial respiration should be used by alternately compressing and relaxing the chest walls with the hands after laying the calf on its side.

2. Apply tincture of iodine to the navel at birth, and dust with boric acid power. If a long cord is attached to the navel, swip it off about 2" from the body before applying iodine. The navel cord should not be tied bur allowed to drain.
3. Udder most conditions the calf will be on its feet and ready for suckling within an hour. Some assistance at this stage is useful. Much infection can be prevented, if an attendant cleans the udder before the calf nurses.
4. Be sure the calf gets first milk (colostrums) at least for 48 hours. The antibodies present in colostrums protect the calf against disease and has a laxative effect. The rate of milk feeding should be about 10 % of the calf's weight per day, upto a maximum of 5-6 litres per day. I scouring occurs, the milk allowance should be reduced to ½ or less until the calf recover.
5. If possible, follow weaning system (to remove the calf from the dam). Usually the calf is separated permanently from its mother after the first feeding because it simplifies management and reduces the food and labour costs for rearing. At present, there is a great variation in practice regarding the best time to remove the calf from the dam. Some dairymen allow the calf to remain with its dam for 2 or 3 days or until the milk is suitable to put in the regular supply. It probably makes little difference as to when the calf is removed from its dam.
6. The calf is best maintained in an individual pen or stall for the first few weeks. This allows more careful attention to individuals. After about 8 weeks of age, it may be handled with a group.
7. Take body weight of the cow, if possible, and identify the calf by tattooing.
8. At the age of 15 days, 30-40.cc. of H.S. serum should be inoculated into the calf.
9. Dehorn the calf at an early age preferably within 15 days.
10. Teats of the udders of heifer in excess of four are usually best removed. Frequently limited amounts of milk may be secreted by extra teats creating difficulty at milking time.
11. At the age of 3 months, the calf should be vaccinated against anthrax and 15 days, thereafter it should be vaccinated against B.Q.

Environmental Stress Management

Environmental temperatures affect dry matter and water consumption of cows and buffaloes, which subsequently affect animal productivity. The animals should be provided *ad libitum* water during hot-dry and hot-humid months so that the requirement of milk synthesis can be met. The roughage intake of cows during summer reduces due to more heat of fermentation generated in rumen from fibrous feed. In fact, heat also reduces total DM intake. Therefore, animals should be fed lush green fodder and adequate concentrate during summer. Crossbred cows can resist the rigours of high temperature for longer periods without adverse effect on dry matter intake, milk production and the production of fat, protein and lactose, if *adlib* water and green fodder are made available during hot-dry months of May-June.

- Provision of wallowing tank for buffaloes during summer and hot-humid season further improves their reproductive behaviour and milk production.
- Through adoption of eco-friendly housing system (Kuccha floor, sand bedding) problems of hoof diseases can be minimized. Besides, introduction of forced water and fan cooling can sustain the body temperature of crossbreds cow at a temperature levels ranging between 38.4 to 38.6^{0}C. The average body temperature of cows can be reduced from 39.62 to 38.40^{0}C in hot-humid season during day time (Singh and Mehla, 1999). The process of sustaining body temperature close to normal range 38.4 to 38.8^{0}C increases average daily milk yield of crossbred cows by 2.86 and 2.26 Kg in hot-dry and hot-humid season, respectively.
- In winter season, adequate protection from the cold stress also improves milk productivity by 2.6 Kg/day/cow. Buffaloes have remarkable capacity to adopt themselves to the most adverse climatic conditions from 4 to 40^{0}C. Appropriate nutritional/ feeding approaches, like offering the fresh feeds during evening/ night or cool hours should be adopted. The lactating animals should be offered succulent green fodder along with high amounts of concentrate. The animal should be offered adequate salt and sodium bicarbonate to maintain the sodium and potassium levels of blood.

Milking management

- Lactating animals should be milked completely and at regular milking intervals. For complete letdown of milk, proper and adequate milking stimulus should be given to buffaloes. Washing with lukewarm water improves milk letdown time. Improper preparation of the lactating animal leads to incomplete evacuation of milk, which in turn increases the amount of residual milk and decreases the intensity and amount of milk secretion.
- If more number of animals are to be milked in a organized dairy farm, use of single cloth for washing the udder and teats should not be done, as it spreads pathogens between cows. The towel cloth should never be dipped in bucket after it has been in contact with a cow.
- Hands of the milder, his dress and milking instruments should be clean and properly sanitized. It is the duty of every milker to regularly inspect the udder, teats and milk for any injury/ abnormality. Any change should be recorded and treatment followed.
- It has been observed that comfortable and congenial environment during milking leads to more milk yield from the animals than that of roughly handled and excited ones (Release of oxytocin is inhibited in stressed animals). Therefore, attempt should be made to make milking a pleasant experience for the cows to ensure more milk flow. Overcrowding of animals in milking place should be stopped, as it also causes stress.

Tips for clean milk production

- Production of clean milk is one of the most important factors in dairy industry.
- Animal housing should be clean and free from any contaminants.
- Milking place should be separate and suitably comfortable.
- Washing of teats/udder before milking.
- Animal should be healthy and free from any disease. Milk drawn from a healthy animal already contains some bacteria.
- Milker hand should be clean/properly washed.

- Milker should be healthy and free from any infection or disease.
- Milking machine, milking utensils/collection vessels should be clean to lower the bacteriological counts of milk.
- Storage tank of milk should be washed with cleaning detergent daily.
- Milk should be stored at 4^0C immediately till milking operations are over.
- A clean and good quality muslin cloth may be used to remove foreign particles of milk.
- Milk tankers should be cleaned at regular intervals and milk transport to the plant should be within 1 hour of milking.
- Milk with high Somatic Cell Counts (SCC) or mastitis should be discarded. Cows producing such milk require immediate attention for mastitis control.

Concetrate feeding

Concentrate is used to supplement roughages to meet milk production requirement and is essential even for maintenance, when poor quality roughages are fed. The grain should be grinded to atleast ¼ of the raw size so that it may not pass off undigested in dung. To further enhance digestibility and palatability, concentrate mixture can be made wet with water and sweetener (Gur) for atleast 4-6 hrs. before mixing with dry feed hay. The ingredients of the concentrate mixture should be of standard quality and free from fungus (aflatoxins), weeds, moulds, and dust.

- Concentrate mixture is given at the rate of 2.5 kg per kg milk for animals yielding milk of high fat percentage, in addition to maintenance ration.

Milk production (kg)	Concentrate (kg)
5.0	2.0
10.0	4.0
15.0	6.0
20.0	8.0

- Concentrate mixture is given at the rate of one kg per 1.5-2.0 kg milk for buffaloes.

- The detailed composition of the concentrate is given below:

Composition of the Feed Materials	Parts
Maize	16%
Barley/wheat/oats or combination	15%
G.N. Cake (oiled)	18%
Mustard Cake (oiled)	8%
Cotton seed cake	7%
Wheat bran	15%
Deoiled Rice bran	8%
Mineral Mixture (BIS standard)	2%
Common salt	1%
BIS Standard for Feed Quality	
Crude Protein not less than	20%
Crude Fibre not more than	10%
Acid Insoluble Ash not more than	2.50%
Crude Fat not less than	4.50%
Moisture not more than	10%

Buffaloes

Milk production (kg)	Concentrate (kg)
5	2.5
10	5
15	7.5
20	10

- The amount of concentrate mixture can be altered based on the type of feed i.e., green or straw and the dry matter content. However, more grain intake relative to the forage often result in off-feed problems, metabolic acidosis and decline in milk production.

Rations for dairy cows weighing 400 kgs with 10 kg milk yield	
Green fodder (25% DM)	10 kg
Wheat Bhusa	4 kg
Concentrate mixture	5 kg
Or	
Green Berseem (12% DM)	12 kg
Wheat Bhusa	5 kg
Concentrate mixture	5 kg

Cow- 450 LW, 20 kg milk (4% fat)

A ration on a leguminous fodder, such as berseem as the chief roughage is given below:

Feedstuffs	Quantity	DM	TDN	CP
Berseem fodder, kg*	80	9.6	6.144	1.344
Concentrate, kg	6.5	5.85	4.095	0.819
TDN 70%				
CP 20%				
Total nutrients, kg		15.45	10.239	2.163

*10 kg of berseem should be replaced by wheat/rice straw, equivalent to its DM for avoiding 'bloat' condition, and to keep the animal warm during winter, as straw generates more heat during fermentation.

Maintenance of lactation

High protein die with highly degradable protein is avoided at the initiation of lactation. An extra allowance of 1-1.5 kg concentrate mixture over and above the calculated amount for a period of 2 months can be given to encourage the cows to produce more milk. Increasing the bypass protein of the diet without increasing the total protein intake can prove economically beneficial to high yielding animals.

The composition of the concentrate mixture is given below:

Ingredients	Percentage Part
1. Ground Nut/Cotton Seed/Mustard Cake	33
2. Maize grain/Oats/Wheat	31
3. Wheat bran/Rice Bran	33
4. Mineral mixture	2
5. Common salt	1

Feeding during dry period

During lactation, the animal exhibit heat symptoms and passes through the various stages of reproductive events and becomes pregnant. During the last 2-3 months of pregnancy, a concentrate supplementation over and above maintenance is given at the rate of 1-2 kg/cow/day and 1.5-3.0 kg/buffalo/day with the composition as described above. The requirement of the buffaloes differs from that of cattle as they are heavier in body weight than cattle, have more feed capacity (0.5%), possess better capacity to utilize crop residue and have more fat in milk. Therefore, buffalo is less temperamental with respect to feeding of crop residue based diets.

Type of fodder and feeding

- The fodder can be fed fresh as such or in preserved form like hay or silage. Non-leguminous fodder substantially meets the maintenance requirement but is limiting in protein content while leguminous fodder are rich in protein, calcium and phosphorus but is limiting in terms of dry matter (and thereby TDN) because of high moisture content. Therefore, a combination of both leguminous and non-leguminous fodder is best to meet the maintenance and production requirement of animals.
- Split feeding day and night during summer and hot-humid months improves milk production. Non-availability of water restricts the total DM intake of lactation animals and could limit peak milk yield. The reports indicate that even a one pound increase in peak yield translates into a 200 pound increase in milk production over the entire lactation.
- Portable and clean water should be provided *adlib* during summer months, as it is one of the most essential input for milk production.
- Lactating animal feed should contain at least 17% crude fibre. The low fibre diet along with high intake of concentrate during hot-humid season leads to drop in milk fat per cent, a condition called "low fat syndrome". The changes occur due to altered ratio of Acetate: Propionate as a result of less feed intake and more of concentrate. On the other hand, high fibre and low quality fodder always limit intake of animals, and this is very true during hot-humid conditions. The quantity of crop residues offered during hot-humid season should be minimum to relieve the animal of extra heat load, as a result of higher heat of fermentation from crop residues. This can also increase the energetic efficiency for milk production.

❑❑❑

Chapter 11

Livestock By-product Management to Increase Farmers Income

D.N. Singh, R. Sirohi and Yajuvendra Singh

Department of Livestock Production Management, College of Veterinary Science and Animal Husbandry, Uttar Pradesh Pandit Deen Dayal Upadhyaya Pashu Chikitsa Vigyan Vishwavidhyalaya Evam Go Anusandhan Sansthan, Mathura

India is bestowed by nature with a vast livestock resources comprising of 299.9 million total Bovine population (Cattle-190 million, Buffalo-108 million, Mithun- 0.29 million and Yak-0.07 million), 65.06 million sheep, 135.17 million goats, 10.29 million pigs and 729.2 million poultry (DAHD&F, 2014). India has one of the largest livestock population in the world. It accounts for around 58% of the world buffalo population and 14.7% of the cattle population (Rais and Kuruvilla,2016). India is bestowed with vast livestock wealth and it is growing at the rate of 6% per annum. The contribution of livestock industry including poultry and fish is increasing substantially in GDP of country, which accounts for more than 40% of total agricultural sector and more than 12% of GDP (Jayathilakan, 2012). This contribution would have been much greater had the animal by-products been also efficiently utilized. Efficient utilization of by-products has direct impact on the economy and environmental pollution of the country. In recent years, there has been wide spread and increasing interest throughout the world in creating newer channels of utilization for the by-products of the dairy, meat and skin industry along with dung & urine for preparation of valuable product, such as Panchgavya, Jeevamrit and Gau-mutra ark, etc. for betterment of socio-economic status of farmers as well as for healthy environmental issues.

The economic growth of a country is directly related with energy, renewable as well as non-renewable. The non-renewable energy resources are limited, and excessive dependence on them not only causes environmental degradation but also escalates the cost of their production/extraction, leading to higher prices for the consumers. During the past few years, India has shown a significant growth in development of renewable energy sources, raising their share to 12 per-cent in the total electricity generation in the country (Mishra and Singh, 2013). Biogas is one of the renewable sources of energy. It is obtained as a by-product of the process called anaerobic digestion. It contains about 60 per cent methane (CH_4) and 40 per cent carbon-dioxide (CO_2). The green-house gas emissions from the livestock farms can be reduced following anaerobic digestion approach of converting cattle dung into bio-energy. Thus, this process can be widely applied for the production of the biogas on a large scale. Moreover, the resulting methane can be utilized for electricity generation, lighting, heating and cooking.

A. Dairy Industry Byproduct

In recent years, there has been widespread and increasing interest throughout the world in creating newer channels of utilization for the by-products of the dairy industry. A dairy by-product may be defined as a product of commercial value produced during the manufacture of a main product. Skim milk, buttermilk, ghee residue and whey are the main dairy by-products. Utilization of dairy by-products improves plant economy, makes valuable nutrients available for humans and reduces environmental pollution originating from dairy waste. Conversion of edible substances into non-food items is not ordinarily justifiable, especially in countries where there is an overall shortage of milk supplies. It has always been realized that economic disposal of by-products is an essential perquisite to profitable dairying. Each and every component of milk must be judiciously processed into edible form for the obvious reason of its unique nutritional value. These by-products are, therefore, receiving increasing attention for their proper utilization and help in income generation for the farmers.

In some countries, like India, the most of problems associated with the production and utilization of dairy by-products are: a low per capita availability of milk, higher proportion of buffalo milk, poor quality of raw milk, lack of organized manufacture of products, lack of adequate technology, high cost of new technologies, lack of in-house R&D, lack of proper infrastructure, lack of indigenous equipments and plants, etc. Before setting up a by-product factory, it is important to consider the economical aspects of the plant, because sometimes the cost of manufacture of the by-product may be more as compared to the by-product and, therefore, the setting up of the by-product plant is not economically feasible. But with advancement in science and technology as also the automation of plants, the economic feasibility of these can be improved.

In India, skim milk is mostly utilized either for standardization purposes or preserved in spray dried form. Only a very small quantity of skim milk, mostly of substandard quality, has to be used as by-product. Whey and Its by-products In India, there has been a tremendous increase in the production of cheese and coagulated milk products resulting in a proportionate increase in whey. Buttermilk is the by-product obtained during the manufacture of butter. The exact amount of buttermilk production in India is not estimated. In addition, a substantial amount of lassi (sour buttermilk) is also produced during the manufacture of makkhan directly from fermented milk (curd). Total annual production of buttermilk in India is estimated at 35 million tonnes. Sweet cream buttermilk resembles skim milk in gross chemical composition and is usually admixed with bulk of skim milk for further spray drying or even product manufacture in dairy plants. Desi buttermilk, on the other hand, has long been an important domestic beverage in India. It has high nutritive and therapeutic value. It also finds its way in the preparation of a host of items, such as kadhi, dhokla and idli. Also a number of state dairy federations and private plants sell salted and spiced buttermilk in 200 ml pouches. Surat-based Sumul does business out of selling buttermilk (chhach) in and around the city."Sumul chhach" in 500ml packs reaches practically every nook and corner of Surat, covering over 850 retail outlets.

By-products of Indian dairy industry

The dairy byproduct utilization also provides source of income by different value addition methods:

Main Product	By Product	Processing method	Products Made
		Pasteurization	Flavoured milk
		Sterilization	Sterilized flavoured milk
1. Cream	Skim milk	Fermentation	Cultured Buttermilk
		Fermentation and Concentration	Concentrated sour skim milk
		Concentration	Plain and Sweetened

			Condensed skim milk
		Drying	Dried skim milk or Skim milk powder or Non Fat Dry Milk NFDM)
	Coagulation		Cottage cheese & edible casein
2. Butter	Butter Milk	Fermentation and Concentration	Condensed buttermilk
		Concentration and drying	Dried buttermilk
		Coagulation	Soft cheese
3. Cheese, Paneer & Chhana	Whey	Fermentation	Whey beverage, Yeast whey
		Concentration	Plain and sweetened condensed whey, whey protein concentrate, whey paste, lactose
		Drying	Dried whey
		Coagulation	Ricotta cheese
4. Ghee	Ghee residue	Processing	Sweetmeat, Toffee, Sweet paste

B. Dung & Urine

Fecal matters (dung) & urine of livestock is a most important source of bio-fertilizer, Dung brick preparation & pest repellent, but at the same time cow's urine, cow's horn and a dead body of a cow can be used for preparing effective bio-fertilizer. In our country, farming and agricultural cultivation, as per the traditional age-old system, used to be done, with cowdung amongst others serving as manure.

Cowdung is a very good source for maintaining the production capacity of soil and enhances the microbial population. Cowdung has been considered as a Gold Mine due its wide applications in the field of agriculture, energy resource, environmental protection and therapeutic applications. It is also used as a co-product in agriculture, such as manure, bio-fertiliser, bio-pesticides and pest-repellent. Several Products has been launched by the manufacturing companies, such as soap, toothpaste, floor cleaners, hair oil, incense, shaving cream and face wash from the cowdung to earn money. The soap contains dried and pulverised cowdung, orange peel, lavender powder and gooseberries, the company says. The toothpaste is made of dung, ghee, and urine. It is now readying a line of cosmetic products and medicines as well.

Panchgavya : Historically, Maharshi Vashishtha served the divine "Kamdhenu" Cow and Maharshi Dhanvantari offered to mankind a wonder medicine "Panchgavya" (a combination of cow urine, milk, dung, ghee and curd). In Sanskrit, all these five products are individually called "Gavya" and collectively termed as "Panchgavya".

Biogas : Gobar has also been successfully used to produce biogas (methane) and generate electricity for consumer use. Biogas is used in cooking, for lighting in homes and streets. It can be used for driving self-combustion engines for various uses, like running a generator to produce electricity. The slurry (residue) could also be used for production of manure, which when spread on crops acts as an excellent fertilizer. Dung for Biogas and its slurry for manure is providing renewable cooking energy and slurry for compost.

Therapeutic uses of cow dung

i) **Skin tonic :** Mixed with crushed neem leaves and smeared on skin - good for boils and heat rashes.

ii) **Tooth polish :** Toothaches gets removed, so instead of toothpaste which is made of chemicals & dead bones of animals it is a good alternative. Through many experiments on cowdung the famous Italian scientist Prof. G.E. Bea God has proven the fresh cow dung kills the germs of Malaria and Tuberculosis.

iii) **Bio-enhancer :** Bio-enhancers are substances, which do not possess drug activity of their own but promote and augment the bioactivity or bioavailability or the uptake of drugs in combination therapy. Such bio-enhancers have been earlier isolated only from plant sources. It has been found that cow urine also act as a bio-enhancer and increases the efficacy of the antibiotics against infectious agents alongwith anti-cancerous property.

C. Livestock slaughter by-product

Meat sector in India plays an important role in providing livelihood to rural people, sustaining livestock production and contributes a valuable foreign exchange to the country. Livestock by-products include all parts of a live animal that are not part of the dressed carcass. The by-products provide many of the raw materials used to make various products (Daniel et al, 2011). Hides and skins are tanned and processed into leather for shoes, purses, clothing, car seats, and other items while intestines can be used as food containers (sausage cas-ings). Other by-products can be used for pharmaceutical, cosmetic, household, and industrial products. Inedible animal by-products include hide or skin, hair, horns, hooves, teeth, fats, bones, ligaments and cartilage, feet, glands, blood, and lungs. These are the primary raw materials used in the manufacture of a broad assortment of industrial, household, cosmetic, pharmaceutical, and medical supplies, in addition to such products as lubri-cants, plastics, soaps, glycerin, and gelatins (Alicia, 2012).

Conclusions

Now-a-day's our society, in which there is great demand for appropriate nutritional standards, is beset by rising cost and often decreasing availability of raw materials together with much more concern about environmental pollution, leading to the consequence that there is much occupation with recovery and recycling of wastes. The use of different by-product of livestock, such as dairy, dung & Urine and meat industries by-product & their importance should be promoted extensively by starting awareness program & educating the farmers to improve their income as well as to improve their socio-economic status.

References

1. 19th Livestock Census (2012). All India Report, Department of Animal Husbandry, Dairying and Fisheries, Ministry of Agriculture, Government of India, Krishi Bhawan, New Delhi.

2. K. Jayathilakan & Khudsia Sultana & K. Radhakrishna & A. S. Bawa (2012). Utilization of by-products and waste materials from meat, poultry and fish processing industries: a review J Food Sci Technol (May–June 2012) 49(3): 278–293.

3. Mishra, R. and Singh, S. (2013) Sustainable energy plan for a village in Punjab for self-energy generation. International Journal of Renewable Energy Research, 3(3): 640-646.

4. Mohammad Rais and Sherin Kuruvilla (2016). Meat Processing in India: Science, Technology, Policy and Skill Development. *Journal of meat science and technology* : 4(2): 53-61.

5. Ramachandra, T.V. and Shruthi, B.V. (2007) Spatial mapping of renewable energy potential. Renewable and Sustainable Energy Reviews, 11: 1460-1480.

6. Sharma BD (2003). Modern abattoir practices and animal by-products technology, Jaypee Brothers Med. Publ., (P) Ltd.

7. Sharma BD and Sharma K (2011). Outlines of Meat Science and Technology, Jaypee Brothers Med. Publ., (p) Ltd. pp. 360.

8. Singh, M.P. (2008) Organic waste creates power and fertilizer. Journal of the International Association on Electricity Generation, Transmission and Distribution, 19-20(1): 18.

❑❑❑

Chapter 12

Low Input Managemental Practices for Upliftment of Small, Poor and Landless livestock Owners

Rajneesh Sirohi, Yajuvendra Singh and D.N.Singh

Department of Livestock Production Management, College of Veterinary Science and Animal Husbandry, Uttar Pradesh Pandit Deen Dayal Upadhyaya Pashu Chikitsa Vigyan Vishwavidhyalaya Evam Go Anusandhan Sansthan, Mathura

---

Agriculture plays a pivotal role in the Indian economy. Although its contribution to gross domestic product (GDP) is now around one sixth, it provides employment to 56 per cent of the Indian workforce. Also, the forward and backward linkage effects of agriculture growth increase the incomes in the non-agriculture sector. The growth of some commercial crops has significant potential for promoting exports of agricultural commodities and bringing about faster development of agro-based industries. Thus, agriculture not only contributes to overall growth of the economy but also reduces poverty by providing employment and food security to the majority of the population in the country and thus, it is the most inclusive growth sectors of the Indian economy.

The structural reforms and stabilization policies introduced in India in 1991, initially focused on industry, tax reforms, foreign trade and investment, banking and capital markets. The economic reforms did not include any specific package specifically designed for agriculture. In the post-reform (since 1991) period, India has done well in some indicators, such as economic growth, exports, balance of payments, resilience to external shocks, service sector growth, significant accumulation of foreign exchange, Information technology (IT) and stock market, improvements in telecommunications, etc. However, there have been exclusion problems in the country. In other words, real development in terms of growth shared by all sections of the population has not taken place. We have problems of poverty, unemployment, inequalities in access to health and education and poor performance of agriculture sector. One of the excluded sector during the reform period was agriculture which showed low growth and experienced more farmers' suicides. There are serious concerns on the performance of agriculture sector in the country. The post-reform growth was led by services. Commodity sector growth (agriculture+industry) has not been higher in the post-reform period as compared to that of 1980s. Particular worry is agriculture sector which showed lower than 2% per annum in the decade of mid-1990s to mid-2000s. There are also concerns on food security and livelihoods.

Small holdings agriculture is important for raising agriculture growth, food security and livelihoods in India. It may be noted that Indian agriculture is the home of small and marginal farmers (80%). Therefore, the future of sustainable agriculture growth and food security in India depends on the performance of small and marginal farmers.

Agricultural Census data shows that there were about 121 million agricultural holdings in India in 2000-01. Around 99 million were small and marginal farmers. Average size has declined from 2.3 ha. In 1970-71 to 1.37 ha. In 2000-01, small and marginal farmers account for more than 80% of total farm hhs. But their share in operated area is around 44%. Thus, there are significant land inequalities in India.

Farmers earn income from various Sources, viz. crop cultivation, horticulture, dairy, poultry, fisheries, other allied activities, non-farm activities, and wage employment. During the last 30 years, the income disparity between farmers and non-farmers has increased. In 1983-84, the average income of a farm household used to be about a third of that of a non-farm household. By the year 2oo4-o5, this statistic had reduced to one-fourth. There was some improvement during the subsequent period, upto 2o13-t4, due to agriculture growth'. It is an indisputable fact that while governmental interventions bring some short term improvements in agricultural productivity and incomes or even green and white revolutions, so to speak, the improvements do not sustain. The uncertainties of prices (both, input and output) and markets, coupled with adverse impact of policy action and climate change, take over before long and farm households sink back into poverty, indebtedness, and distress.

Fundamentally, there are three ways in which income of farmers may be enhanced,viz.,increasing the gross income, reducing the costs, and stabilizing the income.

Diversification can be a major game changer. When we talk about diversification, it is mostly about high value crops. It can be of three types, viz. product (high value enterprises), process (precision farming), and time diversification (delinking from seasonality). Bumper production ofcrops can lead to a sharp fall in prices. This can be prevented by changing seasonality.

How to reduce post-harvest losses in high value crops, is an important issue. Wastages in fruits, vegetables, fish, etc. need to be reduced by creating storage, cold chain, and market infrastructure. States need to be brought on board for addressing the above issues. Exercises similar to that of Madhya Pradesh, which has prepared a roadmap for doubling farmers' income, need to be taken up. The exercise should start at the block Ievel and then go upto the district and state level.

Reducing Costs through Low Input Agriculture

The cost of cultivation has been on the rise' eroding the profits' Lowering the costs without compromising on the output can increase the net income'. It is possible to do so, as there is a general tendency on the part of farmers to apply overdose of fertilizers and pesticides' expecting higher yields'. Organic farming, low external input, sustainable agriculture' precision fu.Lirrg, etc. are being promoted with a view to reducing chemical use' These intervention, however, remained sporadic and limited to a few geographies.

Reducing Costs through the Farming Systems Approach

Complementary relations that could exist among farm enterprises are rarely exploited, as farmers have been increasingly depending on purchased inputs and preferring solo enterprises rather than a mix of them. It has been ,"po, t.d from one of the NABARD sponsored projects that through better by-product management and enterprise portfolio expenditure on purchased inputs can be minimized'. By growing tree species and horticulture crops on the bunds and including livestock, one can derive additional income while obtaining green leaf manure and fodder. This is especially important for rain fed areas, where crop Season is of 3_4 months arrd ih" Iand remains fallow during the remaining period of the year. Integrated farming system (IFS) is an innovative and unique approach to promote efficient land use and animal management techniques based on biophysical resources, particularly of small and marginal farmers.

In spite of the advantages of farming systems, their adoption by farmers is not high due to limitation of available production technologies, biophysical or geophysical constraints, labour and input market constraints, financial and credit constraints, social norms, inter-temporal trade-offs, policy constraints, and constraints to knowledge or skills.

Income Enhancement through Diversification

Diversification can be a major game changer. Diversification can be of three types, viz. product (high value enterprises), process (precision farming), and time diversification (delinking from seasonality to prevent price crash with bumper crop). Diversification towards high value crops is required to improve both income and resource use efficiency. Similarly, diversification towards livestock, poultry and non-farm activities is considered ideal, especially for small holders who do not possess adequate land to generate enough income for the family. Diversification of agriculture offers food and nutrition security, income growth, diversification of sources of income, poverty alleviation, employnnent generation, judicious use of land and water resources, sustainable agricultural development, and environmental improvement.

Income Enhancement through Professionalization

Since farming in India is almost always the hereditary occupation of a family, learning how to farm is nearly always limited to traditional practices passed on through generations. But can modern agriculture be practised without proper skilling and professionalization of the farmers who have to organize resources, collect and leverage information, take crucial decisions and bear the risks? Farming is increasingly transforming into a skilled job with agricultural markets evolving in the digital space, consumer preferences going global, all entrepreneurial functions demanding technical and managerial skills and value chains becoming sophisticated.

Present initiatives in farmers' training, such as farmers' field schools

Life Long Learning for Farmers (LgF), etc, are limited to a few locations in a few states. There are several training arrangements in the country. But there is a need for a unified training system, catering to all types of trainings. Besides, there can be distinct modules in school curriculum that teach about our agricultural traditions and practices.

Stabilizing Income and Risk Management

Farmers face three basic risks: yield, price, and idiosyncratic risks. The yield risks are: weather and input risks. Weather risks include late onset of monsoon, low and untimely rainfall. Major input risks are on account of fertilizer, pesticides, labour, farm machinery, irrigation, credit, information, and seed. The price risks are related to output marketing which include price volatility, non-operational Minimum Support Price (MSP) system, and discrimination in price realization. Idiosyncratic risks are farmer related, such as health issues of the farmers, access to non-farm employment opportunities, access to public distribution, and employment guarantee programmes.

Co-operative society is an organization of group of people with collective responsibilities and thoughts for the development of needy, especially under-privileged. "A co-operative is an autonomous association of persons united voluntarily to meet their common economic, social and cultural needs and aspirations through a jointly-owned and democratically-controlled enterprise." It is based on the values of the development of agriculture, forestry, banking, credit, agro-processing, storage, marketing, dairy, fishing and housing and its network covers 85 per cent of rural households. It occupies a key position in agricultural development with support in resource and input use, harvesting of water resources, marketing channels, storage facilities, distribution channels, value addition, market information and a regular monitoring network system. Co-operatives are also engaged in economic activities, like disbursement of credit, distribution of agricultural inputs (seeds, fertilizers, and agrochemicals), etc. Co-operatives have inherent advantages in tackling the problems of poverty alleviation, food security and employment generation. It is considered to have immense potential to deliver goods and services in areas, where both the public and private sector have failed. By and large, co-operatives (except a few large ones) are "local institutions", addressing "local needs", employing "local talent", and led by "local leaders". A situation is emerging, wherein there is a possibility of people migrating back to rural areas, as the co-operatives exhibit vast potential for generating self-employment opportunities at grassroots.

Since its formal launch in 1904 in India, the Indian Co-operative Movement has played very important role in the Indian economy, especially in the development of the agriculture and rural sectors combining the strengths of both, public and private sector specially in supporting the small and marginal farmers and weaker sections. Immediately after Independence in 1947, the Sector was recognised by the government as a third economic sector to serve as a balancing factor between the private and public sectors. The government had even considered the co-operative sector as a 'Co-operative Commonwealth'. In this way co-operatives developed as a special sector combining the strengths of both, the public and private sectors, especially serving the needs of small and marginal farmers and weaker groups. At present it is the largest Movement in the world. Self-help, self-responsibility, democracy, equality, equity and solidarity which helps in Co-operatives are democratically-managed economic institutions with social objectives providing every kind of services that the members need based on the principles of the Co-operation.

Normally, a livelihood is known by any set of economic activities through which a household meets its basic needs and earns some cash income. When carried out on a repetitive basis, these tend to become a "way of life". The vast majority of people make a living through self-employment or wage-employment in the informal sector. In broader way, the livelihood comprises of people, their capabilities and means of living including food, income and assets. The tangible assets are income and stores, while the intangible assets are claims and access. The livelihoods should be sustainable environmentally and socially. The livelihood of farmers in India largely depends on agriculture and allied agricultural activities and the agriculture depends on land, water, Agri-inputs, credit, market, Govt policies and knowledge base.

Presently, with about 40% of the population living in poverty, livelihood security for the rural poor farmers continues to be a cause of concern in India. As a majority of the rural population is dependent on agriculture for their livelihood, increasing agricultural production through active involvement of the poor and weaker sections of the society is the most appropriate solution.

Small and fragmented land holdings, heavy soil erosion resulting in depletion of soil productivity, inefficient use of water resources, out-dated agricultural production technologies, un-availability of agricultural credit and lack of infrastructure for post-harvest management and marketing of agricultural produce, are responsible for lower yield and income.

Livestock is another source of income for small farmers. However, over 75% of the animals are uneconomical due to severe genetic erosion, inadequate feeding and health care. With lower crop and livestock productivity, the employment opportunities in the farming and other related sectors are reduced further, leading to reduction in farm wages, seasonal employment, malnutrition and migration.

The role of small farms in development and poverty reduction is well recognized (Lipton, 2006). The global experience of growth and poverty reduction shows that GDP growth originating in agriculture is at least twice as effective in reducing poverty as GDP growth originating outside agriculture (WDR, 2008). Small holdings play important role in raising agricultural development and poverty reduction. Broadly, agricultural development policies over time can be divided into four sets of policy packages: (a) institutional reforms; (b) public investment policies; (c) incentive policies; and (d) reforms and globalization policies.

The proportion of socially disadvantaged groups, such as Scheduled Castes (SCs) and Scheduled Tribes (STs) is higher among marginal and small farmers than that of medium and large farmers. Around 22% of semi-marginal and marginal farmers are from SCs compared to 7.8% in medium and large farmers. SCs have more than half of their holdings of less than half a hectare. Similarly, 15.6% of small farmers belong to STs compared to 14.9% among medium and large farmers. The distribution of land ownership among STs is better than SCs. However, the quality of STs land is probably of the lowest quality. Social identity of farmers is also seen to mediate access to economic resources and outcomes. Even after accounting for quantity and quality of land owned by socially deprived classes, their access to information, marketing, credit and publicly provided inputs and extension services are lower. This shows that they possibly suffer from discrimination in the delivery of public services as well as market (NCEUS, 2008).

The country's dairy sector is dominated by smallholders, and contracting with a large number of them involves transaction costs for the processors. The processors do not have much choice but to take milk from smallholder producers. The problem of the higher cost of contracting with small producers is overcome by contracting with a single person in the village-often an agent-who acts as an intermediary between the processor and producers (Birthal et al, 2008).

National Dairy Development Board covers 1,40, 227 village level societies and 14 million farm families, of which 4 million are women. It has a daily procurement of 22 million liters of milk8. *Amul* Pattern of dairy co-operatives have contributed immensely to the fact that India has progressed from a milk-deficit country to emerge as the largest milk-producing nation in the world. In the process, they have generated millions of days of employment for the rural poor and improved their socio-economic condition.

Self-Help groups and group approach: The women's self-help group (SHG) movement particularly SHG-bank linkage programme has spread all over the country. As mentioned above, there are two successful models in the country. One is Andhra Pradesh model and the other is Kerala model. These programme's interventions and processes have resulted in a sustained process of empowerment of its women members. The real power of the SHG-bank linkage model (SBL model) lies in the economies of scale created by Self Help Group (SHG) Federations (comprising 150"200 SHGs each). This is evident, for example, in bulk purchase of inputs (seeds, fertilisers, etc.) and marketing of outputs (crops, vegetables, milk, NTFPs, etc). Government of India has now started National Rural Livelihoods Mission (NRLM) in 2011. There is a clear understanding that the SBL programme can only be successful, if it is tied up with livelihood programmes, such as improved agriculture, dairying, marketing, etc.

The adoption of multiple farm enterprises in an integrated manner can ensure a substantial income generation to sustain the livelihood of farmers over the meagre income from self-standing enterprises. The integrated farming system, once very popular among the farming communities started loosing its importance after green revolution in late-1960s and then further declined drastically after the economic liberalization in early 1990s. The focus of present government is on doubling farmers' income by 2022. The partial budgeting, economic estimation of manure and urine from animal components and factors associated with total income from different enterprise combinations have shown the directions for policy-makers, extension functionaries and progressive farmers to prepare strategies for doubling farmers' income. Only livestock component would provide the facilitating inputs to enhance the income of farm families within a short period of five years in a synergistic mode. The adoption of IFS is the right approach in this direction and should be supported through institutional, extension, policy and marketing interventions in a system approach.

References

V. Kumar, K. G. Wankhede, H. C. Gena (2015) Role of Cooperatives in Improving Livelihood of Farmers on Sustainable Basis. *American Journal of Educational Research.* 3(10): 1258-1266.

Monograph : Doubling farmers income by 2022 by NABARD.

Chand, R., PA Lakshmi Prasanna and Aruna Singh (2011), "Farm size and productivity: Understanding the strengths of smallholders and improving their livelihoods", Economic and Political Weekly, Vol.46, Nos. 26 and 27.

S.Mahendra Dev (2012) Small Farmers in India:Challenges and Opportunities http://www.igidr.ac.in/pdf/publication/WP-2012-014.pdf

□□□

Chapter 13

Sustainable Economic Model of Goat Farming

A.K. Dixit
ICAR-Central Institute of Research on Goats, Makhdoom, Farah, Mathura

Introduction

India has the second largest goat population in the world. It is a home to 135.173 million goats making about 15 per cent of the world goat population in 2012 (FAO STAT accessed in April 2016). Country stood first in goat milk production, second in goat meat production and second in goat skin production in the world. In recent past, the goat population in the country has declined from 140 to 135 million between 2007 and 2012 livestock census periods. The growth rate of goat population in India was about 2.5 per cent during 2007 to 2012 in spite of higher slaughter rate and annual mortality. Goat sector witnessed significant increase in output of its products like meat, milk and skin.

The goats and its products contribute Rs. 38,590 crore annually to the national economy (Table 1). This accounts for 8.4% to total value of output (at current prices) from livestock sector in 2010-11. Goat meat alone contributes about Rs. 22625 crore (59%) to total value of output from goat sector followed by milk (Rs.9564 crores), by-products (Rs.3005 crore), manure (Rs.1535 crore). The sector also generates gainful employment to about 1.5 per cent of country's total workforce in rural area.

Table 1: Contribution of goats to livestock value of output

Items	Production (000 tons)	Value (in crores)
Meat	905	22625.00
Milk	4782	9564.00
Fiber	0.06	15.00
By-products	601.06	3005.28
Manure	10233.79	1535.07
Blood	103.04	206.08
Skin	149.07	1490.70
Increment in stock (Million heads)	0.7423	148.46
Total		**38590**
Value of output from livestock at current price (crores)		459051
Share to value of output from livestock sector		8.41%

Source: Author's estimates based on National Accounts Statistics (CSO) methodology

Population Dynamics

There is significant growth in population of goat in India during the last three decades. As per 19th livestock census, 2012, goat population in India has increased from 95 to 135 million between 1982 and 2012(Table 2). The highest increase in goat population was recorded 16% during 1982 to 1987. About 13% increase has been recorded between 2007 and 2003.Growth in goat population is demand- driven. In urban areas, demand for livestock products rises faster than the other food groups, when income starts to increase. The Goat population has declined by 3.82% over the previous census, attributed to mainly high rate of slaughter, effect of consumer shift resulting pressure on small ruminants, shrinking grazing lands and migrations. Compound annual growth has been worked out for different sets of census periods. Annual growth in goat population was recorded about 3 per cent during 1982 to 1987. However, it has declined to 0.27% during 1997 to 2003 but further increase and maintained about 2.5% during 2003 to 2007. A negative annual growth (-0.78) was recorded between 2007 and 2012.

Table 2: Trends in goat population

Census year	Goat Population (million)	Periods	% increase/ decrease	CAGR (%)
1982	95	-	-	-
1987	110	1987-82	15.79	2.96
1992	115	1992-87	4.55	0.90
1997	123	1997-92	6.45	1.26
2003	124	2003-97	1.34	0.27
2007	140	2007-03	13.01	2.48
2012	135	2012-07	-3.82	-0.78

Source: Basic Animal Husbandry Statistics, 2015

Ownership Pattern of Goats and Nutritional Security

In South Asia, small ruminants contribute enormously towards promotion of livelihoods security and as an insurance cover to cope with crop failures particularly for rural landless, small and marginal farmers. Goat farming is also increasingly being taken up by peri-urban poor population due to easy market access and as a cheap source of nutritional security for the household. Information provided in table-4 compiled from Input survey of Agriculture Census done in 1996-97, 2001-02 and 2006-07, which indicated that the significance of small ruminants among landless, marginal and small farmers has continued to be strong to meet their nutritional requirement and subsidiary income. More than 76% of goats are possessed by the marginal and small landholdings. The share of goat ownership has improved with marginal category by 2% between 2001-02 and 2006-07. It is worthwhile to mention here that small and marginal together constitute about 83% of total land holdings. The ownership share of large category in total goats is maintained 2 to 4%, during the different survey periods. The inference from analysis suggest consolidated efforts with effective road map for marginal and small landholders for improved goat production technologies for higher milk and meat production.

Table 4: Distribution of goats according to land holding size (million nos.)

Land Categories	1996-97	2001-02	2006-07
Marginal (<1.0)	51.5 (53.8)	60.4(52.6)	54.8(56.7)
Small (1.0 - 1.99)	18.8(19.7)	24.6(21.4)	18.8(19.4)
Semi-Medium (2.0 - 3.99)	13.4(14.0)	17.0(14.8)	12.9(13.3)
Medium (4.0 - 9.99)	8.1(8.5)	9.6(8.4)	7.5(7.8)
Large (10 and above)	3.9(4.0)	3.3(2.9)	2.7(2.8)
All groups	95.7(100.0)	114.9(100.0)	96.7(100.0)

Source: Input survey, Agricultural Census, Govt. of India
Figures in Parenthesis are % to all group

Trends in Goat Meat (chevon) Production

Goat meat is one of the important staple red meats in human diets without any social restrictions. Goats are an important nutrient source, particularly for people in the technologically developing regions, situated mainly in the tropics (Casey, 2009). Goat contributes 16 per cent to country's total meat production however, poultry is having lion share (45%). However, share of goat meat production is shown overall increasing trends. Country's goat meat production has increased from 0.398 to 0.914 million tons with an annual growth of 7.17% between 2003-04 and 2014-15 (Table 6) .However, highest growth was recorded (11.6%) during 2007-08 to 2012-13. It was lowest even declined between 2012-13 and 2014-15.As there was increase in goat population, the number of goat slaughter per year has also increased from 41 to 80 million between 2003-04 and 2014-15.

Table 5: Trends in goat meat production in India

Year	Goat population (Million)	No. of goat slaughter (Million)	% to total goats	Avg. yield (per animal)	Total goat meat production (Million ton)	CAGR (%)
2003-04	124.36	40.85	32.85	9.64	0.398	-
2007-08	140.54	77.32	55.02	11.00	0.488	4.16
2012-13	135.17	87.61	64.81	10.74	0.941	11.57
2014-15	133.42	80.06	60.01	11.42	0.914	-1.44

The share of number of slaughter animals to total goat population was recorded 33% in 2003-04 reached 65% in 2012-13 and further declined to 60% in 2014-15. The goat population for the years 2014-15 was extrapolated on the basis of annual growth in goat population between 2007 and 2012. Average carcass yield has also improved from 9.64 kg to 11.42 kg. The impressive growth in meat production in the country resulted exclusively due to increase in number of animals slaughtered. Productivity of most meat producing species is low and need attention.

Why Goat Farming

The advantages of goat farming are as follows:

1. Goat farming needed low initial investment.
2. Less housing requirement and management problems.
3. Small body size, docile nature, high prolificacy, survives on low grade ration and small gestation period are some important attributes of goat production.
4. Less risk in goat farming compared to other livestock species.
5. No religious restriction against goat slaughter and meat consumption.
6. The goat meat is more lean (low cholesterol) and relatively good for health.
7. Goat milk is easy to digest because of small size of fat globules and non-allergic.
8. Goat is more economical on free range grazing under semi-arid conditions.
9. Goat is a very good converter of poor roughages into high value output i.e. meat, milk and fiber.
10. Goat is best suited animal to varied climatic conditions.

Economics of Goat Rearing : Sustainable Model under Field Condition

Goat can be reared under wide agro-climatic conditions due to its wide adaptability characteristics. There are 28 descript breeds of goats in India spread across the country. Barbari is one of the best commercial breeds and best suited and adapted to the climate of the

South- western semiarid zones of Uttar Pradesh and such other semi-arid areas. Small size, clean habits and high prolificacy are some of the characteristics, which make this breed most preferable among commercial goat farmers.

Production and productivity parameters of Barbari breed : Some facts

S.No.	Particulars	Values
1.	Name of the breed	Barbari
2.	Management	Semi-intensive
3.	Birth weight (kg)	1.75
4.	Weight at the time of weaning (60 days)	9.00
5.	Weight at 9 month (kg)	20-22
6.	Age at first pregnancy (months)	7-8
7.	Multiple birth (%):	
	(i) Generally deliver single kid in first kidding	1
	(ii) Kidding in 2nd onward	
	Single:	30
	Twince:	60
	Triplet:	10
8.	Kidding interval (months)	6-7
9.	Lactation length (days)	90
10.	Average milk yield (kg/day)	0.800
11.	Duration of concentrate, etc. feeding for adult doe (@ 250 g/goat/day)	365
12.	Duration of concentrate, etc. feeding for kid (@250 g/kid/day)	180
13.	Kids mortality (%)	10-15
14.	Kidding rate	1.5
15.	Value of home grown prepared concentrate feed (Rs./kg)	12
16.	Expenditure on goat health (Rs./goat/year)	60
17.	Age of kids sale (months)	9-10
18.	Sale price of kids (Rs./kg body weight)	200
19.	Value of goat milk (Rs./kg)	25

Note: The requirement of green and dry fodder will be met through grazing.

Goat which is known as poor man's cow has now becoming a symbol of prosperity in rural India. Goat rearing plays an important role in livelihood security of millions of landless, marginal and small farmers. Starting of dairy farm with cows and buffaloes has become an expensive business as it requires high capital cost in the beginning. Therefore, goat farming is now preferred small scale business among resource poor farmers. A farmer initiate goat rearing with 50 goats of Barbari breed require a capital of about Rs.6.5 lakh. Goat rearing at small scale may utilize family labour (women labour) efficiently and the problem of malnutrition in women and children may also be solved.

Economic analysis of goat unit of 50 does

A. Expenditure (Rs.)

a) Capital cost

i)	Goat shed	1,25,000.00
ii)	Equipment	20,000.00
iii)	50 Barbari goats @ Rs.6000/- per goat (pregnant)	3,00,000.00
iv)	2 Breeding buck @ Rs.8000/- per buck	16,000.00
	Total capital cost	4,61,000.00

b) Recurring cost

i) Feed cost (concentrate feed) 1,08,540.00
Adult does, bucks and kids (@ 250-300 gram per adult goat & kid per day for 200-220 days)

ii) Health management cost (@Rs.80/animal/year) 10,560.00

iii) Labour (imputed value of grazing) @ Rs.4000/month 48,000.00

Total recurring cost 1,67,100.00

Gross cost 6,28,100.00

B. Income (Rs.)

i)	Sale of kids (76 kids of 22 kg body weight at 9 month @ Rs.225/kg/live weight)	1,18,800.00
ii)	Value of 52 adult goats at the end of year	3,16,000.00
iii)	Depreciated value of shed (@10% per year)	1,10,500.00

iv)	Sale of milk (after feeding kids)	21,600.00
v)	Value of goat manure and others	10,000.00
	Total income	9,14,100.00
	Net income	2,86,000.00
	Net income per month	23,834.00
	Net return per doe	5,720.00

It is clear from economic analysis that if a poor farmer start goat rearing with a unit of 50 goats and adopt scientific practices, he may earn net income about Rs.2. 86 lakh annually. Per goat per year net income would be around Rs.5720.

Marketing of Kids

Marketing is an important aspect of any production process. Livestock marketing including goats in the country is highly unorganized. As the goat farmers are illiterate, middlemen exploit them. There is incessantly increasing demand for meat and breeding goats in the country. Sale price of live goats are directly proportional to the market price of goat meat. Farmer should plan to maximize their sale at the time of festivals, like ID, Holi, Durga Puja and Dasshera to realize 2-3 times higher price. The main marketable products include the fattened kids, culled animals, breeding animals, manure and milk. Potential buyers, like big retail meat outlets and wholesale traders should be identified to bypass middlemen.

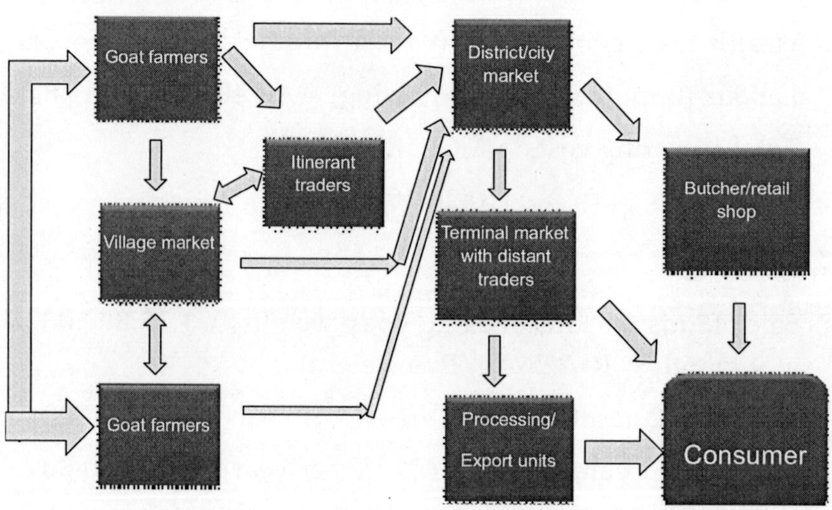

Marketing Tips

- Avoid desperate/ distress selling.
- Goat farmers should be able to negotiate for prices that are commensurate with the quality of the animal.
- Form the group or farmers can come together as a group to strengthen their bargaining power.
- Be aware about market trends (supply and price).
- Produce good quality goats in the right quantities (optimum production).
- Grading for better realization.
- The farmer can sell directly or sell at an auction to avoid middlemen.
- Goat markets should be regulated similar to food grains markets for smooth and effective marketing of goats.

❑❑❑

Chapter 14

Adoption of Traditional Indigenous Practice to Maintain Livestock Health

Rajesh Mandil and Atul Prakash

Department of Pharmacology and Toxicology, College of Veterinary Science and Animal Husbandry, Uttar Pradesh Pandit Deen Dayal Upadhyaya Pashu Chikitsa Vigyan Vishwavidhyalaya Evam Go Anusandhan Sansthan, Mathura

According to National Dairy Development board (NDDB, 2012), livestock population in India is 512.1 million, out of which total bovine population is 299.1 million, goat-135.2 million and sheep is 65.1 million. Livestock sector play significant contribution towards employment (8.8% of the population in India), economy (16% to the income), livelihood (2/3rd of rural community) and welfare of small and landless farmer of the country. Livestock sector contributes 4.11% GDP and 25.6% of total Agriculture GDP, and 20.5 million people depend upon livestock for their livelihood. Growth in this sector may contribute in poverty alleviation of the country. Approximately 70% of livestock population in India is reared by 67% of small, marginal farmer and by the land less people. Livestock sector significantly contributes in our daily life in the form of food, fibers and skins, draft, dung, and animal waste materials, sport as well as social security (Annual Report 2016-17, Department of Animal Husbandry, Dairying and Fisheries, Ministry of Agriculture and Farmers Welfare, Govt. of India).

Due to subtropical climate of the India, livestock are more prone to several infectious and non-infectious diseases, namely mastitis, foot and mouth disease (FMD), surra, bloat, diarrhoea, ephemeral fever, indigestion and parasitic infection, which are substantially affected the farmer's income. Lack of access to modern veterinary facilities to every village/area and/or input high cost in treatment and, delay in treatment to these diseases resulting high mortality may responsible for huge economic loss of farmers, hence, people of rural area relied to use of ethno-veterinary medicine (EVM), which are more readily available and cheaper (Kudi, 1999). In-addition, indiscriminate and non-judicious use of antimicrobials and other veterinary drugs resulted residues of these drugs are excrete in the milk and other animal products which create serious problems of drug resistant in animals and human beings. The presence of drug residues results in development of drug resistant micro-organisms that are difficult to treat and the world is looking for safer herbal alternatives. According to WHO, about 80% people in developing countries rely on indigenous practices for prevention and treatment of diseases in both, humans and animals (Jabbar et al., 2005). India has rich heritage of medicinal plants and farmers of our country use locally available medicinal plants and spices for their animals during suffering from infectious diseases, instead, of routine allopathic treatment regimen.

Plants based practices (Ethno-veterinary practices) has been used by livestock owners since time–honored, where they have their own ways to identify, classify, diagnose and treat animals. India is at the advantage, as it is one of the world's 12 mega diversity countries having about 8% of global plant genetic resources which can be the potent source of herbal medicines (Sri Balaji and Chakravarthi, 2010). Ancient ethno-veterinary literature suggests that the tribal, non-tribal and rural population have been using wild ethno-flora since long for curing diseases of the pet/domesticated animals. Ethno-veterinary medicine deals with people's knowledge, skills, methods, practices, and beliefs about the care of their animals. Indigenous practices (ITK) makes the use of phytotherapy, apitherapy, milk and dairy products, clay, rabbit fat, lard, manual removal of Ixodidae from body of animals, use of fly larvae in cleaning of suppurating wounds, insect repellent action either by rubbing parts of some plants and ashes over animal body or by lightning fire on pasture. Butter, whey, jaggery, curd, and wheat flour serves a vehicle for administration of herbal drugs. ITK formulation administered mostly orally in the form of decoctions, topical as external spray of through fumigation. Dose of medicaments were determined based on body size of animal and availability of plants and response shown by animals and a dose, therefore, it was differed from place to place due to lack of knowledge in farmers about a dose. Most of the ITK preparation made from spices and regional available plants. Almost all the parts of plants are used for the preparation of EVM products, which includes leaves, bark, stem, root, seeds, flowers, and fruits. They can be used as an antimicrobial, antidiarrhoeal, ecto and endo-parasiticides, used against skin infections, to improve production of productive animals, etc.

Based on available scientific literature, here we are discussing some of commonly used indigenous practices:

S. No.		Common protocol followed in allopathic treatment	Ethnoveterinary practices
A.	**Infectious diseases**		
1	Foot and mouth disease (FMD)	Oxytetracycline - 10mg/kg-i.v. or Ceftriaxone -12 mg/kg -i.m., Flunixin meglumine – 1.1 -2.2 mg/kg-i.m., supportive like Ca-borogluconate-i.v., Glucocorticoid (Mishra et al., 2015), Multivitamin preparation etc.	• 1% citric acid or alum solution or potassium permanganate or Methylene blue used for mouth and foot washing. • Juice of sour fruits or lemon for washing of ulcerated tongue, foots and mouth twice a day. • Application of neem or babool leaves paste with mustard oil on foot lesions. • 10 gm Boric acid (Suhaga) + 100 gm jaggery/honey/glycerin mixture applied in mouth and tongue. • Paste of Babool with Jamun bark or paste of peach leaves or Bantulsi for foot lesions. • Banana paste (*Musa paradisiacal*) + sugar candy + water to be given to animal twice daily to fast cure of blisters and sore(s). • Oral feeding or topical application of *Nicotiana tobaccum* (Tobacco) leaves over foot lesions. • *Cuscuta reflexa* Roxb. (Amar Bel) paste of the plant applied twice a day to the affected parts. • *Dalbergia sissoo Roxb.* (Shisham) leaf paste mixed with churning curd & used over the lesions (Malla and Chhetri, 2012). • *Calotropis gigantea* (Safed aak) root decoction applied on the infected foot thrice daily for 3-4 days to control foot rot disease (Rao et al., 2014).
2	Haemorrhagic Septicaemia (HS)	Oxytetracycline– 10mg/kg- iv., or Sulfadimidine – 100 mg/kg-i.v., or Procaine Penicillin – 30-45 thousand IU/kg- i.m., or Trimethoprim sulfadoxine – 3ml/45kg bw i.m., or Tilmicosin 10mg/ kg s.c., or Florfenicol – 20 mg/ kg i.m. (Mishra et al., 2015).	• Provide steam of oil of menthe-20ml, oil of Eucalyptus-20ml, oil of Camphor- 20ml and ammoniac salt- 20gm mixed in hot water. • *Arisaema tortuosum* Schott. (Bagh Janchra) rhizome is crushed to extract the juice and fed to animal. • *Capsicum annuum.* (Shimla mirch) fruit is powdered and boiled for few minutes. This soup fed to animal (Santhivimalarani & Pavadi, 2014). • Chopped leaves of *Solanum incanum* (Indian rennet) mixed with water and then sieved and applied in nose (Yibrah, 2014). • Boiled tamarind and camphor levees applied on

		Antipyretic to reduce fever, Avil/Cadis.in 5-10 ml im.	affected part twice daily for one week. • Crushed seed of *Vernonia amygdalina* Del (bitter leaf) mixed with water and filtered and applied by oral feeding and smeared on nose.
3	Black quarter (BQ)	Penicillin (LA) – 40,000 IU/ kg Bwt. i.m., Antiserum (Mishra et al., 2015). Meloxicam-5.0 ml im., Avil -5 ml, im	• *Musa paradisiaca* (banana) or *Tamarindus indica* (tamarind) or *Aegle marmelos* (wood apple/ Bael) leaves topically applied on femur bone to cure BQ (Pushpangadan et. al., 2016). • *Acalypha indica* (Kuppi, khokli) leaf juice is extracted and fed to the animal (Giday & Teklehaymanot, 2013). • Wash the wound area once daily with potassium permanganate solution (1:10,000, 0.01%)
4	Anthrax	Penicillin – 20,000 IU / kg - i.m. bid, or Streptomycin – 8-10 g /day in 2 doses i.m., or Oxytetracycline – 5 mg / kg / day i.v., Antiserum – 100-250 ml daily for 5 days (Mishra et al., 2015).	• leaf juice of *Aloe trichosantha* Berger applied oral and nasal route (Giday & Teklehaymanot, 2013). • *Acalypha indica* L (Kuppi, khokli) Whole part > juice extract > fed to animals suffer from anthrax. • Homogenized juice extracted from root of date palm (*Balanites aegyptiaca* (L.) Del) with water and fed orally to animals. (Giday & Teklehaymanot, 2013). • Combination of tulsi (*Oscimum sanctum*), neem (*Azadarichta indica*), longa (*Curcuma longa*), punarnava (*Boerhavia diffusa*) and amrita (*Tinospora cordifolia*) act as natural antimicrobial agents
5	Actinobacillosis	Potassium iodide – 6-10 g/ day for 7-10 days orally, Sodium iodide – 1 g/12 kg i.v. (single dose), Streptomycin – 5 g/day for 3 days i.m., Isoniazide – 10 mg/ kg bw for 3-4 weeks i.m. (Mishra et al., 2015).	• Grinded seed powder of Ipomea sp. (Behaya) mixed with water and then fed orally (Yibrah, (2014). • *Calotropis procera seed* crushed and squeezing with butter and fed to animal (Gidey *et. al.*, 2012).

B.	**Parasitic infections**		
1	Endoparasites	Ivermectin – 0.2 mg/ kg s.c., or Albendazole – 7.5 mg/kg orally,or Febantel – 7.5 mg/ kg orally, or Levamisole – 7.5 mg/kg orally or Parenterally, or Piperazine-citrate -2-3 g/10 kg bw (Mishra et al., 2015).	• Oral Administration of 20-30ml mustard oil with 10-15gm common salt for 2 days with repetition after 21 days; Extract of 250gm radish leaves with 10-15gm common salt orally (Sharma and Tiwari, 2008). • 250-500ml whey with 10-15gm common salt orally; Onion or garlic extracts 30ml with 10-15gm common salt orally; Catachue powder 10-15gm with common salt 10-15gm to be given orally; • *Butea monosperma* (Dhak)-seed powder mixed with salt and water and orally given to animal twice a day for deworming (Nigam et al., 2010). • Leaves powder of *Azadiruchta indica* (Neem) mixed with jaggery or buttermilk and orally administered to animals (Nag et al., 2007). • Leaves of *Solanum sisymbrifolium lam* (Wild tomato) mixed with garlic or salt given orally for endoparasites. • 40-50 grams of Aloevera sap given to sheep and goats and repeat one month after for endoparasite removal (Nag et al., 2007). • Decoction made from roots and leaves of *Adhatoda vesica* Nees. given orally to calves for elimination of intestinal worms (Khan *et. al.*, 2012). • Tuber juice made from *Dioscorea deltoidea* Wall. ex Griseb. (Baniatakari, Harvish) and administered 5-7 teaspoons twice a day to treat roundworm infestation in sheep (Mala & Chhetri, 2012). • *Artemisia vulgaris* (Black mugwort) & *A. absinthium* (White mugwort) leaves used as fly repellant and antihelminthic. • Approximately 4.0 liters extract made from Leaves of *Vitex negundo* (Nirgundi)+ Aloe vera (Gheekumari) + Neem seeds + *Andrographis paniculata* (kalmegh/kariyat)+ Calotrophis (aak/madar) by taken of 1 kg each ingredients and ground well mix with little water and filtered. Oral administration of 100 ml and 30 ml of above filtered mixture is enough for large and small ruminants for removal of endoparasites.
2	Fluke infection	Oral administration of Triclabendazole –	• Powder obtained from stem bark (*Schima wallichii*, DC., Korth. Chilauni,

		10-12 mg/ kg or Albendazole - 7.5-10 mg/ kg or Netobimin – 20 mg/kg or Closantel – 10 mg/kg or Oxyclozanide – 18.7 mg/ kg (Mishra et al., 2015).	Kanak, Makrisal) used for treating liver flukes in animals (Malla & Chhetri, 2012). • Rhizome of *Dryopteris filix mas* (male fern) used gainst *Taenia saginata, Taenia solium* and flukes (Mishra et al., 2015)
3	Ectoparasiticides	Several types of chemicals like carbamate (aldicarb, propoxur), chlornated hydrocarbon (DDT, BHC, aldrin), organophosphate (Diazinon, malathion), synthetic pyrethroids (cypermethrin, deltamethrin, permethrin, Flumethrin-1%), formadidine (amitraz-12.5% w/v-2-3ml/1lit water applied externally) and macrocyclic lactones (ivermectin, melbemycin, doramectine) are in use.	• Leaves of *Clerodendrum inerme* (Sankuppi/ glory bower) used for ectoparasiticides; Leaves of *Ocimum sanctum* (Tulsi) used for scabies infection; *Allium sativum* bulb paste is use for ectoparasite • Extract or paste of Neem leaves or bitter guard (Karela) or peach leaves applied or sprayed on skin against ectoparasites. • Leaves paste made from *Annona squamosa* L. (sharifa or sitaphal) a pplied over the infected area; *Butea monosperma* Taub (palash or tesu or dhak) gum exudates is very effective in ectoparasite infestation (Nag et al., 2007). • leaves of *Azadirachta indica (neem)* mixed with jaggery or buttermilk and orally fed to animals to expel endo parasites (Satapathy, .KB., 2010). • Leaf juice of *Allium cepa* (pyaz), *Cryptolepis buchanani* (kala bel) is applied externally on site of insect bite (Lakshminarayana and Narasimha Rao, 2015) • Neem leaves + tulsi leaves+ garlic+ turmeric powder+ sitaphal seeds-20g each, ground well and boiled in 200 ml of neem oil and applied over the body surface of large and small animals.
C	**Plants and EVM practices used for reproductive**		
1	Abortion		• Shivlingi (*Bryonopsis laciniosa*) seed powder mixed with pure ghee is given orally to pregnant animals for abortion (Nigam et al., 2010). • Sclerotium of *Claviceps purpurea* (Ergot) is used for uterine stimulant, oxytocic and abortifacient (Sharma and Singh.1989). • Decoction made form leaves of *Cissus quadrangularis* (Hadjora) along with pepper and garlic and kept into cervix to relieve dystocia (Raikwar and Maurya, 2015). • Dhaniya/Coriander (*Coriandrum sativum*)

			fruits to be given 3-4 times after pregnancy for successful conception
2	Retention of placenta	Manual removal of retained placenta. In general immediate post-partum, administration of PGF_2 alpha, oxytocin or calcium Administered locally (intrauterne) or systemically antibiotics.	• Root decoction of *Triumfetta pentandra* (Diamond burbark/ chikti) is used to overcome retention of placenta • Dried leaves of Bans (*Bambusa arundinacea*) mixed with lukewarm water and fed to animal twice a daily; Gular Fruits (*Ficus glomerata*) orally fed to the animal twice daily (Nigam et al., 2010) • Leafs of sugarcane (*Saccharum officinarum*) is also helful for easy expulsion of placenta after calving (Nigam et al., 2010). • Roots powder (Ashwagandha; *Withania somnifera*) + seed powder (*Hyoscyamus niger*) + leaf powder (*Bambusa arundinacea*)+ Gur + ginger powder (Zingiber officinale) mixed together and boiled in milk to make decoction and it is given to animal twice a day to cure retard placenta (Nigam et al., 2010).
3	Prolapse of uterus	Epidural anaesthesia, Cleaning of uterus with mild antiseptic like chlorine or quaternary ammonium compound Antibiotics– terramycin/ aureomycin/oxytocin/pituitrin hormone	• Crushed bulb of onion 1 Kg daily or powder of onion seeds for 3–5 days is effective in prolapse of uterus (Nigam et al., 2010). • Keep the animal in a slightly slanting place in such a way that keeping the head part in a lower level for a week. • Clean the prolapse mass with any antiseptic lotion. Lift the prolapse mass by placing both hands, and make a paste by mixing the Lajwanti (*Mimosa pudica*) leaves powder or whole plant with goat's milk it fed orally to animal at least three times at 12hrs intervals.
4	Repeat breeding	Hormonal treatments (prostaglandins E_2) and ciprofloxacin and Tinidazole (Bogan et al., 2008). Provide optimal nutrition during the transition period and during early lactation	• Leaves of bara gokhru (*Pedalium murex*) or *Chinaberry tree/ Bakain* (*Melia azedarach* or Ragi/ Finger millet (*Eleusine coracana*) are using for treatment of repeat breeding and sterility of animals
	Anoestrous	Provide high energy diet, mineral supplements along with maintenance of optimal nutrition during the transition	• Anoestrous problem in large animals solved by feeding of chicken egg (07 pieces/ per day/week) or *Kala*" banana)(one dozen along with 400 g sugar/2 days). • 100 g paste made from *Gurhal* (*Hibiscus rosasinensis*) flower's bud and old

		period and during early lactation and reduced sucking. Hormonal treatments with prostaglandins, gonadotrophin-releasing hormone (GnRH) or progestagens or FSH/PMSG PMSG (Folligon) + GnRH (eg. Receptal)	sugarcane *(Saccharum sinense)* jaggery and fed to animals for 15 days. • *Asok* (Ashoka, *Saraca asoka*) tree's bark (100 g) grounded well and fed to the cattle. • *Asok* tree (Ashoka, *Saraca asoca*) bark (200 g) boiled with 1 litre milk and drenched with water to animals everyday and this treatment should continued to 15-20 days. • A mixture made with the extract of bark of peepal *Aswatha (Ficus religiosa)* and gruel and is to be fed for 10-15 days. (De Amitendu et al., 2004)
	Mastitis	Administration of intramammary or systemic antibiotics or a combination of both. β-lactams (amoxicillin, ceftiofur, cephapirin, cloxicillin, hetacillin, and penicillin) and a lincosamide (pirlimycin) etc.	• Washing of teats with 1% boric or 0.1% potassium permanganate or 1% alum solution before and after milking (Sharma and Tiwari, 2008). • Application of paste of marigold (Genda) on udder and teats as it has anti-inflammatory action. • Exposure to smoke of bark of *Lyonia ovalifolia* (Ovalleaved staggerbush) grinded and mixed with *Quercus leucotricophora* (Blackjack oak). • Application of rhizome of *Curcuma domestica* (Common turmeric) mixed with oil of *Brassica campestris* (Field mustard). • Animals are also fed with mixture of crushed bark of *Bombax ceiba (Cotton tree)* and seeds of *Glycine max* (Soybean) in water (Phondani *et al.*, 2010) • Ash of *Cocculus pendulus* (Moonseed) mixed with cow's milk fat for feeding; Application of lukewarm water with salt on all teats and udder. • A paste made from haldi rhizome powder (*Curcuma longa*), rock salt and pure ghee and fed to the animal to cure the swelling of teats. • 50 g sodium bicarbonate mix with lemon juice and water up to 200 ml and fed oraly to animal. • 2-3 petals of Aloe vera, 50 g turmeric powder and 10 g limestone-all the ingredients grounded and mix well and applied over the teats thrice daily for one week.
	Milk Fever	Injection of calcium borogluconate, vitamin D and minerals supplements etc.	• 1 kg Calcium hydroxide (lime/chuna/khadiya) powder mix with 20 litres of water and keep it overnight. Collect 200 ml of supernatant and add 200 ml of fresh water and feed the animal daily to prevents calcium deficiency.
	Cough and cold	Antihistamines avil, Antibiotic-broad	• 100 g tulsi leaves and 100 g Basak leaves (*Adhotoda vasica*) are boiled with water

		spectrum and antipyretic-paracetamol, etc.	Extracted mixture mix with one teaspoonful honey and oraly fed to animals. • *Golmorich* (Black pepper, *Piper nigrum*), *Adarak* (Ginger, *Zingiber officinale*) and garlic (*Allium sativum*) and ghee used to make paste, one part of the paste fed to the animal and other part is topically applied over head and neck (De Amitendu et al., 2004). • An extract prepared from 3-4 leaves of *Tejpata* (*Cinnamomum tamala*), 50 g *Adarak* (Ginger, *Zingiber officinale*) and peepal (*Ficus religiosa*) leaves and drenched to the animal along with water (De Amitendu et al., 2004). • Extract of *Tulsi* (*Ocimum sanctum*) and *Basak* (*Adhatoda vasica*) leaves are mixed with ghee, *Adarak* (*Zingiber officinale*) and molasses and fed to the cattle (De Amitendu et al., 2004).
E	Gastrointestinal disorders		
	Diorrhea / dysentery/loose motion	General treatment schedule is given for 5-7 days i.e. Sulphonamide 100-300 mg/kg or pthalylsulphathiazole-100-150 mg/kg orally/parenterally. Or Tetracycline 4-8 mg/kg or furazolidine 10-20 mg/kg Metronidazole-200-400 mg tid orally for dogs Diphenoxylate or atropine, Fluid therapy (ringer lactate, normal saline or glucose saline-iv etc.	• 250-500 gm Jaggery, 50 gm salt and 20 ml lemon extract orally; ½ Kg rice gruel, 50 gm kaolin, 30 gm salt and 250 gm jaggery for oral administration to animal (Sharma and Tiwari, 2008). • 500 gm oat flour, 250 ml rice water, 50 gm kaolin, 250 gm jaggery in 1 L whey (Sharma and Tiwari, 2008). • Use of Shisham leaves powder 100 gm, bael fruit powder 25 gm with ½ kg barley (Jowar) flour and ½ kg jaggery to administer 100 gm orally 2 times for 3-5 days. • Jawar (*Sorghum vulgare*) seed flour mixed with whey and this paste given to animal twice a day to cure loose motion. • *Cannabis sativa* (Bhang) leaf powder mixed with whey and water is given to animal twice a day to cure loose motion (Nigam et al., 2010). • Tender leaves of pomegranate + guava + jamun + dried ginger 50 g- grind and mix with 100 g jaggery to divided into three bolus dose and fed to animals one bolus at a time till recovery.
	Bloat/ tympany /colic	Fluid therapy, Pethidine hydrochloride-1 mg/kg, Atropine sulphate, Tranquilizers-Chloral hydrate-30-60 g orally	• Oil of *Phoenix dactylifera* (Date palm) with charcoal, seeds of *Piper nigrum* (Black pepper), linseed oil with ginger, turmeric and asfoetida, bark decoction of *Syzygium caryophyllatum* (Jambolan) and *Ficus glomerata* (Goolar). • Colic- Oil of *Phoenix dactylifera* (Date palm) in combination with *Tamarindus indica* (Tamarind) juice.

		Purgatives-liquid paraffin linseed oil-500-1000ml Phenargan(5%)-15-20 ml i.m. Easily digestible laxatives foods-bran mash and linseed mashed with 60 g common salt. Surgical removal of impaction mass, etc.	• Oral treatment with mixture of 100gm onion, 100gm garlic, 30gm asfoetida, 5gm black pepper in 250ml mustard oil • 60ml Turpentine oil and 30gm asfoetida in 500ml linseed oil orally. • Put a green neem stick approx. 1 inch thick in mouth horizontally and tie it with the help of rope behind the horn so that animal will chew and release the gas (Phondani *et al*., 2010). • *Amaranthus viridis* (Chaulai) seeds powder mixed with water and given orally twice a day to cure tympany (Nigam et al., 2010) • Paste ready by mixing of Ajwain seeds (*Trachyspermum ammi*), Adrak (*Zingiber officinale*), Hing (*Ferula asafoetida*) and kali mirch powder (*Piper nigrum*) with water and orally administered to animal to cure bloat or tympany (Phondani *et al*., 2010) • Wood ash 100g+ 60g Sodium chloride orally fed to animals twice daily. • 50-60 g sodium bicarbonate administered orally to large animals.
	Indigestion	Livertonic, Vitamin-B complex, Digestant, oral administration of magnesium sulphate to correct acidosis. Administration of 3-4 L rumen fluid collected from healthy ruminants etc.	• An oral dose of chiraita, dry ginger, crushed mustard seed 30gm each, ammonium salt 15gm, black salt 15gm, rock salt 15gm in 250ml molasses; • 30gm Black salt, 30gm asfoetida, 15gm roasted cumin seeds (Jeera) powder, 15gm aniseed (Saunph) powder, 15gm thymol (Ajwayan) powder and 5gm cardamom seed (Elaichi) powder in 500ml water orally (Sharma and Tiwari, 2008). • Dhania (*Coriandrum sativum*) seed power mixed with leaf powder of henna (*Lawsonia inermis*) and water kept in overnight and next day it is given to animal twice a day to cure loose motion.
	Constipation	Mineral oil- liquid paraffin, Vitamin B complex, Livertonic, Magnesium sulphate 30-60 g orally, Calcium therapy orally or parenterally Fibrous diet, enema water with soap or glycerine, neostigmine or carbachol, etc.	• Oral administration of castor oil 500ml; Magnesium sulphate 500gm in 1L water orally; • Dried juice or leaf pulp and root of aloevera act as purgative and anti-colic; Poppy leaves (Kali dhaturi). • 50gm salt, 30gm black salt, 15gm asfoetida, 50gm aniseed powder, 30gm cumin seed powder, 5gm cardamon seed powder in 500gm jaggery given orally (Sharma and Tiwari, 2008).

F	Pyrexia/fever		
		Asprin, salicylate or paracetamol, Steroid (dexamethasone), multivitamins, Broad spectrum antimicrobial tetracyclines/ cefalosporins, etc.	• Decoction of leaves of basil (Tulasi). • Dry powder of *Tinospora cardiofolia* (Gelo) @25-30gm per day 3-5 days orally • Solution of 15gm sodium bicarbonate (Meetha soda), 15gm nausadar, 15gm salicylic acid, 50ml potassium nitrate, Chiraita powder 30gm with 250gm molasses mixed with 250ml water orally; • Saunth 30gm tulasi leaves 10gm with 250 500gm jaggery given orally (Sharma and Tiwari, 2008) • Bolus consisting of whole plant part of *Leucas aspera* (Thumbai) and rhizome of *Piper longum* (Long pepper) • Fruit juice of *Tamarindus indica* (Tamarind) ready in water used for dehydration and pyrexia; • *Coriandrum sativum* (Coriander) leaves juice used for dehydration and pyrexia.
G	Wound		
1	Burn	Fluid and electrolytes supplementation for prevention of dehydration and shock. Local application of emollients Local analgesics, Tannic-acid/ iodoform ointment Silversulphadiazine/ silvadene Antibiotics-paracenterally, etc.	• Apply cold water or ice on burn. • Apply olive oil or coconut oil on affected area • Apply equal parts of lime water and linseed oil on burn • Bael-pulp (*Aegle mormelos*) mixed with water and filtered and added sore milk. This product applied twice a day to on burned area of the animal; • *Aloe barbadense* (Ghikumari) pulp mixed with sore milk and water and, applied twice a day to cure burns of the animal. (Nigam et al., 2010). • Paste made from Alsi seed (*Linumusitatissimum*) powder, gur powder, lime water and seed oil (*Linum usitatissimum*) applied on the affected portion of the animal twice a day to cure burns due to fire, • Paste prepared from Ber (*Zizyphus jujube*) leaf powder and Alsi oil (*Linum usitatissimum*) *and* applied on the affected part of the animal to cure burn (Nigam et al., 2010).
2	Wound/ Cut on hooves/ Yoke gall	Cleaning of wound-Acriflavin lotion or hypertonic saline solution (5-10%) Apply antiseptic cream/ powders/iodoform, triple-sulpha /neosprin powder, antibiotic-penicillin	• Apply extract or paste of indigo plant leaves (Neelkhuri) on wound. • Paste of peach leaves or basil leaves. • Extract or paste of neem or babool leaves or bark • *Annona squamosa* (Sharifa) leaf paste mixed with lime, and, this paste applied on the wound and bandaged to cure foot disease (Nigam et al., 2010). • Paste of turmeric, alum with jaggery applied on closed wound.

			• Oral feeding of milk with turmeric and jaggery suitable for close wound treatment; Wet/dry fomentation with lukewarm water with common salt or magnesium sulphate use for maturation of wound. • Apply ice on cut to check bleeding and then apply paste of indigo leaves on cut followed by bandaging • Apply neem oil with turmeric and lukewarm jaggery • Apply sesame oil/Til oil with turmeric powder
3	Maggoted wound	Remove the maggot with the help of forceps Lorexane cream application, etc.	• Paste made from leaves or fruit of Custard apple applied on wound. • Fly repellant-neem oil applied over the wound area. • Turpentine oil application or daily application of paste of fresh *Anona* leaves fly repellant and antiseptic. • Paste made from Karonda (*Carissa carandas*) root and coconut Nariyal oil (*Cocas nucifera*) is applied twice a day on maggot wound • *Hyoscyamus niger* oil (Khurasani Ajawayan) applied on the wound with the help of cotton twice a day to remove the maggot from the wound • Ratanjot (*Jatropha curcas*) milky sap applied on the affected parts and shoulder of animal thrice a day to cure maggot wound or yolk sore, respectively • *Mimosa pudica* (Lajwanti) fresh leaf paste fed to animal with 1 to 2 chapattis, twice a day to cure maggot wound; • Root (*Datura metel*) powder is uses by farmers to the animal twice a day to check bleeding of any part of the body due to maggot infection (Nigam et al., 2010). • Pain and discharge from ear Put mixture of 50ml mustard oil with 5 gm garlic in it after boiling and straining it.
H	**Fungal infection**		
		Ringworm infection -treatment is Amphotericin B – 0.4 1.5 mg/kg Bwt. for 10-40 days i.v. Itraconazole – 3 mg/kg Bwt. orally BID for 3-4 months, Potassium iodide –	• 50ml Juice made from leaf of *Solanum indicum L.* (Badi Kateri, Vanabharra) and fed twice a day for treating ringworm in cattle. • Juice obtained from stem bark of *Massachisia* Buch.-(Bilaum) and fed to animals orally to treat ringworm in animals. • Topical application of leaf paste made from *Clausena dentate (Willd.)* kattu on the affected

		6-10 g daily orally for [illegible] days, Sodium iodide – 1 g/ 12 kg Bwt. intravenous (1 dose), Griseofulvin 5-10 mg/ kg orally SID for 3-6 weeks.	parts.
I	**Fracture healing**		
		Fracture treatment includes-reduction, retension and immobilization Analgesics, muscles relaxants and antimicrobials, Calcium and vitamin- D preparations, etc.	• Application of seed paste of *Eleusine coracana* (Ragi) and *Lens culinaris* (Lentil) at the fractured site. • Paste made from milled seeds of *Vigna mungo* (Black gram) and *Cynodon dactylon* (Bermuda grass) to cast off as plaster over fractured bone followed by support with bark of *Betula utilis* (Bhojpatra) or *Zanthoxylum armatum* (Winged prickly ash); • Bark of *Butea monosperma* (Palash) and *Cissus quadrangularis* (Hadjora) used for bone settling (Raikwar and Maurya, 2015). • In cases of joint swelling or joint pain- powdered mixture of 10-15 gm of snails shell, 10gm aloevera, 10gm Moringa, 25 gm red ochre heated in 200ml of castor oil or mustard oil and cooled and applied 2-3 times daily on affected part. • Chironji (*Buchanania latifolia*) bark powder mixed with cow milk and filtered it and administered orally twice a day during backbone fracture. • *Lannea coromandelica* (Jhingar) plants roots (25 gm) ground with cow urine and pasted on the broken bone every day for a hour 15 to 30 days. Strips of 'tusharu' wood (*Debregeasia dealbata*) used for supporting the fractured bones of animals. The strips tied together with the help of cloth (Samal et.al., 2003). • Hot fomentation is given with *Akanda* leaves (*Calotropis gigantea*) along with ghee. Luke warm paste made from Garlic (*Allium sativum*) and ghee and applied on the affected part (De Amitendu et al., 2004).

Based on above scientific information on EVM-practices, suggesting animals diseases can be treated effectively by application of indigenous knowledge and home available plants ingredients, which reduced the treatment cost, use of antibiotics, chemical drugs and their residues in the animal products and microbial resistance.

References

1. Annual Report 2016-17, Department of Animal Husbandry, Dairying and Fisheries, Ministry of Agriculture and Farmers Welfare, Govt. of India.

2. Bogan Randy, L., Murphy, M. J., Stouffer Richard, L. and Hennebold, Jon D. (2008). "Prostaglandin Synthesis, Metabolism, and Singanlling Potential in the Rhesus Macaque Cropus Luteum Throughout the Luteal Phase of the Menstrual Cycle", Endocrinology, 149: 5861-5871.

3. De Amitendu, H P S Arya, Babulal Tudu and A Goswami.2004. Indigenous technical knowledge in animal husbandry. Livestock Research for Rural Development 16(8).

4. Giday, M. and Teklehaymanot, T. (2013). Ethno-botanical study of plants used in management of livestock health problems by Afar people of Ada'ar District, Afar Regional State, Ethiopia. Journal of Ethno-biology and Ethno-medicine. 9(8): 1-10.

5. Gidey, Y., Mekonen, T., Gebrerufael, G. and Samuel (2012). An ethno-veterinary survey of medicinal plants used to treat livestock diseases in Seharti-Samre district, Northern Ethiopia. African Journal of Plant Science. 6(3): 113-119.

6. Khan, M.A., Khan, M.A. and Hussain, M. (2012). Ethno-Veterinary Medicinal Uses of Plants of Poonch Valley Azad Kashmir. Pak. J. Weed Sci. Res. 18(4): 495-507.

7. Kudi, A.C., Umoh, J.U., Eduvie, L.O. and Gefu, J. (1999). Screening of some Nigerian medicinal plants for antibacterial activity. Journal of Ethno-pharmacology. 67: 225-228.

8. Lakshminarayana, V. and Narasimha Rao, G. M. (2013). Ethno-veterinary practices in northcoastal districts of Andhra Pradesh, India. Journal of Natural Remedies. 13(2): 109-117.

9. Malla, B. and Chhetri, R.B. (2012). Ethno-veterinary practices of some plant species by ethnic people of parbat District, Nepal. Kathmandu University Journal Of Science, Engineering And Technology. 8(I): 44-50.

10. Mishra, D.P., Sahu, R.K., Mishra, N. and Behera, A.K. (2015). Herbal treatment for common diseases in ruminants: an overview. Journal of Livestock Science. 6: 36-43.

11. Nag, A., Galav, P. and Katewaa, S.S. (2007). Indigenous animal healthcare practices from Udaipur district, Rajasthan. Indian journal of Traditional Knowledge. 6(4): 583-588.

12. National Dairy Development board (NDDB, 2012).

13. Nigam, G and Sharma, N. K. (2010). Ethno-veterinary plants of Jhansi district, Uttar Pradesh. Indian Journal of Traditional Knowledge. 9(4): 664-667.

14. Phondani, P.C., Maikhuri, R.K. and Kala. C. P. (2010). Ethno-veterinary uses of medicinal plants among traditional herbal healers in alaknanda catchment of Uttarakhand, india. Afr. J. Trad. CAM. 7(3): 195-206.

15. Pushpangadan, P., Ijinu, T.P., Bincy, A.J., Anzar, S., Aswany, T., Chitra, M.A. (2016).Traditional Medicine in livestock management. J. Traditional and Folk Practices. 04(1): 43–49.

16. Raikwar, A. and Maurya, P. 2015. Ethno-veterinary medicine: In Present perspective. Int. J. Agric.Sc & Vet. Med. pp. 44-49.

17. Rao, M.L.S., Ramakrishna, N. and Saidulu, Ch. (2014). Ethno-Veterinary Herbal Remedies of Gujjars and Other Folklore Communities of Alwar District, Rajasthan, India. International Journal of Ayurveda and Pharma Research. 2(1): 40-45.

18. Samal, P. K., Shah, A., Tiwari, S. and Mehra, B. Agrawal. D. K. 2003. Indigenous animal health care practices in Indian Central Himalaya: Empirical evidences. Indian Journal of Tradional Knowledge. 2(1): 40-50.

19. Santhivimalarani, S. and Pavadai, P. (2014). Ethno-veterinary practices among tribes of Kolli hills in Tamil Nadu, India. Int. J. Pharm. Sci. Rev. Res. 28(2): 267-271.

20. Satapathy, K.B. (2010) Ethnoveterinary Practives in Jajpur District of Odisha. Indian Journal of Traditional Knowledge. 9(2): 338-343.

21. Sharma, M.C. and Tiwari, R. 2008. Successful use of indigenous technical knowledge for curing livestock diseases. In VIII annual conference of Indian Society of Veterinary Pharmacology and Toxicology, pp 20-23.

22. Sharma, P.K. and Singh, V. (1989). Ethno-botanical studies in North West and Trans Himalayas, V Ethno-veterinary medicinal plants used in Jàmmu and Kashmir, India. J Ethno-pharmacol. 27: 63–70.

23. Sri Balaji, N. and Vikrama Chakravarthi, P. (2010). Ethno-veterinary Practices in India-A Review. Veterinary World. 3(12): 549-551.

24. Yibrah, T. (2014). An ethno-veterinary botanical survey of medicinal plants in Kochore district of Gedeo Zone, Southern Nations Nationalities and Peoples Regional State (SNNPRs), Ethiopia, Journal of Scientific and Innovative Research. 3(4): 433-445.

□□□

Chapter 15

Advances in Reproductive Management of Dairy Animals

Atul Saxena

Department of Veterinary Gynaecology & Obstetrics, College of Veterinary Science and Animal Husbandry, Uttar Pradesh Pandit Deen Dayal Upadhyaya Pashu Chikitsa Vigyan Vishwavidhyalaya Evam Go Anusandhan Sansthan, Mathura

Poor reproductive performance remains one of the primary reasons for involuntary culling of dairy cows globally. Roughly one third of dairy cows culled annually due to reproductive problems. Culling of animals, that fails to conceive cause an economic loss to dairy farmer. Low fertility results in reduced herd milk production, increased cost associated with multiple inseminations and increased number of replacement heifers needed to maintain herd size. An increase in trend of pregnancy rate has been reported in United State dairy industry and this reversal is because of use of modern biotechnological and managemental tools. Pregnancy rate is the product of the estrous detection or submission rate (for dairies using timed artificial insemination) and the conception rate. It is a measure of how quickly cows that are eligible to become pregnant (i.e. after the voluntary waiting period) actually become pregnant. Thus improved fertility means use of technologies to improve submission rates.

This paper will discuss some of the reproductive management tools that have resulted in reducing the reproductive culling.

Approaches for improving estrus detection rate

With the increase use of AI, the detection of estrus is put on by the livestock owner which has often been faulty. The fault in estrus detection results in wrong time of AI resulting in failure of fertilization and increased chances of repeated breeding and infertility. Correct identification of animals in estrus improves fertility in the herd. The following will help in improving estrus detection:

- Use of CCTV and its recording
- Use of computerized assisted program for maintaining herd record (Herdsman software)

Application of Synchronization techniques

The major difficulty in obtaining optimum reproductive performance is failure to detect estrus in a timely and accurate manner and therefore, in modern dairy practices controlled breeding program are used. The control of breeding can be done with the use of PG, progesterone and GnRH either alone in various combinations.

Use of PG following ovarian palpation

The program is based on the fact that upon rectal examination, if a cow is found to have a responsive CL will be treated with PG injection. Such program could be set up on weekly or bi-weekly schedule in farm. With these programmes, all cows eligible for breeding after the voluntary waiting period (50 to 55 days) are palpated on a given day of the week. Cow with a CL receive PG and are observed for heat three times daily on 2,3,4 and 5 day post-injection. Cows exhibiting standing behavior are inseminated. Cows without a CL and those not observed in heat following the initial PG injection are examined again during the week. The program continues on a routine basis and cows remain on the program until diagnosed pregnant or until a specific number of repeat inseminations have been attempted.

Use of prostaglandin without ovarian palpation

7 - day program : As error in detection of CL is possible, hence, this option is adopted. Although with this program additional doses of PG is required as some of the cows, which do not have a CL also receive a PG, however, this error is less costly than failure to administer PG to eligible cattle possessing a CL. Thus, all cows were injected with PG on a given day of the week. Cattle observed in heat are inseminated and those not seen in heat are re-injected on the same day of the following week. This system is repeated on the third week after which a veterinarian examines the cow. This practice is frequently called as Monday morning program, since administering PG on

Monday will induce most heats between Wednesday and Saturday. Thus, all insemination will occur on weekdays.

11- days or 14 days program : All eligible cow after the voluntary waiting period receive PG and observed for heat two to five days after injection and inseminated. Cows that don't exhibit heat are re-injected 11 days later. At least three such attempts are followed after which the non-responder animals were examined.

Targetted breeding program : Cows are administered PG prior to the end of the voluntary waiting period. The purpose is to synchronize (setup) cows into stage of the cycle, when they are most likely to respond to the breeding shot of PG administered 14 days later. At the initial PG injection cow exhibiting estrus are not inseminated. A voluntary waiting period (usually 50–55 days post partum) is established and cows are listed chronologically according to calving dates. Those cows within 14 days of the end of the VWP are administered the setup shot. Fourteen days later the cows receive the first breeding injection of PG and are observed for heat two to five days after injection and inseminated accordingly. Cows that do not exhibit heat are re-injected 14 days later, observed for heat and inseminated. Injections are continued at 14–days intervals until estrus is exhibited.

Modified targated breeding (GnRH + PG system) : eligible cows receive PG 21 days before the end of the voluntary waiting period (VWP). This is followed by a GnRH injection 14 days later and a second PG injection 7 days after the GnRH injection. During the three days following the last PG injection cows are inseminated based on observed heat. Cows not observed in heat by 72 hours post-PG injection are inseminated between 72 and 80 hours. Thus, all cows are inseminated.

Ovsynch program (GnRH–PG-GnRH Program–Timed AI) : The program includes injection of GnRH seven days later with PG. The first injection of GnRH affects follicular growth by causing either ovulation or luteinization of the dominant follicle and prevents estrus until after the PG injection, which causes the corpus luteum or luteinized follicle to regress. A new dominant follicle forms and is available to be ovulated by the second GnRH injection given 48 hours after the PG injection. The program synchronizes follicular development and ovulation and allows effective timed AI 16-18 hr of the last injection. Some important points to consider with this program is (1) Timing of first GnRH injection is not critical, however, the time of second injection is critical so that insemination could take place at reasonable time of day (2) The program should not be used for heifers (3) If a cow exhibits estrus before the completion of the hormonal treatments, she should be inseminated and remaining injection should not be administered (4) Program will be useful for cows that simply do not express estrus after several attempts with PG (5) The program is also useful in herds, where cattle are not turned out for a heat detection on a routine basis.

Pre-Synch : It is a modification of ovsynch in which two PG injections 14 days apart are administered 14 days before initiation of the first GnRH injection of ovsynch. This Sync program improves first service conception rate compared to ovsynch and is a good strategy for programming animals to receive their first postpartum timed AI by day 50-55 postpartum. The system provides better conception with ovsynch. The only advantage of this synch system is that because of long duration re-synchronization can not be planned.

Heat–Synch : This is an alternative to Pre- Synch or ovsynch in which 1.0 mg of estradiol cypionate (ECP) is administered 24 hours after the PG injection of ovsynch to induce ovulation rather than administering GnRH 48 hours after PG. The system results in similar reproductive performance to Presynch, but is not effective for synchronizing anovular animals. The system is less costlier compare to Pre-synch.

3. Sperm pre-selection (sex sorted sperm)

The selection of desired sex is one of the determining factors in increasing the genetic progress and farmer profitability in dairy cattle. With the advancement in research, separation of the Y sperm from the X is possible due to the differences on the DNA content of these spermatic cells (X sperm has about 4% more genetic material than Y) by flow cytometry. Advances in sex sorting of sperm using flow cytometry have enabled its incorporation into commercial reproductive management. The technique (sex sorted sperm) is being used for artificial insemination (AI) with estrus detection, timed artificial insemination (TAI), embryo transfer with superovulation (ET) and timed embryo transfer (TET).

The encouraging results of sex semen in breeding heifers has placed it's used in genetic improvement program involving use of heifers.

Further, the average female calves weigh about 2 kg less at birth than male calves. Thus, reducing the possibilities of dystocia in first calf heifers. Because of increased production of female calf as a result of sex selection technology, older female can be spared from regular breeding programme and can be used for cross-breeding with beef animals. The cross bred beef produced animals grow faster and have an economical impact in beef industry.

Production of male calves from best cows using embryo transfer will further assist in semen bank and AI programme. Although the embryo produced with the superovulated cow will be less (low sperm concentration), however, this application of the technique is still the best.

Herd expansion could occur more quickly and possibly without purchasing females which is very valuable from a biosecurity standpoint, and possibly from a genetic standpoint, too.

Early methods of pregnancy diagnosis

A large percentage of cows fail to conceive following insemination or lose embryos prior to rescuing CL function (Pereira *et al.*, 2013). Theoretically, these cows could be detected in estrus and be re-inseminated 21 to 24 days after their first insemination. However, as stated above, not all these cows will exhibit estrous behavior and those that often go undetected resulting in less than 50% of open cows being detected in estrus 21 to 24 days after insemination. These cows have been called "phantom" cows (Lucy *et al.*, 2004). Therefore, if a pregnancy specific signal could be detected during early pregnancy, it could be used to identify failed conceptions and allow for re-insemination of open cows at 21 to 24 days intervals.

Discovery of interferon tau (IFN- τ) as the conceptus signal responsible for rescuing CL function in ruminants (Bazer *et al.*, 2009) have made it possible for the detection of open animals that fails to cycle even before day 21-24 post-insemination. However, the difficulty of interferon tau is that it do not come in blood and present locally in the uterus. Subsequent study has confirmed that the interferon tau cause expression of interferon stimulating gene (ISG) in the peripheral blood leukocytes which can be detected, when these open animals are having their second or third follicular wave. Advantage of this can be helpful in re-inseminating these open cow by day 21-24.

Cows detected open at day 18 to 20 after insemination would receive injection of a luteolytic dose of PGF and be bred on detected estrus or receive TAI accompanied by a GnRH injection 48 to 72 h after the PGF injection.

These methods are expensive and time consuming, hence, use of ultrasound will be helpful in the present scenario.

Use of ultrasound for accurate prediction of uterine and ovarian events

Palpation of uterine contents per rectum is the most widely used method for pregnancy diagnosis in dairy cattle. The technique can be performed reliably after day 30 of pregnancy however requires a skilled veterinarian. Moreover, there is risk of pregnancy loss, especially during early stage of pregnancy. Risks of transfer of infection to animals and examinee are always there. Use of ultrasound in dairy industry has made it possible for the earliest and accurate pregnancy diagnosis. The technique also provides quick result. The further advantage of the technique include: (a) presence of twins (b) viability of fetus (c) sex of fetus (d) ovarian structure.

Ultrasound scanning of non-pregnant uterus is helpful in determining the stage of the oestrous cycle or diagnose pathologic conditions of the uterus. During the follicular phase, the endometrium becomes oedematous, increasing its thickness, and the anechoic vascular zone is more easily visualized (Griffin and Ginther, 1992). The content of the uterine lumen typically absent during the luteal phase, whereas a small amount of fluid may be present during the follicular phase (Barlund *et al.*, 2008). However, to further clarify the stage of the oestrous cycle, observation of the ovaries is required.

Inflammatory conditions of the uterus can be detected which could not be possible by rectal examination. Ultrasound is considered the second method of choice after cytological examination in diagnosing the inflammatory condition of the uterus. Ultrasound is helpful in diagnosing mucometra, pyometra and abscess of the uterine wall. The ecographical difference between mucometra and pyometra is the ecogenicity of the uterine content. Whereas, the sterile mucus has an anechoic appearance, the purulent content shows a certain degree of ecogenicity, depending on the amount of purulent material in the mucus (Quintela *et al.*, 2006). Abscesses in the uterine wall will appear to have a hyperechoic content surrounded by a wall of certain ecogenicity (Quintela *et al.*, 2009).

The structure that can be visualized through US of a normal cyclic ovary is follicle and corpus luteum. The follicle is anechoic spherical structure and can be found in variable numbers and size (Griffin and Ginther 1992). The advantage of US compared with rectal palpation is that the subjectivity inherent in the estimation of size and content can be eliminated, as the follicular fluid can be visualized and the diameter can be measured. This makes it possible to detect the presence of a cohort of follicles, dominant follicles or pre-ovulatory follicles.

To determine the stage of the oestrous cycle of a cow, visualization of CL and estimation of its stage is important. Ultrasound (US) is believed to be the most accurate method for detecting the presence of a CL in a bovine ovary. Many of the CL, which is embedded in the ovary could not be palpated by rectal examination and hence use of US facilitates such detection and increase efficiency of detection of CL. Moreover, haemorrhagic and cavitary CL (cystic CL) with a soft consistency may be confused with follicles (Hanzen *et al.*, 2000; Quintela *et al.*, 2006) and US helps in detection of the same.

The size of the CL may also be used to estimate its age. Perez-Marín (2009) indicated that the CL increases in size until about day 8 post-ovulation, maintains a constant size until about day 16 post-ovulation and decreases after this period.

Knowledge about the ovarian cycle and follicular dynamics together with US examination of the uterus and ovarian structures (number and size of follicles, existence of a cavity and size of CL) allows us to estimate the stage of the oestrous cycle of a cow. The size of the dominant follicle is helpful in treating condtions of delayed ovulation and anovulation.

Cystic ovarian follicles (COF) are an important cause of subfertility in dairy animals. COF are follicles with a diameter of at least 2 cm that are present on one or both ovaries in the absence of any active luteal tissue and that clearly interfere with normal ovarian cyclicity (Vanholder *et al.*, 2006). There are two types of COF depending on the wall thickness: follicular cysts have a wall thickness <3 mm and luteinized cysts have a wall thickness >3 mm (Tebble *et al.*, 2001; Vanholder *et al.*, 2006). Ultrasound examination of ovarian cysts allows us to distinguish follicular and luteinized cysts much more efficiently than rectal palpation (Douthwaite and Dobson, 2000).

Many non-pregnant animals do not show heat, or their heat is not detected which significantly increases the days open (Roelofs *et al.*, 2010). An early pregnancy diagnosis facilitates the detection of non-pregnant cows and enables them to be treated for a new insemination (Romano *et al.*, 2006).

Ultrasound helps in detection of embryonic vesicle as an anechoic zone with slightly dilated uterine horn. Inside the embryonic vesicle, the embryonic mass can be located (Griffin and Ginther, 1992; Quintela *et al.*, 2006). Once the embryo is visualized, its viability can be confirmed by checking the heartbeat frequency.

The accuracy of the diagnosis of non pregnant animals is 100%. As embryonic loss usually occurs in the second month of gestation and hence, certain degree of false positive occurs.

The diagnosis of twins is important for dairy farms as the risks of pregnancy losses, freemartinism or dystocia are higher than in single pregnancies (Eddy *et al.*, 1991; Silva del Rio *et al.*, 2009).

An embryo resorption can be ultrasonographically recognized by the following characteristics: the amount of alantoid fluid is lower than expected for the gestational age; there is a presence of membrane fragments freely floating in a cloudy fluid, an absence of embryo/foetus, an absence of heartbeat. The existence of one or several of these signs are indicative of gestation loss (Gnemmi, 2004; Quintela *et al.*, 2006).

Foetal malformations can be detected after approximately 55–60 days of pregnancy. Most large organs of the head, thorax, abdomen and pelvis were visible with ultrasound during the first 4 months (Rajamahendran *et al.*, 1994). Alterations of the normal anatomy, as for example, ascites, umbilical cord alterations, etc., are indicative of reduced foetal viability, so it may be appropriate to induce abortus to avoid increasing the days open.

Colour Doppler

The black and white US is helpful in understand the reproductive physiology and hence, the development of reproduction management systems in the cow. To gain more precise information on the physiological status of the ovaries, the local blood flow in individual ovarian follicles and CLs can be observed using colour Doppler US. The technique is based on the Doppler Effect that establishes that when an US bunch with a given frequency finds a flow of erythrocytes, part of the US bunch is reflected towards the probe with modified frequency, higher if the interface is approaching to the probe and lower, if it is moving away. Therefore, by measuring the apparent change of frequencies between emitter and receiver, the blood flow velocity can be determined (Herzog and Bollwein, 2007).

A colour Doppler image shows the area, where a blood flow is detected, so the amount of colour represents the volume of blood present in the examined structures rather than its flow rate.

The growth, atresia and ovulation of the follicle and CL functionality can be assessed by colour Doppler US. The flow is maximum in the dominant follicle and reduced in the subordinate follicles with simultaneous reduction in size (Acosta *et al.*, 2005). The atretic follicle was characterized by a lack of detectable blood flow and a progressive decrease in diameter. There is an increase in the blood flow in the mature follicle following LH surge that reflect the process of ovulation (Acosta *et al.*, 2003) .The CL is one of the most highly vascularized organs and receives the greatest rate of blood flow per unit of tissue of any organ in the body (Wiltbank *et al.*, 1988). During its initial development (48–120 h), a gradual increase in the blood flow around the CL matches with an increase in its volume and in the serum progesterone concentration (Acosta *et al.*, 2003), which suggests that local blood flow in the CL is related to its potential to produce and release progesterone.

In the process of spontaneous luteolysis, blood flow in the CL was observed to increase during the days 16–17 of the oestrous cycle, concomitant with an increase in plasma levels of 14-dihydro-15-keto-prostaglandin F2á (PGFM) and was followed by a decrease in plasma progesterone concentration 1 day after (Miyamoto *et al.* 2005; Shirasuna *et al.*, 2008; Shirasuna, 2010).

References

1. Acosta TJ, Hayashi KG, Matsui M, Miyamoto A, 2005: Changes in follicular vascularity during the first follicular wave in lactating cows. *J Reprod Dev* 51: 273–280.

2. Acosta TJ, Hayashi KG, Ohtani M, Miyamoto A, 2003: Local changes in blood flow within the pre-ovulatory follicle wall and early corpus luteum in cows. *Reproduction* 125: 759–767.

3. Barlund CS, Carruthers TD, Waldner CL, Palmer CW, 2008*:* A comparison of diagnostic techniques for postpartum endometritis in dairy cattle. *Theriogenology* 69*:* 714–723.

4. Bazer FW, Spencer TE, Johnson GA, Burghardt RC, Wu G. 2009. Comparative aspects of implantation. *Reproduction*, 138: 195-209.

5. Douthwaite R, Dobson H, 2000*:* Comparison of different methods of diagnosis of cystic ovarian disease in cattle and assessment of its treatment with a progesterone-releasing intravaginal device. *Vet Rec* 23*:* 355–359.

6. Eddy R, Davies O, David C, 1991*:* An economic assessment of twin births in British dairy herds. *Vet Rec* 129*:* 526–529.

7. Gnemmi G. 2004*: Atlante di ultrasonografia ginecológica buiatrica. Ed. Le Point Veternaire, Milano, Italy, Pp 127.*

8. Griffin PG, Ginther OJ, 1992*:* Research applications of ultrasonic imaging in reproductive biology. *J Anim Sci* 70*:* 953–972.

9. Hanzen CH, Pieterse M, Scenzi O, Drost M, 2000*:* Relative accuracy of the identification of ovarian structures in the cow by ultrasonography and palpation per rectum. *Vet J* 159*:* 161–170.

10. Herzog K, Bollwein H, 2007*:* Application of doppler ultrasonography in cattle reproduction. *Reprod Dom Anim* 42*:* 51–58.

11. Lucy MC, McDougall S, Nation DP. 2004. The use of hormonal treatments to improve the reproductive performance of lactating dairy cows in feedlot or pasture-based management systems. *Anim Reprod Sci*, 82/83: 495-512.

12. Miyamoto A, Shirasuna K, Wijayagunawardane MP, Watanabe S, Hayashi M, Yamamoto D, Matsui M, Acosta TJ, 2005*:* Blood flow: a key regulatory component of corpus luteum function in the cow. *Domest Anim Endocrinol* 29*:* 329–339.

13. Pereira RV, Caixeta LS, Giordano JO, Guard CL, Bicalho RC. 2013. Reproductive performance of dairy cows re-synchronized after pregnancy diagnosis at 31 (±3 days) after artificial insemination (AI) compared with re-synchronization at 31 (±3 days) after AI with pregnancy diagnosis at 38 (±3 days) after AI. *J Dairy Sci*, 96: 7630-7639.

14. Quintela LA, Díaz C, Becerra JJ, Herradón PG, 2009*: Atlas de ecografía en la vaca. Ed. Quintela L.A., Spain, Pp. 205.*

15. Quintela LA, Díaz C, Herradón PG, Peña AI, Becerra JJ, 2006*: Ecografía y reproducción en la vaca. Ed. Servicio de publicaciones e*

intercambio científico of the University of Santiago de Compostela, Santiago de Compostela, Spain, Pp 92.

16. Rajamahendran R, Ambrose DJ, Burton B, 1994: Clinical and research applications of real-time ultrasonography in bovine reproduction: a review. *Can Vet J* 35: 563–572.

17. Roelofs J, López-Gatius F, Hunter RHF, van Eerdenburg FJCM, Hanzen CH, 2010: When is a cow in estrus? Clinical and practical aspects *Theriogenology* 74: 327–344.

18. Romano JE, Thompson JA, Forrest DW, Westhusin ME, Tomaszweski MA, Kraemer DC, 2006: Early pregnancy diagnosis by transrectal ultrasonography in dairy cattle. *Theriogenology* 66: 1034–1041.

19. Shirasuna K, 2010: Nitric oxide and luteal blood flow in the luteolitic cascade in the cow. *J Reprod Dev* 56: 9–14.

20. Shirasuna K, Yamamoto D, Morota K, Shimizu T, Matsui M, Miyamoto A, 2008: PGF2á stimulates endothelial nitric oxide synthase depending on the existence of bovine granulose cells: analysis by co-culture system of endothelial cells, smmonth muscle cells and granulose cells. *Reprod Dom Anim* 43: 592–598.

21. Silva del Rio N, Colloton JD, Fricke PM, 2009: Factors affecting pregnancy loss for single and twin pregnancies in a high-producing dairy herd. *Theriogenology* 71: 1462–1471.

22. Tebble JE, O'Donnell MJ, Dobson H, 2001: Ultrasound diagnosis and treatment outcome of cystic ovaries in cattle. *Vet Rec* 31: 411–413.

23. Vanholder T, Opsomer G, De Kruif A, 2006: Aetiology and pathogenesis of cystic ovarian follicles in dairy cattle: a review. *Reprod Nutr Dev* 46: 105–119.

24. Wiltbank MC, Dysko RC, Gallagher KP, Keyes PL, 1988: Relationship between blood flow and steroidogenesis in the rabbit corpus luteum. *J Reprod Fert*, 51: 3–520.

□□□

Chapter 16

Augmenting Productivity Through Assisted Reproductive Technique in Dairy Animals

Anuj Kumar, Vikas Sachan and J.K. Agarwal

Department of Veterinary Gynaecology & Obstetrics, College of Veterinary Science and Animal Husbandry, Uttar Pradesh Pandit Deen Dayal Upadhyaya Pashu Chikitsa Vigyan Vishwavidhyalaya Evam Go Anusandhan Sansthan, Mathura

Reproductive inefficiency is one of the most important causes of economic losses in animal industries and it is realized throughout the world. Despite of the remarkable advancement that has been made in the field of reproductive physiology in recent years, infertility due to low conception rate and high embryonic mortality rate remains a major problem. On the other hand, there is an increasing necessity to produce animals with high genetic potential and to increase the productivity of animal unit instead of increasing the number of animal herds to achieve high quality and quantity production.

To meet future needs and to be able to sustain agricultural production, agricultural research and its applications need to use all emerging technologies, one of which is the modern reproductive biotechnologies. The various assisted reproductive techniques have been developed and refined to obtain a large number of offspring from genetically superior animals or to obtain offspring from infertile (or subfertile) animals in addition to disease control.

The various recent available assisted reproductive techniques, which may be helpful in improving the current status of livestock reproduction are :

1. Multiple Ovulation and embryo transfer (MOET)
2. Semen Sexing

3. Cloning
4. Artificial Insemination.

Multiple Ovulation and embryo transfer (MOET)

The term MOET was coined by Nicholas and Smith (1983) to consider embryo transfer and related technology in the context of optimizing genetic improvement of cattle. Multiple ovulation and embryo transfer (MOET) is often referred as the Assisted Reproductive Technology (ART) that is "to the female", while AI is "to the male", i.e. a method of producing more offspring from a genetically valuable female than would be possible by natural breeding. Embryo transfer technology is an important tool to improve livestock at faster rate as well as gives an opportunity to utilize the genetic contribution of both male and female at the same time. By MOET the selection intensity in females can be doubled in elite herds, thus increasing the possibility of producing high yielding bulls and heifers.

Embryo Transfer (ET)

It is removal of embryos from biological dam (donor) and placement into a surrogate mother (recipient) for development of viable calf. It is rapid method for multiplication of desired germplasm and practiced throughout world for production of breeding bulls. Surgical methods for embryo collection and transfer are increasingly replaced by non-surgical methods, which are much more practical and less expensive in selection programmes.

Benefits of Embryo Transfer

- Traditionally, cows produce only one calf per year. ET allows the production of many offspring within a year from a single donor cow.
- ET can increase the genetic potential of a herd in a relatively short period of time.
- ET can increase milk production in dairy herds.
- ET can increase weaning weights in beef and dairy herds.
- ET allows other producers to take advantage of superior genetics because frozen embryos can be shipped almost anywhere.
- ET preserves superior genetics for future generations due to embryo freezing.

Limitations of Embryo Transfer

- Expensive
- Labor intensive
- Requires trained personnel

Selection of Donor Cows

- High milking ability
- High growth rate
- Outstanding reproductive capacity

Hormonal status of donor cow

In donor cows in which **progesterone conc. is 3ng/ml** prior to superovulation, (SOV) such donar shows better ovarian response to SOV treatment :

- **Estrogen conc. :** At luteal phase 1-6pg/ml
- At estrus 10-15pg/ml (Cows $\leq$ 10-15pg/ml not be selected).

Recipient Cows

- Normal reproductive efficiency
- Normal genetilia
- The recipient cow must be able to maintain her pregnancy to term and produce an adequate milk supply for her calf.
- Should have completed at least 2 gestations.
- **Hormonal status**. In recipient progesterone concentration is more important than estrogen.
- At estrus - 0.1 to 0.8 ng/ml(P4 conc)
- 9 to 16 days-4.5ng/ml (cow $\leq$ 4.5ng/ml should not be selected)

Estrous Synchronization

Correct uterine environment is very critical for embryo survival. Synchronization refers to the process of programming a group of animals (recipient) to come in estrus at approximately same time as the donor animals, which is being superovulated. Optimally 12 hours of variation in synchrony is a good acceptable limit. However, it should not exceed beyond thirty six hours. This is a management technique that makes use of hormones to control or reschedule the estrous cycle. Out of most protocols available, the most commonly used protocol in cattle and buffalo is by use of Prostaglandin $PGF_2\ \alpha$ which is based on the fact that it shortens the lifespan of corpus luteum. Two $PGF_2\ \alpha$ injections at 11 or 12 days apart synchronizes estrus in 90% of the animals.

Basis for Synchronization of Estrus

- Manipulate life span of CL
- Manipulate growth of follicles and timing of ovulation

The crucial steps of ET

1. Donor cows of good pedigree animals are treated with hormones (FSH and LH) to increase the number of eggs released at ovulation (multiple ovulations (MO) or superovulation).
2. Then the cows are artificially inseminated using semen from a proven bull or sexed semen.
3. After 6-7 days, the embryos are flushed out non-surgically using a catheter placed into the uterus. This is possible because, in cattle, there is a delay in embryos becoming implanted in the uterine wall. On average, 4-7 embryos are collected.
4. The embryos may then be implanted into recipient cows, whose oestrous cycle is at the correct receptive stage-usually as the result of hormonal manipulation.
5. Embryos may be frozen and stored, using techniques similar to those applied to semen, (though precise control of the regime is somewhat more critical).

Thus, embryo transfer has the potential to bring about genetic improvement twice as fast as AI alone. Moreover, the use of MOET technique could lead to increased selection intensity and reduced generation intervals, resulting in improving genetic gains. Embryo transfer as a part of other biotechnologies will in principle remain as a bottom line technique of other advance technologies, such as stem cell research, cloning and transgenesis, etc.

Sexing of Sperm

The ability to preselect or predetermine the sex of offspring prior to conception is a highly desired technological tool for assisted female breeding programs specifically for milk production, and in males, for meat production and increasing livestock numbers. The current technology is based on the well-known differences in amount of DNA of X- and Y-sperms. The technology uses modified flow cytometric instrumentation for sorting X- and Y-bearing sperm.

How sperms are sexed

- The basic principles are simple; the X-sperm contains more DNA than the Y-sperm (approximately 4% more in the case of cattle). Although this difference is small, by attention to details, it is possible to measure DNA content of individual sperm with sufficient accuracy to distinguish between X- and Y-sperm with about 90% accuracy for 50% of the sperm. Therefore, about half of the sperm are discarded as unsexable, and there is a 10% error rate for those sexed with routine procedures.
- The DNA content of sperm is determined using a fluorescing dye, Hoechst 33342 that readily penetrates the sperm cell membrane and binds to the DNA stoichiometrically.
- The fluorescence is measured by a detector and analyzed by computer. Since X-sperm have 4% more DNA, and therefore, bind more dye than Ysperm, they give more fluorescence, which the computer can recognize.
- The basic instrument used is a flowcytometer/cell sorter. It consists of a pump to move the fluid containing sperm pass through detectors. A laser provides the correct wavelength of light to cause fluorescence without damaging the DNA. A powerful computer also is needed to analyze the fluorescence.
- The cell sorting part of the system works as follows: when the stream of fluid exits the flow cytometer, it is broken into small droplets by a vibrator, forming about 70,000 to 80,000 droplets per second. About one-third of the droplets contain a sperm and about two-thirds are empty; a few droplets contain two or more sperm.

- If a droplet contains an X-sperm as analyzed by the computer, a positive electrical charge is added to the droplet; if the droplet contains a Y-sperm, a negative charge is added; and if the droplet contains no sperm, multiple sperm, damaged sperm, or sperm that are indistinguishable relative to DNA content, no charge is given to the droplet.
- As the droplets fall when they exit the nozzle of the flow cytometer (at a speed of about 80 km/h), they pass through electric fields that are positive on one side and negative on the other. Since opposite electrical charges attract each other, the droplets with a positive charge (containing X-sperm) move the negative part of the field, those with a negative charge move towards the positive field, and those with no charge continue straight down. Thus,three streams of droplets are produced that can be collected into three different test tubes, thereby separating the X from the Y-sperm. In practice, about 20% of sperm end up in the X-fraction, 20% in the Y-fraction and 60% are damaged or not sexable for one reason or another.
- The method for detecting and discarding dead and damaged sperm is to add food colouring to the sperm to be sorted. Sperm with a damaged cell membrane become coloured, whereas those with healthy cell membranes exclude the food colouring.

Beltsville Sperm Sexing Technology

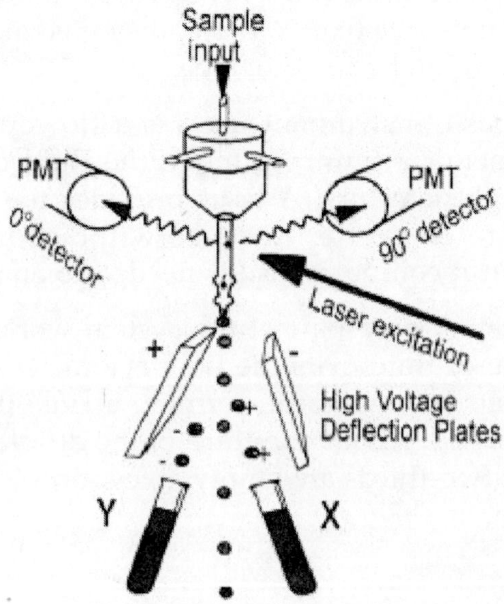

Schematic diagram of a sperm sorter. The electronic signals from the photomultiplier tubes (PMT) are sent to a computer for analysis. Modified from Johnson and Welch, 1999.

The limitations of sexed sperm technology

- The equipment for sexing sperm functions quitewell, but is fairly complicated and expensive, over $350,000 per sperm sorter.
- Skilled operators are required, which results in training costs. Because of these large fixed costs, most sorters are operated in shifts for 14–16 h or more per day.

Low sperm dose insemination

- Typically, a dose of frozen bull sperm for artificial insemination contains $\geq 20\times10^6$ sperm. However, for most bulls, fertility is satisfactory at 10×10^6 sperm, and for some bulls fertility remains high at 2×10^6 frozen sperm per dose.
- Routine operation of a flow cytometer/cell sorter for sexing sperm results in sexing about 10×10^6 sperm/h of each sex.
- Using fewer sexed sperm per dose usually 2×10^6 sperm.

Normality of calves

The calves produced are phenotypically normal. Genetic damage likely is very low, or does not occur at all.

Applications of sexed sperm for cattle

- Because sexed sperm have been used to breed heifers successfully on many occasions, one obvious application is to breed heifers to have female calves. These should result in excellent replacements for beef and dairy herds, since the youngest cattle in any herd with a genetic improvement program are genetically superior to the older cows.
- A major additional benefit is that on the average, female calves weigh about 2 kg less at birth than male calves, so the incidence of dystocia in first calf heifers will be decreased with this application.
- Another application is to obtain male calves from the very best cows in the herd to use as breeding bulls. Sexed sperm could be especially useful to obtain calves of one sex or another for a particular mating, through ET.

Cloning

Cloning is a powerful technique and potentially, it could be used for multiplication of elite animals and minimize the genetic variation in experimental animals. It can be used for the conservation as well as tool for the production of stem cells for therapeutic purposes, as therapeutic cloning. Cloning using somatic cells offers opportunities to select and multiply animals of specific merits. Numerous types of somatic cells are used as donors in somatic cloning, e.g. foetal fibroblasts, adult fibroblasts, granulosa cells, hepatocytes, lymphocytes, etc.

First animal obtained by somatic cloning was a sheep called "Dolly". She was derived from cells that had been taken from the udder of a 6-years old Finn Dorset ewe and cultured for several weeks in the laboratory. Individual cells were then fused with unfertilized eggs from which the genetic material had been removed.

Two hundred and seventy seven of these reconstructed eggs' - each now with a diploid nucleus from the adult animal - were cultured for 6 days in temporary recipients. Twenty nine of the eggs that appeared to have developed normally to the blastocyst stage were implanted into surrogate Scottish Blackface ewes. One gave rise to a live female lamb, Dolly, some 148 days later. Dolly was born on July 5, 1996.

Somatic-cell nuclear transfer
Roslin Technique

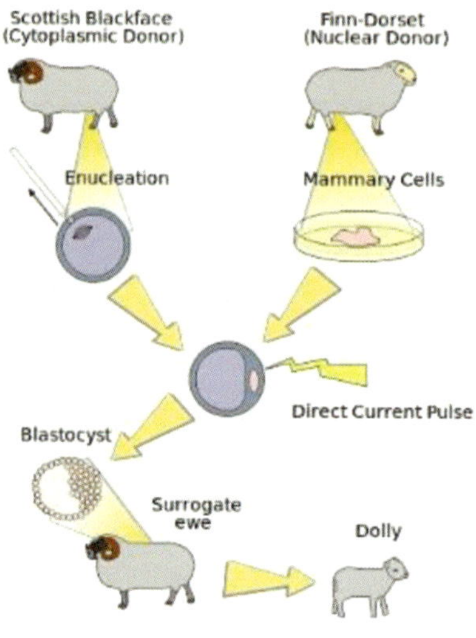

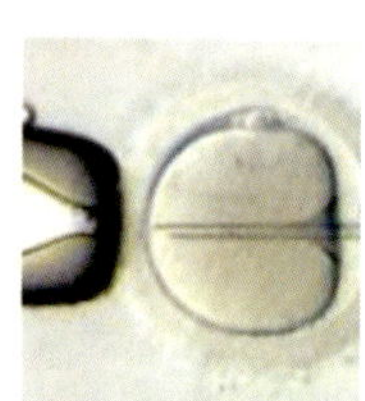

Somatic cell nuclear transfer (SCNT) was used successfully for cloning cattle, pig and goat. Procedure using embryonic stem cells (ESCs) is called Nuclear Transfer-derived Embryonic Stem Cell (NTESC). However, although ESCs were derived for humans and some laboratory animals, derivation of farm animal embryonic stem cells (faESCs) is still unsuccessful. The alternative to faESCs could be embryonic germ cells (EGCs) and spermatogonia stem cells.

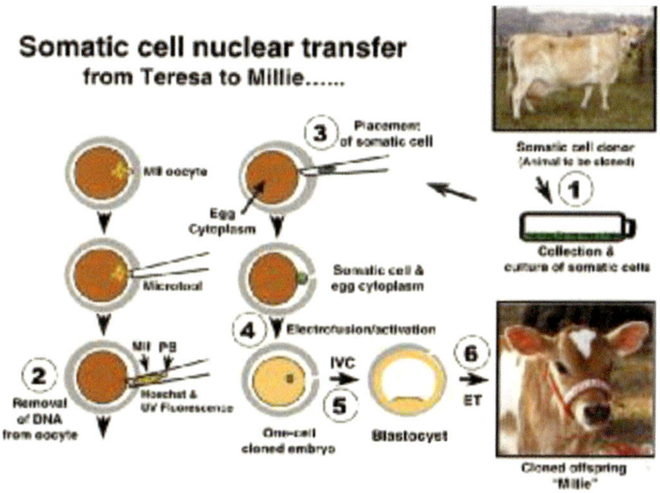

Artificial Insemination

Artificial insemination was the first assisted reproductive technology to be applied commercially for the genetic improvement of animals in the mid-1900s. This technology has now become a practical technology in commercial dairy cattle programs in both, developed and developing countries. Artificial insemination (AI) is the process of collecting sperm cells from a genetically superior male animal and manually depositing them into the reproductive tract of a female.

The first successful insemination was performed by Spallanzani, (1784) in a bitch. Pioneering efforts to AI were begun in Russia in 1899 by Ivanoff. Ivanoff (1922) had studied AI in domestic farm animals, dogs, foxes, rabbits, and poultry. Use of frozen semen (Polge *et al.*, 1949) revolutionized the AI program through worldwide transport of semen. Initially, the AI was used to spread improved indigenous breeds, which were followed by the introduction of crossbreeding, hence, grade up the local low yielder breeds.

The AI technology maximizes the use of outstanding males, dissemination of superior genetic material, improve the rate and efficiency of genetic selection on the male side, introduction of new genetic material by import of semen rather than live animals and thus, reducing the international transportation costs, enabling the use of frozen semen even after the donor is dead and reduces the risk of spreading sexually transmitted diseases.

Various aspects of AI technology have been globally standardized for each species. A large number of AIs are performed globally, more than 100 million cattle, 40 million pigs, 3.3 million sheep and 0.5 million goats are artificially inseminated every year (Boa-Amponsem and Minozzi, 2006).

The conception rate from AI programs in developing countries is relatively low and therefore the desired goal from it has not been achieved, which may be due to the lack of proper management and poor technical skill. The AI will become more effective and economic only, when farmers will have access to considerably better technical and organizational facilities.

□□□

Chapter 17

Use of Ultrasonography in Management of Bovine Reproduction

Anuj Kumar, Vikas Sachan and J.K. Agarwal

Department of Veterinary Gynaecology & Obstetrics, College of Veterinary Science and Animal Husbandry, Uttar Pradesh Pandit Deen Dayal Upadhyaya Pashu Chikitsa Vigyan Vishwavidhyalaya Evam Go Anusandhan Sansthan, Mathura

Introduction

In bovine practice, ultrasonography has become an important diagnostic tool for evaluating the female reproductive system. With the help of ultrasound technology, entire reproductive system can be examined in a non-invasive manner. The quality of the images depends the user's understanding of the interactions between the ultrasound wave and the organ tissue, as well as proper use of the instrument's controls. The objective of this manuscript is to understand some basic principles of ultrasonography, to present its principal uses in bovine reproduction, and the economic benefits of early pregnancy diagnosis.

Principle of Ultrasonography

Images description

The image on the ultrasound screen represents a fine section of an organ, grossly resembling a weakly-magnified histological cut. *The probe, therefore, simulates the passage of a knife, slicing through an organ tissue from top to bottom.* Ultrasonography, thus, presents a flattened two-dimensional image of a finely-cut section of tissue; whereas radiography is a two-dimensional superimposed view of the entire thickness of an animal or of a limb under observation. Ultrasound images are rapidly renewed and images are superimposed one over the other as the probe moves across a tissue surface. The rapid succession of tissue section views gives the impression that the structures are moving like an animated cartoon. When interpreting sectional views of an organ on the screen, it is essential to have a good appreciation of the three-dimensional shape of the organ in space.

Transducer or probe characteristics

The probe is the most delicate component of the ultrasound machine. In the veterinary practices, usual probes have a frequency of 3.5, 5.0 or 7.5 MHz. The ability of the instrument to distinguish between two structures located very close together along the axis of the ultrasound beam is called its axial resolution. The axial resolution is best, when the groups of waves emitted have a short wavelength. Since the number of cycles in each group of waves is set according to instrument design, the only way to shorten their length is to use a probe with a higher frequency. For example, the group of waves produced by a 7.5 MHz probe will be shorter than one produced by a 3.5 MHz probe and will provide better axial resolution.

There are two types of probes: linear and sectorial (Figure 1). In bovine reproduction, linear probes are preferred for transrectal examinations of the ovaries and uterus. This probe has a set row of crystals that are selected electronically to form a rectangular image. The linear probe provides good resolution for tissues located close to the probe. Sectorial probes have one or several crystals, whose position produces a beam in the shape of a pie slice. The advantage of the sectorial probe is that it doesn't require a large surface of contact, and it scans a greater overall surface. The disadvantage is that the visual field and the lateral resolution (i.e. the ability of a system to differentiate between two adjacent structures) are more restricted close to the probe. The sectorial probe is ideal for viewing the small ruminant fetus by transabdominal ultrasound imaging and for ultrasound-guided transvaginal aspiration of bovine follicles.

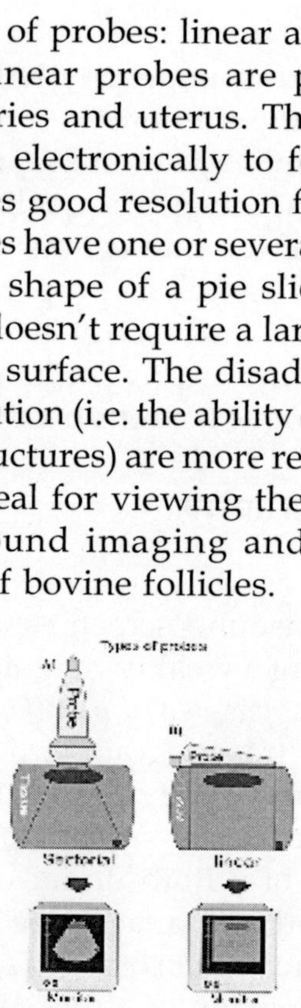

Figure 1: Type of probe

Resolution of an ultrasound image as well as the depth of the tissue observed depends on the frequency and the *focalization* of the scanning beam. With a lower frequency, tissue penetration will be deep, but the resolution will be lower. A higher frequency enables better resolution, but beam attenuation will be greater and it will not penetrate the tissue as deeply.

Images description

The description of ultrasound images is based on an evaluation of the shape, contour, size, and position of the structure being studied, as well as its echogenicity, which depends on the amplitude of the echoes received. An echogenic structure reflects the majority of sound waves back to the probe and thus, appears from white to different shades of grey on the screen. *An anechogenic structure does not produce echoes;* instead, it transmits the waves on to more deeply situated tissues. An example of an anechogenic structure is fluid filled cavity, like follicular fluid, urinary bladder which appears black on the screen. The terms hypoechogenic and hyperechogenic indicate respectively a decrease and an increase in relative echogenicity in comparison with the surrounding tissue, whereas the term isoechogenic is used to describe similar echogenicity with the surrounding tissue.

Echotexture terminology

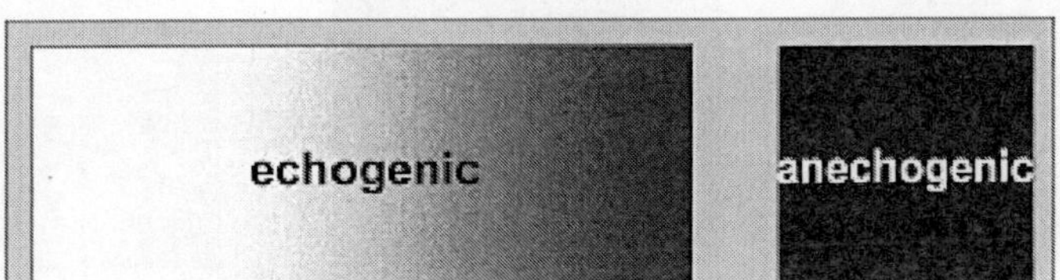

Echotexture terminology of a tissue structure relative to the surrounding tissue

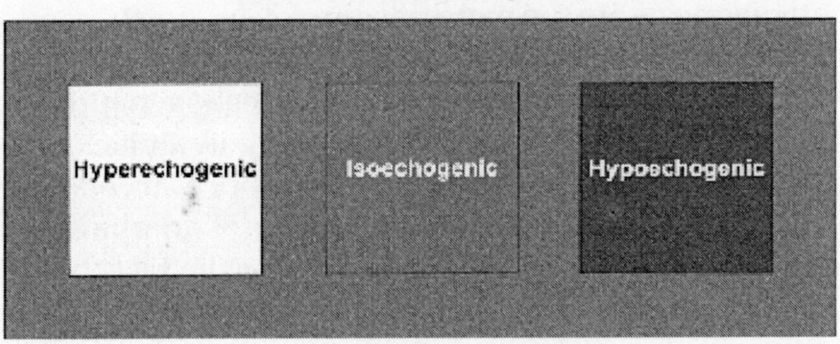

Ultrasound Applications

Ovary and uterus

With the use of ultrasound since 1984, enormous progress has been made in our understanding of folliculogenesis and the development of the bovine corpus luteum. Ultrasound enables us to explain the dynamics of follicular growth in follicles greater than 1 mm in diameter throughout estrous cycle. The same pattern of growth repeats itself approximately every seven days. It starts with the growth of a cohort of many follicles, known as a follicular wave, which includes a follicle that will pursue its growth and will be called dominant while the other follicles of the cohort will regress by atresia. The most common pathological conditions of the ovaries in bovine practice are cystic ovaries (follicular and luteal cysts). These two types of cysts can be differentiated by ultrasonography and treated accordingly. Increased growth of a non-ovulating follicle may lead to development of a follicular or luteal cyst. An ovary is usually considered cystic, when it contains a hollow structure greater than 25 mm that persists for more than 10 days. A follicular cyst can be differentiated from a luteal cyst by its thin wall and uniformly anechogenic follicular fluid.

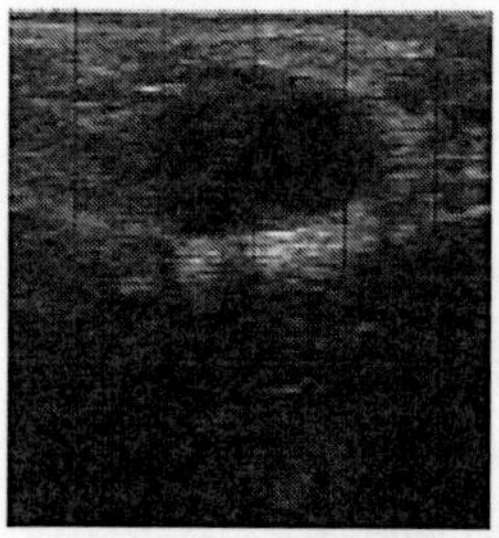

Ovary with follicles

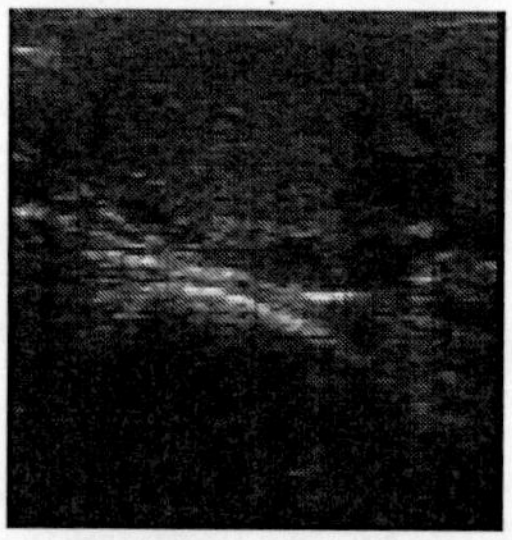

Corpus luteum

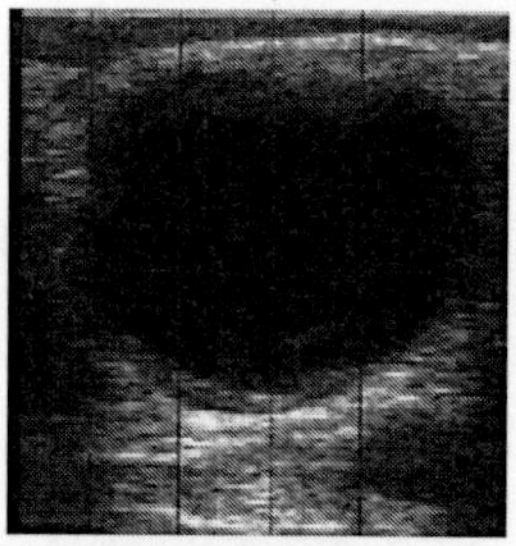

Follicular cyst

The two most frequently observed uterine pathologies in ultrasound diagnosis are the metritis complex (pyometra-endometritis) and mucometra. In the case of endometritis-pyometra, the contents of the uterus may vary in appearance as anechogenic fluid in black, to the presence of echogenic material floating in a black background, to a purulent exudate, that is echogenic in appearance and similar to the surrounding tissue, or isoechogenic. The characteristic of mucometra resembles a pregnancy, except for the fact that there is no embryo/foetus placentomes, or foetal membranes.

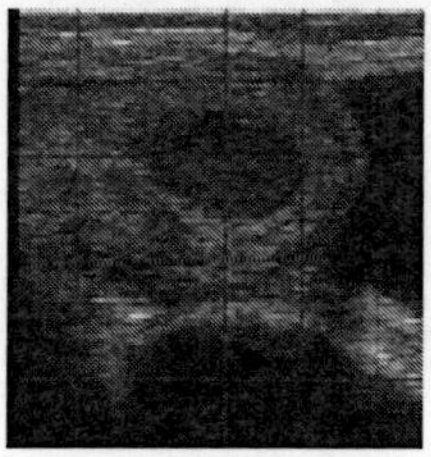
Pyometra

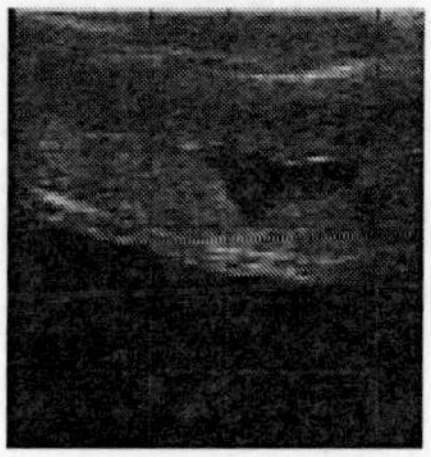
Non-pregnant uterus

Pregnancy diagnosis

Stage of gestation period

Diagnosis of pregnancy in cows is an important part of management of infertile cow in dairy herds. The pregnancy examination is considered essential and economical for livestock owners. Transrectal palpation has been used for the past 50 years to diagnose pregnancy. This diagnosis can be made after 30 to 35 days in adult cows and slightly earlier in heifers. However, it is important to note that the accuracy of early diagnosis by palpation varies according to the skill and experience of the veterinarian. Transrectal palpation in an early phase of pregnancy can be harmful by causing embryonic death as a result of improper handling.

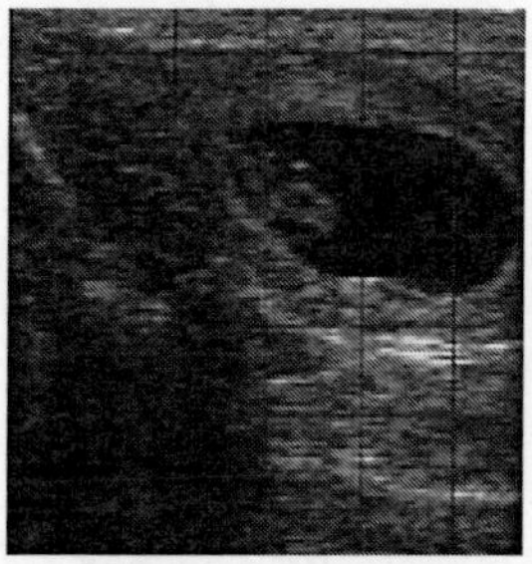
30 days pregnancy

Embryonic death is one of the most important factors associated with dairy cow infertility. It is defined as the death loss of an embryo between the moment of fertilization and the first stages of differentiation, at around day 45 of pregnancy. The majority of embryonic deaths occur before day 25. However, the period, between days 25 and 45 is critical for the fixation of the embryonic membranes to the uterine epithelium and corresponds to the period when early pregnancy examinations are performed on dairy cows.

Ultrasonography is less harmfull and more accurate than transrectal palpation for diagnosing pregnancy in dairy cows before day 35.

Accuracy of the method

Diagnosis of pregnancy by ultrasonography can be made as early as day 25 after insemination. An evaluation of this diagnostic method has demonstrated excellent sensitivity (detection of pregnancy, when the animal is truly gravid): greater than 95% at day 26 post-insemination. Ultrasonography's greatest advantage for the clinician is to diagnose non-pregnant animal as early as possible after insemination. The accuracy increases to 98 and 100%, if the pregnancy diagnosis is performed respectively after day 30 and day 31 post insemination. This excellent characteristic enables veterinarians for management or treatment of non-pregnant animals as quickly as possible.

The accuracy of early pregnancy diagnosis using ultrasonography depends upon many factors. Out of these factors, most important is the stage of pregnancy, when the reproductive examination is performed. Theoretically, with advancement of pregnancy, the amniotic vesicle and the embryo will occupy the more space within the uterus and they will be easy to visualize. Other factor is the position of the uterus in the pelvic canal. There are more false negatives between days 24 and 33 after insemination, when the uterus is located at the cranial part of the pelvic bone. It appears that a complete examination of the reproductive tract is more difficult, when the uterus is located in this position. The cow's parity also has an impact on diagnostic accuracy, which has proven to be inversely proportional to the age of the cow being examined. Diagnostic accuracy is also influenced by the type of instrument and probe used. In bovine reproduction, where it is important to evaluate ovarian and uterine structures in detail, we prefer to use linear probes that produce frequencies of 5 to 7.5 MHz; these give a better resolution compared to probes with lower frequencies.

Embryo's viability characteristics

During pregnancy diagnosis, Embryo viability can be assessed by examine the fetal heart beat. It is generally visible near about at the centre of the embryo starting at day 25 of pregnancy, appearing as a twinkling light with a frequency that varies between 140 and 160 beats per minute.

Another important sign of normal embryonic development is the appearance of the umbilical cord between the uterus and the embryo between days 40 and 45 of pregnancy. Starting on day 45, we may also observe the first movements of the fetus. Finally, the presence of a homogeneous, anechogenic fetal fluid in sufficient quantities within the amnios is another way of confirming that viable fetal development is progressing normally. When the presence of many echogenic particles are noted within the uterine fluid, the veterinarian should question the viability of the embryo and wonder, if embryonic death has occurred. At this time, it is important to review the various signs of embryonic vitality, such as the heartbeat, fetal movement as well as its length in relation to the stage of pregnancy. The presence of a large amount of debris within the amnionic fluid is generally the result of embryonic degeneration. On occasion, it is also possible to observe a dead but nearly intact embryo. However, upon further examination, the embryo's contours may appear irregular and small particles may be found in the immediate surroundings.

Foetal Sexing

The ultrasound diagnosis of the foetal sexing involves three steps: locating and identifying the fetus, verifying fetal viability and determining fetal sex. The clinician first locates the fetus in the gravid uterus. With a complete examination of the two uterine horns, the user will be able to determine the number of fetuses present. During examination, the aspect of the amniotic fluid and the presence of a fetal heartbeat observed to confirm viability. Now the clinician will determine the sex of the fetus in following ways:

Male fetus

At around day 50, the genital tubercle migrates cranially along the median line towards the umbilicus. This migration gradually increases the distance separating the genital tubercle from the tail of the fetus. At around day 58, the genital tubercle reaches its final destination, slightly caudal to the umbilicus. Following this migration, the genital swellings are now in a caudal position in relation to the genital tubercle and have fused together near the median line between days 65 and 70 in the male fetus, a change is observed in the appearance of the genital tubercle. The two-lobed structure observed earlier in the pregnancy gives way to a four-lobed structure following a view of the genital tubercle and the urogenital folds. In the male, the genital tubercle is the origin of the penis, the urogenital folds form the prepuce and the genital swellings form the scrotum. The migration of the testicles toward, the scrotum occurs later and is generally complete by day 140 of pregnancy.

Female fetus

Starting on day 40, as for the male, a vertical lengthening of the genital tubercle and the presence of the urogenital folds can be detected. Between days 50 and 58, the genital tubercle migrates from its initial position between the hind limbs towards the anal region, which is in the opposite direction from that of the male. In the female, the genital tubercle is located under the tail and the genital swellings undergo progressive atrophy starting on day 50, and eventually disappear completely. The genital tubercle is the origin of the clitoris and the urogenital folds form the vulvar labia.

Stage of gestation period for fetal sexing

Ultrasound fetal sexing examination can be done between days 58 and 100 of pregnancy, but best time period is between days 60 and 70. Even though the genital tubercle is already visible at day 45, it doesn't reach its definite position until day 58. Migration may occur more rapidly in certain animals, sometimes enabling definitive diagnosis at day 54 or 55. Clinician ability to establish a diagnosis at the end of the first trimester of pregnancy (90 to 100 days) will depend on the position of the uterus within the pelvic/abdominal cavity and the possibility to reach the gravid uterine horn with the probe. A uterus deep in the abdominal cavity will make the diagnosis more difficult.

Diagnosis of twin/multiple foetuses

Diagnosis of multiple fetuses is generally performed by the veterinarian at the same time as sexing the fetus, after day 57 of pregnancy. By embryo transfer technique, it has become possible to implant two embryos in a recipient. If the presence of twins is confirmed before day 55 of pregnancy, it is then important to do another ultrasound exam after day 60 to determine the sex of the foetuses. If the fetuses are male and female, the owner will then have the opportunity to choose whether to maintain the pregnancy and run the risk of obtaining a freemartin heifer or to terminate the pregnancy.

Abnormal development of fetus

During the ultrasound examination for pregnancy, and especially when determining the sex of the fetus, it is very important to ensure that the fetus is viable and its appearance is normal. It is important to recognize the fetal defects, like siamese twins; schistosomus reflexus; amorphous globosus. Certain acquired or congenital defects may be noted during the ultrasound exam in an older foetus. Among these, it is worthwhile to mention hydrocephalus, fetal ascites and pericardial effusion. These conditions have a very poor prognosis for fetal survival. Before proposing the termination of the pregnancy on the cows presenting these anomalies, it is essential for the veterinarian to do a careful ultrasonographic examination using more than one view and to repeat the scanning more than once to confirm his definitive diagnosis.

Conclusions

The diagnosis of reproductive characteristics can be acquired by examining hundred to thousands of cow by per-rectal examination during a period of time. On the other hand veterinarians who are less experienced in transrectal examination can improve their manual mistake by ultrasonography, along with offering a more accurate and extensive diagnostic service. The use of this diagnostic tool increases the value of a veterinary clinic's services. The use of ultrasound technology is economically advantageous for dairy producers and veterinarians.

❏❏❏

Chapter 18

Renewable Energy – A New Ray of Hope in Minimizing Inputs and in Getting Higher Returns

Yajuvendra Singh, D.N. Singh and Rajneesh Sirohi

Department of Livestock Production Management, College of Veterinary Science and Animal Husbandry, Uttar Pradesh Pandit Deen Dayal Upadhyaya Pashu Chikitsa Vigyan Vishwavidhyalaya Evam Go Anusandhan Sansthan, Mathura

Renewable energy is energy that is collected from renewable resources, which are naturally replenished on a human timescale, such as sunlight, wind, rain, tides, waves, and geothermal heat. Renewable energy often provides energy in four important areas: electricity generation, air and water heating/cooling, transportation, and rural (off-grid) energy services.

Based on the report of Renewable Energy Policy Network for the 21st Century (2016), renewables contributed 19.2% to humans' global energy consumption and 23.7% to their generation of electricity in 2014 and 2015, respectively. This energy consumption is divided as 8.9% coming from traditional biomass, 4.2% as heat energy (modern biomass, geothermal and solar heat), 3.9% hydroelectricity and 2.2% is electricity from wind, solar, geothermal, and biomass. Worldwide investments in renewable technologies amounted to more than US$286 billion in 2015, with countries like China and the United States, heavily investing in wind, hydro, solar and biofuels. Globally, there are an estimated 7.7 million jobs associated with the renewable energy industries, with solar photovoltaics, being the largest renewable employer. As of 2015 worldwide, more than half of all new electricity capacity installed was renewable.

Renewable energy resources exist over wide geographical areas, in contrast to other energy sources, which are concentrated in a limited number of countries. Rapid deployment of renewable energy and energy efficiency is resulting in significant energy security, climate change mitigation, and economic benefits. As greenhouse gas (GHG) emitters begin to be held liable for damages resulting from GHG emissions resulting in climate change, a high value for liability mitigation would provide powerful incentives for deployment of renewable energy technologies. In international public opinion surveys there is strong support for promoting renewable sources, such as solar power and wind power. At the national level, at least 30 nations around the world already have renewable energy contributing more than 20 per cent of energy supply. National renewable energy markets are projected to continue to grow strongly in the coming decade and beyond. Some places and at least two countries, Iceland and Norway generate all their electricity using renewable energy already, and many other countries have the set a goal to reach 100% renewable energy in the future. For example, in Denmark the government decided to switch the total energy supply (electricity, mobility and heating/cooling) to 100% renewable energy by 2050.

Renewable energy systems are rapidly becoming more efficient and cheaper. Their share of total energy consumption is increasing. Growth in consumption of coal and oil could end by 2020 due to increased uptake of renewables and natural gas.

Start of alternate/ renewable energy

- **In 1830**, scientists discovered *photo-voltaic* compounds, which release energy when exposed to light. This discovery eventually led to the development of *solar cells and solar power*.
- **In 1839**, William Robert Grove invented the first *hydrogen fuel cell*, which harnessed electricity from the reaction between hydrogen and oxygen.
- **In the late 1880**, *hydroelectric power* first became commercially available in the United States, and solar power was discovered in Europe. Governments established the first energy departments shortly before the turn of the century.
- **In 1947,** The first nuclear reactor project aimed at energy production was initiated in Brookhaven, New York. At the same time, political tensions between the United States and Middle Eastern countries threatened the U.S. supply of oil.

- **In 1970**, the US Environmental Protection Agency (EPA) was established. Damage to natural areas as a result of *energy harvesting* was one of the first issues addressed by the agency.
- **In 1976**, Congress authorized a committee to examine the potential for the development of electric vehicles, with the goal of reducing dependence on fossil fuels.

Different major types of renewable energy

Most renewable energy comes either directly or indirectly from the sun, however, alternative energy resources can be divided into more specific categories includes:

1. Solar Power

Solar energy, radiant light and heat from the sun, is harnessed using a range of ever-evolving technologies such, as solar heating, photovoltaics, concentrated solar power (CSP), concentrator photovoltaics (CPV), solar architecture and artificial photosynthesis. Solar technologies are broadly characterized as either passive solar or active solar depending on the way they capture, convert and distribute solar energy. Passive solar techniques include orienting a building to the Sun, selecting materials with favourable thermal mass or light dispersing properties, and designing spaces that naturally circulate air. Active solar technologies encompass solar thermal energy, using solar collectors for heating, and solar power, converting sunlight into electricity either directly using photovoltaics (PV), or indirectly using concentrated solar power (CSP).

A photovoltaic system converts light into electrical direct current (DC) by taking advantage of the photoelectric effect. Solar PV has turned into a multi-billion, fast-growing industry, continues to improve its cost-effectiveness, and has the most potential of any renewable technologies together with CSP. Concentrated solar power (CSP) systems use lenses or mirrors and tracking systems to focus a large area of sunlight into a small beam. Commercial concentrated solar power plants were first developed in the 1980s. CSP-Stirling has by far the highest efficiency among all solar energy technologies.

In 2011, the International Energy Agency said that "the development of affordable, inexhaustible and clean solar energy technologies will have huge longer-term benefits. It will increase countries' energy security through reliance on an indigenous, inexhaustible and mostly import-independent resource, enhance sustainability, reduce pollution, lower the costs of mitigating climate change, and keep fossil fuel prices lower than otherwise. These advantages are global. Hence, the additional costs of the incentives for early deployment should be considered learning investments; they must be wisely spent and need to be widely shared". Italy has the largest proportion of solar electricity in the world, in 2015 solar supplied 7.8% of electricity demand in Italy. In 2016, after another year of rapid growth, solar generated 1.3% of global power.

From an environmental perspective, solar power is the best thing going. A 1.5 kilowatt PV system will keep more than 110,000 pounds of carbon dioxide, the chief greenhouse gas, out of the atmosphere over the next 25 years. The same solar system will also prevent the need to burn 60,000 pounds of coal. With solar, there's no acid rain, no urban smog, no pollution of any kind.

2. Wind Power

Wind power is the use of air flow through wind turbines to mechanically power generators for electricity. Wind power, as an alternative to burning fossil fuels, is plentiful, renewable, widely distributed, clean, produces no greenhouse gas emissions during operation, and uses little land.

Airflows can be used to run wind turbines. Modern utility-scale wind turbines range from around 600 kW to 5 MW of rated power, although turbines with rated output of 1.5–3 MW have become the most common for commercial use. The largest generator capacity of a single installed onshore wind turbine reached 7.5 MW in 2015. The power available from the wind is a function of the cube of the wind speed, so as wind speed increases, power output increases up to the maximum output for the particular turbine. Areas where winds are stronger and more constant, such as offshore and high altitude sites are preferred locations for windfarms. Typically full load hours of wind turbines vary between 16 and 57 percent annually, but might be higher in particularly favorable offshore sites.

Wind-generated electricity met nearly 4% of global electricity demand in 2015, with nearly 63 GW of new wind power capacity installed. Wind energy was the leading source of new capacity in Europe, the US and Canada, and the second largest in China. In

Denmark, wind energy met more than 40% of its electricity demand, while Ireland, Portugal and Spain, each met nearly 20%.

Globally, the long-term technical potential of wind energy is believed to be five times total current global energy production, or 40 times current electricity demand, assuming all practical barriers needed were overcome. This would require wind turbines to be installed over large areas, particularly in areas of higher wind resources, such as offshore. As offshore wind speeds average ~90% greater than that of land, so offshore resources can contribute substantially more energy than land stationed turbines. In 2014, global wind generation was 706 terawatt-hours or 3% of the world's total electricity.

3. Hydropower

Flowing water creates energy that can be captured and turned into electricity. This is called hydroelectric power or hydropower. In 2015, hydropower generated 16.6% of the world's total electricity and 70% of all renewable electricity. Since water is about 800 times denser than air, even a slow flowing stream of water, or moderate sea swell, can yield considerable amounts of energy. There are many forms of water energy.

The most common type of hydroelectric power plant uses a dam on a river to store water in a reservoir. Water released from the reservoir flows through a turbine, spinning it, which in turn activates a generator to produce electricity. But hydroelectric power doesn't necessarily require a large dam. Some hydroelectric power plants just use a small canal to channel the river water through a turbine.

Another type of hydroelectric power plant–called a pumped storage plant – can even store power. The power is sent from a power grid into the electric generators. The generators then spin the turbines backward, which causes the turbines to pump water from a river or lower reservoir to an upper reservoir, where the power is stored. To use the power, the water is released from the upper reservoir back down into the river or lower reservoir. This spins the turbines forward, activating the generators to produce electricity.

Advantages of Hydropower

a) Once a dam is constructed, electricity can be produced at a constant rate.

b) If electricity is not needed, the sluice gates can be shut, stopping electricity generation. The water can be saved for use another time, when electricity demand is high.

c) Dams are designed to last many decades and so, can contribute to the generation of electricity for many years/decades.

d) The lake that forms behind the dam can be used for water sports and leisure/pleasure activities. Often large dams become tourist attractions in their own right.

e) The lake's water can be used for irrigation purposes.

f) The build up of water in the lake means that energy can be stored until needed, when the water is released to produce electricity.

4. Geothermal energy

The adjective *geothermal* originates from the Greek roots *geo*, meaning earth, and *thermos*, meaning heat. High Temperature Geothermal energy is from thermal energy generated and stored in the Earth. Thermal energy is the energy that determines the temperature of matter. Earth's geothermal energy originates from the original formation of the planet and from radioactive decay of minerals. The geothermal gradient, which is the difference in temperature between the core of the planet and its surface, drives a continuous conduction of thermal energy in the form of heat from the core to the surface.

The heat that is used for geothermal energy can be from deep within the Earth, all the way down to Earth's core – 4,000 miles (6,400 km) down. At the core, temperatures may reach over 9,000 °F (5,000 °C). Heat conducts from the core to surrounding rock. Extremely high temperature and pressure cause some rock to melt, which is commonly known as magma. Magma convects upward, since it is lighter than the solid rock. This magma then heats rock and water in the crust, sometimes upto 700 °F (371 °C). "Some geothermal systems are formed, when hot magma near the surface (1,500 to 10,000 meters deep) directly heats groundwater." The heat generated from these hot spots flows outward toward the surface, manifesting as volcanoes, geysers, and hot springs. From hot springs, geothermal energy has been used for bathing since Paleolithic times and for space heating since ancient Roman times, but it is now better known for electricity generation.

Low Temperature Geothermal refers to the use of the outer crust of the earth as a Thermal Battery to facilitate Renewable thermal energy for heating and cooling buildings, and other refrigeration and industrial uses. In this form of Geothermal, a Geothermal Heat Pump and Ground-coupled heat exchanger are used together to move heat energy into the earth (for cooling) and out of the earth (for heating) on a varying seasonal basis. Low temperature Geothermal (generally referred to as "GHP") is an increasingly important renewable technology because it both reduces total annual energy loads associated with heating and cooling, and it also flattens the electric demand curve eliminating the extreme summer and winter peak electric supply requirements. Thus, Low Temperature Geothermal/GHP is becoming an increasing national priority with multiple tax credit support and focus as part of the ongoing movement toward Net Zero Energy.

Advantages of Geothermal Energy

a) **Reduce Reliance on Fossil Fuels :** Dependence on fossil fuels decreases with the increase in the use of geothermal energy. With the sky-rocketing prices of oil, many countries are pushing companies to adopt these clean sources of energy. Burning of fossil fuels releases greenhouse gases, which are responsible for global warming.

b) **No Pollution :** This is one of the main advantages of using geothermal energy, since it does not create any pollution and help in creating clean environment. Being the renewable source of energy, geothermal energy has helped in reducing global warming and pollution. Moreover, Geothermal systems does not create any pollution, as it releases some gases from deep within the earth which are not very harmful to the environment.

c) **Direct Use :** Since ancient times, people having been using this source of energy for taking bath, heating homes, preparing food and today this is also used for direct heating of homes and offices. This makes geothermal energy cheaper and affordable. Although the initial investment is quite steep but in the long run with huge cost saving, it proves quite useful.

d) **Job Creation and Economic Benefits :** Government of various countries is investing hugely in creation of geothermal energy, which on other hand has created more jobs for the local people.

5. Bio energy

Biomass is biological material derived from living, or recently living organisms. It most often refers to plants or plant-derived materials which are specifically called lignocellulosic biomass. As an energy source, biomass can either be used directly via combustion to produce heat, or indirectly after converting it to various forms of biofuel. Conversion of biomass to biofuel can be achieved by different methods which are broadly classified into: *thermal*, *chemical*, and *biochemical* methods. Wood remains the largest biomass energy source today; examples include forest residues - such as dead trees, branches and tree stumps - yard clippings, wood chips and even municipal solid waste. In the second sense, biomass includes plant or animal matter that can be converted into fibers or other industrial chemicals, including biofuels. Industrial biomass can be grown from numerous types of plants, including miscanthus, switchgrass, hemp, corn, poplar, willow, sorghum, sugarcane, bamboo, and a variety of tree species, ranging from eucalyptus to oil palm (palm oil).

Plant energy is produced by crops specifically grown for use as fuel that offer high biomass output per hectare with low input energy. Some examples of these plants are wheat, which typically yield 7.5–8 tonnes of grain per hectare, and straw, which typically yield 3.5–5 tonnes per hectare in the UK. The grain can be used for liquid transportation fuels, while the straw can be burned to produce heat or electricity. Plant biomass can also be degraded from cellulose to glucose through a series of chemical treatments, and the resulting sugar can then be used as a first generation bio-fuel.

Biomass can be converted to other usable forms of energy like methane gas or transportation fuels, like ethanol and bio-diesel. Rotting garbage, and agricultural and human waste, all release methane gas - also called landfill gas or biogas. Crops, such as corn and sugarcane, can be fermented to produce the transportation fuel, ethanol. Biodiesel, another transportation fuel, can be produced from left-over food products, like vegetable oils and animal fats. Also, biomass to liquids (BTLs) and cellulosic ethanol are still under research. There is a great deal of research involving algal fuel or algae-derived biomass due to the fact that it's a non-food resource and can be produced at rates 5 to 10 times those of other types of land-based agriculture, such as corn and soy. Once harvested, it can be fermented to produce bio-fuels, such as ethanol, butanol, and methane, as well as bio-diesel and hydrogen. The biomass used for electricity generation varies by region. Forest by-products, such as wood residues, are common in the United States. Agricultural waste is common in Mauritius (sugar cane residue) and Southeast Asia (rice husks). Animal husbandry residues, such as poultry litter, are common in the United Kingdom.

Biofuels include a wide range of fuels, which are derived from biomass. The term covers solid, liquid, and gaseous fuels. Liquid biofuels include bioalcohols, such as bioethanol, and oils, such as bio-diesel. Gaseous biofuels include biogas, landfill gas and synthetic gas. Bioethanol is an alcohol made by fermenting the sugar components of plant materials and it is made mostly from sugar and starch crops. These include maize, sugarcane and, more recently, sweet sorghum. The latter crop is particularly suitable for growing in dryland conditions, and is being investigated by International Crops Research Institute for the Semi-Arid Tropics for its potential to provide fuel, along with food and animal feed, in arid parts of Asia and Africa.

With advanced technology being developed, cellulosic biomass, such as trees and grasses, are also used as feedstocks for ethanol production. Ethanol can be used as a fuel for vehicles in its pure form, but it is usually used as a gasoline additive to increase octane and improve vehicle emissions. Bioethanol is widely used in the United States and in Brazil. The energy costs for producing bio-ethanol are almost equal to, the energy yields from bio-ethanol. However, according to the European Environment Agency, biofuels do not address global warming concerns. Bio-diesel is made from vegetable oils, animal fats or recycled greases. It can be used as a fuel for vehicles in its pure form, or more commonly as a diesel additive to reduce levels of particulates, carbon monoxide, and hydrocarbons from diesel-powered vehicles. Bio-diesel is produced from oils or fats using trans-esterification and is the most common biofuel in Europe. Biofuels provided 2.7% of the world's transport fuel in 2010.

Biomass, bio-gas and bio-fuels are burned to produce heat/power and in doing so harm the environment. Pollutants, such as sulphurous oxides (SO_x), nitrous oxides (NO_x), and particulate matter (PM) are produced from the combustion of biomass; the World Health Organisation estimates that 7 million premature deaths are caused each year by air pollution. Biomass combustion is a major contributor.

The conversion of animal waste, ashes and other minerals into bio-gas encourages onsite energy production and brings the production of bio-energy6 to the farm level, thus providing a way of reducing the agricultural sector's reliance on the combustion of traditional biomass while improving the soil, air quality and human health. Generating methane from manure produced by livestock under controlled conditions could supplement energy needs and, consequently, reduce the direct contribution of methane to climate change; essentially mitigating the use of firewood by relying on a more sustainable energy source.

The multiple benefits of anaerobic digestion are making it an increasingly attractive manure management technology. Other than being adopted at the household level, the system can efficiently be used in medium and large livestock farms. Such larger scale energy production could provide electrification to entire rural communities for local use or for sale to small-scale industries via mini-grids.

The livestock manure may be applied as a solid on pastures and ranges. This results in the generation and release of methane into the atmosphere, contributing to greenhouse gas emissions. At the same time, most rural areas depend heavily on firewood as their primary energy source. If livestock production methods are modified such that a high proportion of the manure generated can be harnessed and fed to an anaerobic digester, methane can be generated under controlled conditions.

In the case of livestock-dependent where production systems are based on grazing land, the use of the system requires concise logistical and management systems. A key constraint in the development of renewable waste substrates as energy resources is their dispersed nature. Large sources of waste substrates are often located at some distance from potential energy production sites. In addition, a significant amount of livestock manure (as much as 25-35 per cent) of total residues may remain unrecoverable.

The collection, transport and processing of renewable waste also poses significant challenges to their use in energy production. For these and other reasons, the technology is best suited to integrated crop-livestock systems at the household level, where families own upto four pigs, heads of cattle and/or poultry animals.

Daily required input and fuelwood equivalent per plant volume

Bio digester size (m^3)	Daily dung feeding (kg)	Use of biogas stove (hour)	Use of biogas lamp (hour)	Wood value replaced (kg)
4	20-40	2-4	8-16	4-8
6	40-60	4-6	16-24	8-12
8	60-80	6-8	24-32	12-16
10	80-100	8-10	32-40	16-20
15	100-150	10-15	40-60	20-30

Bio-gas digesters are generally sized on the basis of local energy requirements and the manure production of the farm. Two main types of technologies exist–the brick bio-digester and the tubular plastic one. The brick bio-digester consists of a fixed dome placed underground. The plant is constructed with local materials: bricks sand and cement and has an estimated lifetime of 20 years. The total size ranges from 4 to 10 cubic metres, depending on the resources available.

The tubular plastic digester is relatively simple and cheap. The average cost of materials is currently around US$150, starting from 3 to 8 cubic metres per bio-digester. The plastic tube is generally installed in a pit in the ground. The waste inlet is installed higher than the outlet and a plastic tank is connected by a PVC tube with a diameter of 21 millimetres linking the gas reservoir to the gas burner. The waste is mixed with water, which drains into a plastic barrel dug into the ground.

Advantages presented by the use of biomass

Renewable biomass energy occupies an important position and plays a decisive role in the present world energy structure. It has the potential to supply about 14 per cent of global energy consumption, however, only 1 per cent of its total energy capacity has been used to date (World Bank, 2009).

Given the recognition of biomass energy as a viable alternative resource, greater efficiency should be sought in its production and use. Future prospects for RETs are also good, with growing acknowledgement of their potential for the environment, price stability, local job creation and energy security. Manure collection is efficient, where the livestock are kept in a pen (stalled) and provided with food and water. This system allows for manual collection. Alternatively, purpose-built pens allow manure to be swept into a drain connected to a bio-gas digester. Biomass resources have attracted much interest and enthusiasm because of five key advantages they hold over fossil fuels and/or other renewable energy sources:

a) Widely available resource

Biomass resources are diverse, widespread and often found in large volumes. In principle, biomass residues exist, wherever trees and crops are grown and wherever food and fiber are processed.

b) Available on demand

Biomass is a form of stored energy and can, therefore, provide energy at all times, without the need for expensive storage devices. In this respect, biomass resources are like fossil fuels and differ markedly from intermittent renewable energy sources, such as solar, wind and hydropower, with their nightly, seasonal or sporadic supply shutdowns.

c) Convertible into convenient forms

Biomass can be provided in all the major energy carriers: electricity, gases and liquid fuels for transportation and space heating. Biomass can, therefore, be used to substitute fossil fuels or other energy supplies needed to underpin poverty reduction, development and growth strategies for the 2 billion people who currently lack access to modern forms of energy, and thereby help reduce forest depletion rates and deforestation.

d) Potential to contribute to greenhouse gas reductions and other environmental objectives

The use of waste resources as an energy source is climate-friendly. In sharp contrast to fossil fuels, their production and use emit little or no carbon dioxide. Instead, the carbon dioxide released, when biomass resources are burned, will be re-absorbed from the atmosphere during biomass regrowth. Modern bioenergy technologies can serve similar ends by replacing traditional cooking fuels with clean, smokeless, efficient and easily controlled liquid and gas alternatives based on renewable biomass.

e) Source of rural livelihoods

Much of the value added and income generation offered by bioenergy systems are retained locally and can help to reduce rural poverty " in sharp contrast to fossil fuel or central electricity production and distribution systems. Indeed, modern bioenergy is widely thought to be a key means of promoting rural development. When biomass is produced in a sustainable manner, it is considered as a renewable energy source that can generate power and heat by combustion or anaerobic digestion. All things considered, the economics of bio-gas digesters suggest that it is a perfect micro-level solution to macro-level issues of climate change, social empowerment and agricultural productivity...

References

1. Aitken, Donald W. (2010). *Transitioning to a Renewable Energy Future*, International Solar Energy Society, January, 54 pages.
2. Nicola Armaroli, Vincenzo Balzani: *Energy for a Sustainable World – From the Oil Age to a Sun-Powered Future*, Wiley-VCH 2011, ISBN 978-3-527-32540-5.
3. Armstrong, Robert C., Catherine Wolfram, Robert Gross, Nathan S. Lewis, and M.V. Ramana et al. The Frontiers of Energy, *Nature Energy*, Vol 1, 11 January 2016.
4. ESMAP (2016). Assessing and Mapping Renewable Energy Resources, The World Bank: Washington, DC.
5. HM Treasury (2006). *Stern Review on the Economics of Climate Change*, 575 pages.
6. International Council for Science (c2006). *Discussion Paper by the Scientific and Technological Community for the 14th session of the United Nations Commission on Sustainable Development*, 17 pages.
7. International Energy Agency (2006). *World Energy Outlook 2006: Summary and Conclusions*, OECD, 11 pages.
8. International Energy Agency (2007). *Renewables in global energy supply: An IEA facts sheet*, OECD, 34 pages.
9. International Energy Agency (2008). *Deploying Renewables: Principles for Effective Policies*, OECD, 8 pages.
10. International Energy Agency (2011). *Deploying Renewables 2011: Best and Future Policy Practice*, OECD.

11. International Energy Agency (2011). *Solar Energy Perspectives*, OECD.

12. Martin Kaltschmitt, Wolfgang Streicher, Andreas Wiese (ed): Renewable energy. Technology, economics and environment, Springer, Berlin/Heidelberg 2007, ISBN 978-3-540-70947-3.

13. Lovins, Amory (2011). *Reinventing Fire: Bold Business Solutions for the New Energy Era*, Chelsea Green Publishing, 334 pages.

14. Makower, Joel, and Ron Pernick and Clint Wilder (2009). *Clean Energy Trends 2009*, Clean Edge.

15. National Renewable Energy Laboratory (2006). *Non-technical Barriers to Solar Energy Use: Review of Recent Literature*, Technical Report, NREL/TP-520-40116, September, 30 pages.

16. Volker Quaschning: *Understanding Renewable Energy Systems*. Earthscan, London, 2nd edition 2016, ISBN 978-113878-196-2.

17. REN21 (2008). *Renewables 2007 Global Status Report*, Paris: REN21 Secretariat, 51 pages.

18. REN21 (2009). *Renewables Global Status Report: 2009 Update*, Paris: REN21 Secretariat.

19. REN21 (2010). *Renewables 2010 Global Status Report*, Paris: REN21 Secretariat, 78 pages.

20. REN21 (2011). *Renewables 2011: Global Status Report*, Paris: REN21 Secretariat.

21. REN21 (2012). *Renewables 2012: Global Status Report*, Paris: REN21 Secretariat.

22. Renewable Power Generation Costs in 2014 (February 2015), *International Renewable Energy Agency*. Executive summary (8 pages). More concise summary (3 pages).

23. REN21 (2016). Renewables 2016 Global Status Report: key findings, Renewable Energy Policy Network for the 21st century.

24. Renewable energy, Wikipedia, the free encyclopedia.

25. Anonymous sources.

Chapter 19

Sustainable Economic Model of Poultry Farming

Amitav Bhattacharya and Pankaj Kumar Shukla
Department of Poultry Science, College of Veterinary Science and Animal Husbandry, Uttar Pradesh Pandit Deen Dayal Upadhyaya Pashu Chikitsa Vigyan Vishwavidhyalaya Evam Go Anusandhan Sansthan, Mathura

The term 'Poultry' refers to all those species of birds which are reared for economic benefit and they should be able to reproduce freely under captivity. Poultry indicates chickens, turkeys, ducks, quails, pheasants, pea-fowls, etc. whether they are alive or dressed. The study of principles and practices involving production, processing and marketing of poultry and its products is called 'Poultry Science'. The study of other species of birds not classified as poultry is called 'Ornithology.' However, in colloquial terms one refers poultry as chicken. Chicken are reared for meat and egg production. Broilers are reared for 4-5 weeks for meat production and layers are reared for 72 weeks for egg production.

The following points need consideration in site selection for construction of a poultry farm:

1. Access to road service
2. Future expansion needs
3. Drainage
4. Exposure of the farm
5. Wind direction
6. Distance between the different sheds/ houses in farm

It is always advisable for a person with no experience in poultry farm to start a broiler farm and rear broilers in cycles with small flock size. Though broiler rearing involves receiving quick output, it is more prone to risks due to high market fluctuations, inclement weather and disease outbreak. On the other hand, a layer farm involves higher investment, slow and gradual returns, high flock size and comparatively lower risk due to lesser market fluctuations, more stable performance at slight changes in environment at temperature and less prone to infections.

Layer rearing

Layers can be reared both in deep litter and cage system. However, cage system is preferable for layers. Broilers are preferably reared in deep litter system in northern India. However, in recent years, the use of Environmentally Controlled (EC) Houses has considerably increased.

Advantages of cage system over deep litter system

1. Increases stocking density
2. Less problem due to cannibalism
3. Easy egg collection
4. Eggs are cleaner
5. Elimination of broodiness
6. Slightly heavier egg weight
7. Slightly lower mortality
8. Slightly increased feed efficiency

Disadvantages of cage system

1. Increased incidence of cracked eggs
2. Difficulty in manure disposal
3. Cage layer fatigue may be a severe problem
4. Protection from excessive heat is a problem, especially in severe summers.

Floor space in deep litter system

Age in weeks	Floor
0-4weeks	0.5 sq. ft.
5-8 weeks	1.0 sq. ft
9-12 weeks	1.5 sq. ft.
above 12 week	2 sq. ft.
Above 18 weeks	2.5 sq. ft

Cage system

A floor space of 24 sq.inches/ bird is adequate upto 6 weeks of age for white leghorn pullet chicks. Thereafter, 36, 45 and 60 sq.inches/ bird are recommended for 14, 18 and 22 weeks of age respectively. A floor space of 60 sq. inches/ bird is recommended for layers.

Feeding

Three types of rations are recommended for layers. During the first 8 weeks, chick starter ration is provided to the chicks. Thereafter, grower ration is provided till 17-18 weeks of age. Then layer ration is provided till 72 weeks of age. It is always advisable to follow the specifications of Bureau of Indian Standards pertaining to the quality of feed.

Techno economic feasibility of rearing 5000 layers under deep litter system

In the beginning, for unit of 5000 birds, 500 additional birds were purchased assuming the mortality rate around 10% (5% during brooding phase & 5% during maintenance phase). The average space requirement for a layer bird is 0.75 sq ft per bird during 0-8 weeks and 2 sq ft per bird from 8 week onwards.

Particular	Amount (Rs.)
Variable Cost for stock maintenance:	
Cost of 5,500 DOFM chicks @ Rs. 40/sexed chick	2,20,000
Cost of feed for 5500 chicks @ Rs. 20/- per kg (5500X8 kg X Rs.20) till laying	880,000
Cost of water, electricity, medicines, etc. till laying (Rs.4/- X 5500)	22,000

Labour (1 labour for 1000 birds) (5 X Rs.3000/- X 5)	75, 000
Total cost	11, 97,000
Non-recurring cost	
Buildings	
One layer shed/poultry house (deep litter system) covering plinth 2 sq. feet each @ Rs. 100/sq. feet (2 X 5000 X 100)	10, 00,000
Cost of brooder house (0.75X5000X100)	3,75,000
Cost of feed store (20′x10′ = 200 sq. feet @ Rs. 100/sq. feet)	20,000
Cost of equipment @ Rs. 12/bird	60,000
Total cost	14, 55,000
Capital required (Variable cost + Non recurring cost)	26, 52,000

Variable cost for stock maintenance is Rs.11,97,000/-.Expenditure on the labour is about Rs.75000/-.

Cost and returns from a unit of 5,000 birds.

Particulars	**Amount (Rs.)**
Recurring cost	
Variable cost	11, 97,000
Cost of feeding 5000 birds (5000 X Rs.24 X 38 kg)	45, 60,000
Cost of water, electricity, medicines (4 X 5000)	20,000
Cost of labour (12 X 5X 3000)	1, 80,000
Total cost	59, 57,000
Income	
Sale of eggs produced by 5,000 layers (300 X 5000 X 4.00)	60,00,000
Sale of 5,000 spent hens @ Rs. 50/bird	2, 50,000
Sale of manure (300 ton X Rs.600)	1, 80,000
Sale of gunny bags (3300 X Rs.15)	49,500
Total income	64, 79,500
Gross income (Total income-Recurring cost)	5, 22,500
Fixed cost	
Depreciation on building @ 5%	69,750
Depreciation on equipment @ 10% per annum	6,000

Maintenance cost of buildings @ 5%	69,750
Maintenance cost of equipment @ 5%	3,000
Interest on fixed capital @ 12% per annum	3, 18,240
Insurance Rs.1.50/- per bird	7,500
Total fixed cost	4, 74,240
Net income (Gross income- Fixed Cost)	48,260

The gross income/returns on the unit from the sale of eggs, culled birds, manure and the gunny bags were Rs. 5, 22,500/- for the cycle period. The net income for the cycle period was Rs. 48,260/-.

Broiler rearing

Deep Litter system

A floor space of 0.8 to 1 sq. ft per broiler is recommended.

EC House

Most of the poultry houses, in India, are conventional or open-sided which means the poultry producers rely on the free flow of air through the house for ventilation. The width of the open-sided poultry house is about 30ft and no more than 40 ft wide. Houses that are wider will not provide ample ventilation during hot weather.

A controlled environment house is one in which inside conditions are maintained as near as possible to the birds optimum requirements. It is a completely enclosed insulted house with no windows. Air is removed from the house by exhausted fans and fresh air is brought in through intake opening, since, air is mechanically exhausted from the environmentally controlled house, rather than removed by natural air movement as in the open-sided house, the width of the enclosed house may be greater than 30 ft. These houses are often 40 to 50ft (12.2 to 16.5m) wide.

Feeding

Three types of rations are recommended for broilers. During the first 7 days, pre-starter ration is provided to the chicks. Thereafter, starter ration is provided till 21 days of age. Then finisher ration is provided till they are sold. It is always advisable to follow the specifications of Bureau of Indian Standards pertaining to the quality of feed.

Techno economic feasibility of rearing 5000 broilers under deep litter system

Keeping in view the 6 weeks cycle, the total production of broilers will be 260000 broilers in a year.

Capital investment for poultry farm (broilers) of 5,000 chicks

Particulars	Amount (Rs.)
Recurring cost	
Cost of day old chicks @ Rs. 17/ chick (52 X 5000 X 17)	20,000
Cost of feed @ Rs. 27/- per kg (5000X52 X 2.7 XRs.27)	1, 89, 54,000
Cost of water, electricity, medicines (Rs.4/- X5000 X 52)	10, 40,000
Labour (1 labourer for 2000 birds) (15 X Rs.3000/- X 12)	5, 40,000
Total cost	2, 49, 54, 000
Non recurring cost	
Buildings Pens (7 X 5000 X 1 X 100)	35, 00,000
Cost of feed store (20'x10' = 200 sq. feet @ Rs. 100/sq. feet)	20,000
Cost of equipment @ Rs. 10/bird (10 X 7 X 5000)	3, 50,000
Total cost	38, 70,000
Capital required	
Building & Equipments	38, 70,000
Cost of 30000 day old broiler chicks	5, 10,000
Feed for 30000 broilers (30000 X 2.7 X 27)	21, 87,000
Cost of electricity, water, medicines. etc. (30000 X 4)	1, 20,000
Labour cost (15 X 1.5 X 3000)	67,500
Total	67, 54,500

Income generated from the broiler farm

Particulars	Amount (Rs.)
Sale of 260000 birds of 1.5 kg @ Rs. 70/bird	2, 73, 00,000
Sale of 1275 ton manure @ Rs.600/-	7, 65,000
Sale of 11375 gunny bags @Rs.15/-	1, 70,625
Total	2, 78, 35,625
Gross income (Total income- Recurring cost)	28, 81,625
Other expenses	
Depreciation on building @ 5 % pa	1, 76,000
Depreciation on equipment @ 10% pa	35,000

Maintenance cost on buildings @ 5%	1, 76,000
Maintenance cost on equipments @ 5%	17,500
Interest on fixed capital @ 12%	7, 38,900
Insurance @ 0.50 paisa	1, 30,000
Total	73,400
Net income (Gross income- Other expenses)	16, 08,225
Net income / bird	6.19

□□□

Chapter 20

Sustainable Economic Model for Backyard Poultry Farming

Amitav Bhattacharya and Pankaj Kumar Shukla
Department of Poultry Science, College of Veterinary Science and Animal Husbandry, Uttar Pradesh Pandit Deen Dayal Upadhyaya Pashu Chikitsa Vigyan Vishwavidhyalaya Evam Go Anusandhan Sansthan, Mathura

The total poultry population of India is 729.2 million numbers (Livestock Census, 2012). About 95% of the poultry of India comprises of chicken followed by 3% ducks and 2% other species. Out of the total poultry population of India, the backyard poultry population in rural and urban areas is 67.89 million and 4.3 million respectively. Rural backyard poultry, though still contributing nearly 30% to the national egg production, is the most neglected one. This is in spite of the fact that their poultry eggs and meat fetch a much higher price than that of commercial poultry.

Commercial chicken production is capital intensive and is generally concentrated in and around urban areas. There is a wide disparity in consumption of the poultry products between urban and rural population. Around 75% of country's population living in the rural areas has limited access to the protein rich poultry products. Protein deficiency is quite common in the diets of rural people. Adoption of rural poultry farming may ameliorate the high incidence of protein hunger in growing children and pregnant women. For the poorest of the poor and the landless, the major issues are food security and risk spreading through subsidiary income, which is not addressed by the commercial sector. Backyard poultry, needs hardly any infrastructure for rearing small size flock. Besides income generation, rural backyard poultry provides nutrition supplementation in the form of valuable animal protein and empowers rural youth and women socially and economically. It has also been noticed that the demand for rural backyard poultry is quite high in tribal areas.

It has been seen that the commercial birds have poor immunity against common poultry diseases. As production is inversely proportional to the viability traits, the nutrients absorbed are mostly diverted for growth in commercial chicken. On the other hand, indigenous birds reared in rural areas are resistant to many diseases and pests. Unlike the local breeds maintained in villages, the commercial breeds require high level of input pertaining to feed and healthcare to maintain production and check mortality.

One of the major inputs required for commercial poultry is feed. Over the years, procuring quality fed at an optimum price has been a major hurdle in profitable commercial poultry farming. On the other hand, the birds reared under backyard system requiring low input technology can easily sustain on kitchen wastes, insects, worms, leaves, etc. Further, commercial poultry production under intensive system of production causes environmental pollution and large scale intensification of poultry rearing is often debatable from the environment point of view. Thus, the concept of 'Backyard poultry farming or Family Poultry Farming' is gaining momentum in African, Asian and Latin American countries. Around 80% of the poultry production in Africa is based on low input scavenging or backyard system. In developed countries, extensive rearing of poultry is gaining momentum, as it is more close to organic poultry and acceptable in terms of poultry welfare.

Several Government institutes *viz.*, CARI, Izzatnagar, DPR, Hyderabad, CPDO, SAUs in many states have been propagating improved varieties resulting from various types of cross-breeding of native chicken with exotic breeds and distributing them to the farmers for backyard rearing over the last two decades. Chabro is one of them. This has been developed by Central Poultry Development Organization (CPDO). These birds have better productivity levels as compared to indigenous birds in terms of egg and meat production and can be reared easily with low input in the challenging rural conditions of India. However, the private firms *viz.* Kurolier produced by Keggfarms, Delhi, Indbro brown layer and Rainboo rooster from Indbro Research and Breeding farm Hyderabad, Satpuda Desi from Yeswant Agrotech Pvt Ltd, Jalgaon District of Maharashtra are also interested to commercialize the native germplasm because of the premium price fetched by the native chicken in the market and 10 % market share that exists for native chicken in Poultry meat industry. Over the last few years, DUVASU, Mathura has been supplying day old chabro (multicoloured) chicks to cater to the needs of farmers, rearing poultry for meat production under rural production system.

Newly developed low input technology birds by government institutes

Low input strains	Source	Utility
Giriraja	Veterinary College, Hebbal, Banglore	Egg and meat
Swarndhara	Veterinary College, Hebbal, Banglore	Egg
Vanaraja	Directorate on Poultry Research, Rajendranagar, Hyderabad	Egg and meat
Grampriya	Directorate on Poultry Research, Rajendranagar, Hyderabad	Egg
Gram laxmi	Veterinary College, KAU Mannuthy, Kerala	Egg
Krishna – J	Veterinary College, Jabalpur, M.P	Egg
Gramalakshimi	Veterinary College, Mannuthy, Kerala	Egg
Kalinga Brown	CPDO, Bhubaneswar, Odisha	Egg
Hitcari	Central Avian Research Institute, Izzatnagar	Egg and Meat
Cari shyama	Central Avian Research Institute, Izzatnagar	Egg

As mentioned, birds reared under backyard system requiring low input technology can easily sustain on kitchen wastes, insects, worms, leaves, etc. The quantity of scavenger feed base of village varies according to seasonal rainfall, changes in the environment, agricultural practices, socio-economic status, ethnic groups, etc. If the feed base is lesser than the flock biomass, there may be large scale mortality. On the other hand, the survivability of the birds will be better, if the feed base is more than the flock biomass. Further, some birds may travel longer distance to scavenge while others may not. Certain birds have better scavenging ability than others. Hence, it is important, the scavenger feed base is monitored from time to time thereby assessing the gap between the availability and requirement. During the lean period, the birds may be supplemented with different nutrients. Many a times, the house hold wastes are imbalanced. It is quite natural that the quality of scavenger feed base of a village will vary round the year. During lean period, the birds can develop various mineral and vitamin deficiencies. Hence, the birds may be fed on supplemental feed during this period. The requirement of supplemental feed may vary between 20-60 g/bird/day. During the laying period, the birds may be provided with marble chips or stone grit @ 5-7g/bird/day for better egg shell quality. In addition, the quality of scavenger feed base may be improved by including different unconventional feed ingredients *viz.* maggots, termites, worms, etc.

Three types of rearing units are used for raising poultry under low input technology. The type of unit depends upon the availability of capital and space.

Free range or extensive system: A huge space is allocated for the birds and the birds feed on seeds, insects, herbs, etc. provided the birds are protected from natural enemies and parasitic infection. Space provided is generally 1 acre for 100 birds. A flock of 10-20 birds may be left scavenging around the house during day time. They may be given kitchen wastes, sorghum, maize bran etc as supplementary feed. Many a times, the birds may have to move long distances for feed and water. The birds are kept in small houses or shelters at night to protect them from predators.

Semi-intensive system: It is generally adopted, where the availability of space is limited apart from outside run. This system was once popular for laying and breeding flocks on the assumption that it imparts physical stamina to the birds. Space provided upto 6 weeks of age is 0.09 m^2 per bird. In this system the birds are generally provided with 20-30 square yards/ bird of outside run. Sometimes, the run may be divided to provide 10-15 square yards per bird of outside run on either side of the house. This may help the birds to avail fresh grounds. Further, the size of semi-intensive unit depends upon the number of birds, availability of space and capital. However, in all cases the maximum density is 500-750 birds/ha of land.

Folding unit system: The birds are confined to a small run and the position is changed every day. This enables the birds to avail fresh grounds. One of the major disadvantages of this system is water and supplementary feed has to be brought by the labourer to the fresh grounds. Generally, a unit for 25 hens is most commonly used. Around 1 square foot/ bird of floor space and a run of 3 square feet/ bird of run are allowed. So, a unit of 5′X20′ is sufficient for 25 birds. The bird house will be 5′X5′ and the rest is run.

Over the years, it has been observed that one of the major reasons for failure of different backyard programs is early chick mortality. In the rural areas, lack of technical knowledge in poultry management develops conditions for loss in backyard poultry farming. Vaccination for New Castle disease may curtail the loss caused due to early chick mortality in backyard poultry. Further, as already mentioned, monitoring the scavenger feed base throughout the year will effectively optimize the egg and meat production.

Economics of production of indigenous chicken under extensive system

	Cost (Rs./bird)
Non-recurring expenditure	
Construction of poultry sheds	50
Equipment	5
Total non-recurring expenditure	55
Recurring expenditure	
8-week old birds	50
Feed	
Medicines and vaccines	10
Labour, electricity, etc.	3
Miscellaneous	5
Total recurring expenditure	68
Income	
Eggs, Rs. 2/egg	84
Live birds, Rs. 110/ kg	138.23
Litter, Rs. 20/ quintal	5
Gunny bags, Rs. 5/ bag	
Total income	227.23
Gross profit Rs. 227.23-68	159.23

Net profit may be calculated by deducting the depreciation values of the non-recurring expenditure and any interest for loan taken from the bank.

Economics of Rural Poultry Unit- for meat (20 chabro birds under backyard system)

Fixed cost will depend on the type of night shelter provided to the birds

Recurring cost	
Cost of 4 week old birds 20 nos. Rs. 80/ bird	1600
Cost of feed -3 kg / bird upto 60 days Rs. 20/ kg for 20 birds	1200
Sub total	2800
Income	
Sale of birds 20 birds @ Rs. 150/ bird	3000
Gross profit	200

❑❑❑

Chapter 21

Sustainable Economic Model for Quail Farming

Amitav Bhattacharya and Pankaj Kumar Shukla

Department of Poultry Science, College of Veterinary Science and Animal Husbandry, Uttar Pradesh Pandit Deen Dayal Upadhyaya Pashu Chikitsa Vigyan Vishwavidhyalaya Evam Go Anusandhan Sansthan, Mathura

Coturnix quails, popularly known as bater in Hindi, belong to the Class Aves, Family- *Phasianidae* and genus *Coturnix*. They were introduced in Unites States by bird fanciers around 1870. They are also known as Pharaoh's quail, Eastern Quail, Asiatic quail, Japanese Grey Quail, Common quail, Stubble quail, King quail, Japanese King Quail, Red-throat quail, Japanese migratory quail, etc. They are hardy and easy to handle and within reasonable limits can adapt to varied environments. Its ability to produce 3-4 generations per year makes it an interesting laboratory animal. Because of low volume, low weight, short generation interval and high acceptability as a source of egg and meat, the commercial quail farming has occupied a very significant position in poultry production activities in several thickly populated countries, like Japan, Hongkong, Singapore and France. Japanese quail were introduced to Indian farmers during early 80's and its small size and different taste made it a delicacy. The weight of the eggs is approximately 10 g (6.7 -13.7g), which is about 7% of the hen's body weight. At hatch, quail chicks weigh 7-8 g and by 5 weeks, the females weigh 150-180 g and males weigh 120-150 g. The female is characterized by long and pointed feathers with black speckles on the throat and upper breast. The males have rusty brown throat and breast feathers. Sexually active males have a cloacal gland, a bulbous structure located at the upper edge of the vent, which discharges a white foamy material.

The initial production potential of Japanese quail was 130 g body weight at 6 weeks of age with a feed conversion ratio of 3.6-3.8.

Presently, strains weighing 180- 200 g at market age at 4 weeks of age with a FCR of 2.4-2.6 and livability of 88-92 per cent are available. For breeding, a sex ratio of 1M: 3F is adopted widely and the total hatchability varies from 63-72 percent. Floor space allowance given is 45cm^2 per chick at day old which is gradually increased to 180 cm^2 at four weeks. Breeder and layer quails are provided with a floor space of 225-250cm^2 depending on body size on deep litter. Commercial meat type Japanese quail are mostly reared under deep litter system only and both deep litter and cage rearing systems are in practice for rearing layer/ breeder quail.

Japanese quails lay smaller eggs than chicken but are prolific layers. Some females lay as early as 5 weeks of age depending upon the day length. The average age at first egg is about 50 days and they are in full production by about 60 days of age. Under favourable environment, they produce for long periods averaging 250 or more eggs per year. *Coturnix* is similar in sexual development and egg production to high producing strains of chicken. Approximately 65% of all chicken eggs are laid in the morning, whereas 75% of quail eggs are laid between 3 PM and 5 PM and 20% of the eggs in darkness. *Coturnix* eggs are multicoloured ranging from dark brown, blue and white to buff, each heavily mottled with black, brown and blue. Individual hens lay eggs of a characteristic shape, size and colour pattern. The first egg of a sequence is smaller than succeeding eggs in contrast to that in chicken.

Domestic quails reproduce throughout the year. Special care should be taken during collection and handling of hatching eggs, as they are thin shelled and breaks easily. For optimum fertility, the parents should be 10-24 weeks of age. Hatchability is maximum in eggs of 8-24 weeks age. One male should mate to 1-3 females and eggs should be collected for hatching 4 days after the introduction of males to females. Fertility in mass mated females although continues for approximately 10-12 days after males are removed, it decreases sharply after 3 days. Fertility reduces, when they are more than 6 months old. Hatchability of fertile eggs reduces with age in old females. Ageing has no effect on fertility of males. It takes about 17 days for quail eggs to hatch. Hatchability of quail eggs decreases at a fairly constant rate about 3% per day during storage. Age of parent stock has a pronounced effect on hatchability.

Eggs are transferred to hatcher on 14th day or earlier. Chicks are removed on the 18th day of incubation. Both battery and floor system of brooding and rearing may be employed. Battery brooding is done upto 3 weeks of age. Battery broading appears to be better than floor brooding due to small size of the chick. The starting temperature should be 37^{0}C and gradually reduced (at the rate of 3^{0}C in every 4 days) to 22^{0}C by the end of the third week. For each chick, 75cm^2 of hover and 75 cm^2 of run space is allowed in battery brooder for better performance. The feeder and water space requirement during this period are 2-3 cm and 1-1.5 cm respectively. Males and females should be separated as soon as possible and grown separately. Females are housed in laying quarters around 6 weeks. Continuous light should be provided for the first 48 hours. If the birds are desired to mature earlier, this can be continued. Otherwise 12 hours of light and 12 hours of darkness may be followed during the growing period. Quail broilers are marketed around 5 weeks of age. Eight hours of light and 16 hours of darkness at least 7-10 days before marketing help to improve the condition of quail broilers.

Feeding

For feeding quails efficiently and economically, they can be classified as starter (0-3 weeks), grower (4-5 weeks) and layer or breeder (6 weeks onward) depending upon their growth rate, efficiency of feed utilization, production and reproduction performance.

	Commercial Meat Type			Layer/ Breeder		
	Single Phase	Two Phase		Brooder	Grower	Layer
	(0-5) weeks	Starter (0-2) weeks	Finisher (3-4 weeks)	(0-3 weeks)	(4-6 weeks)	(>6 weeks)
Metabolizable energy (Kcal/kg)	2750	2750	2850	2700	2600	2650
Protein (%)	24	25.5	23.0	22	18	20

The quails are very sensitive to abrupt environmental changes particularly during the first 2 weeks of their life. They need better care during the brooding age. Quails are refractory to Ranikhet disease virus and *Ascardia galli* infection. They are also resistant to 8 strains of Eimeria pathogenic to chicken. *Aspergillus fumigatus* causes brooder pneumonia in quails. This can be checked by adding calcium propionate @ 2 kg/ tone of feed. *Clostidium colinum* causes ulcerative enteritis. It usually follows the outbreak of coccidiosis, aplastic anaemia and infectious bursal disease. Mostly growers are affected at 4-10 weeks of age with 5-10% mortality. Streptomycin, bacitracin and neomycin @ 50-100 kg/tone of feed effectively control ulcerative enteritis. Colibacillosis, mycoplasmosis, coryza, brooder pneumonia and clostridial infections are few diseases noticed in commercials, while fowl cholera, egg bound and fatty liver syndrome have been noticed in breeders.

Economics of rearing Japanese quails for meat

(500 birds every 6 weeks)	
Non-recurring expenditure,	Rs.
Building , 250 sq.cm/ bird, 12.5 sq. m, Rs. 2000 /sq. m	25,000
Equipment, feeders and drinkers	2,500
Miscellaneous	7,500
Total	35,000
Recurring expenditure, per batch, Rs.	
Chicks, Rs. 7/ chick	3,500
Feed, 0.50 kg/ bird, Rs. 30 per kg	7,500
Miscellaneous	2,000
Total	13,000
Cost/ bird assuming 10% mortality, Rs.13,000/450	29
Selling price Rs. 40/ bird, Gross income, Rs.40X450	18,000
Gross profit per batch	5,000
Total Gross profit Rs. 5,000 X 8 =	40,000

The net profit may be calculated by deducting the depreciation on building and equipments from the gross profit.

❑❑❑

Chapter 22

Biochemical Markers for Prediction of Livestock Production Diseases

Shanker Kumar Singh

Department of Veterinary Medicine, College of Veterinary Science and Animal Husbandry, Uttar Pradesh Pandit Deen Dayal Upadhyaya Pashu Chikitsa Vigyan Vishwavidhyalaya Evam Go Anusandhan Sansthan, Mathura

The production diseases of the dairy animals are the manifestation of the animal's inability to cope with the metabolic demands of high production. Over the past several decades dairy cows have undergone intensive genetic selection, which has increased milk yield to a level where the demand for nutrients from the diet and body tissue reserves often results in ill-health and infertility. Production diseases may be considered 'as a man-made problem' resulting in 'a breakdown of various metabolic systems due to high production and modern intensive husbandry practices. More recent definitions of production disease have been informed by the influence of high production and management on 'factors, such as animal behaviour, immunity and gene expression', thus, the definition has been expanded to include not only 'metabolic and nutritional diseases' but diseases of 'infectious and genetic nature'. It is important to state that both, production and environmental factors are equally implicit in the onset of production diseases, as it has been stated that 'triggers for production disease likely lie at the interface between environmental stressors and productivity'.

A pivotal time in the life of a dairy cattle occurs during a period 3 weeks prior to through 3 weeks after calving, called transition period, is a very crucial period for occurrence and / or induction of production diseases in dairy cattle. In late gestation, the demands of the pregnant uterus are high, but the demands associated with early lactation are much greater. The change from a gestational non-lactating to a non-gestational lactating state adversely affects the both, metabolic and immune status dairy animals. During this period, dairy animals undergo physiological stress preparing for and recovering from parturition and hence, face tremendous metabolic and physiologic changes challenging the homeostatic mechanisms of the body. The dramatically altered metabolism of transition animals also associated with reduced dry matter intake (DMI), negative energy balance (NEB) and oxidative stress. In addition to the metabolic changes seen in the transition animal, both neutrophils and lymphocytes functions are also impaired. These dynamic changes seem to be central to the metabolic disturbances, which favour the establishment of infection in the postpartum cow. Diagnosis of clinical diseases and disorders with estimation of chemical changes in blood, urine, or milk of dairy cattle has existed for almost 100 yr. Evidence in the scientific literature that clinical health disorders, such as milk fever and ketosis were related to changes in blood and urine chemistry began appearing in the 1920s and 1930s. In recent past we begun to realize the value of analytes measured in these fluids for both individual cow and herd level disease detection and monitoring. At present time, various methods of predicting the occurrence of metabolic diseases in advance, so that control strategies could be considered and implemented in livestock for the augmentation of productivity are in common practice. The laboratory measurement of certain components of blood, urine, or milk can reflect the nutritional status of the animal, with or without the presence of clinical abnormalities. Therefore, by monitoring certain components of the blood, urine, or milk on a regular basis, it can be possible to predict the occurrence of production disease in a dairy herd. We would theoretically be able to detect the qualitative and quantitative adequacy of the diet of cows expected to produce a certain quantity of milk or return to estrus within a desirable length of time following parturition:

Metabolic Indicators and Energy Balance

Energy balance is one of the chief critical nutritional factors impacting on animal health, lactation and reproductive performance. Traditionally, changes in energy balance were monitored via body weight and body condition score changes over time. This method may not be a sensitive enough tool, when dealing with the transition cow. However, body condition score monitoring is still an important management tool, especially in assessing body condition changes with lactational performance.

When rapid changes in energy balance status may not be detectable from changes in body condition score, high values of non-esterified fatty acids (NEFA) indicate negative energy balance. Presently, NEFA have become the mainstay in determination of energy balance and are considered a sensitive indicator of energy status of dry cows in the last month of gestation. Serum NEFA concentration is the result of adipose tissue fat mobilization in response to negative energy balance. Circulating NEFAs are absorbed and metabolized for energy by the liver and other tissues. NEFA concentration cut-points are known to be associated with a higher risk of postpartum diseases, higher risk of poorer reproductive performance, and lower milk production. Serum NEFA concentration can be used to as predictors of displaced abomasums in dairy cows. In cows with LDA, mean NEFA concentration began to deviate from the mean in cows without LDA 14 days before calving. The data from Michigan State University Clinical Nutrition Laboratory suggest that NEFA concentrations above 0.4 (Close-up dry) and 0.6 (Fresh) mEq/L (mmol) are associated with 4 and 5-fold increase of disease risk, respectively. Albeit, the association of elevated pre-and postpartum serum NEFA concentrations with subsequent negative disease, production and reproduction effects at both the individual animal and herd levels has been reported, but so far no rapid cow-side test is available for this important energy metabolite. Thus, measurement of NEFA concentrations is still expensive on a per-sample basis, and future development of a rapid, inexpensive cow-side test for blood NEFA concentrations will allow its routine use on commercial dairies. Similar to NEFA, an increase in peripartum haptoglobin has been implicated as an indicator of early-lactation disease, such as metritis and has been associated with reduced milk yield and risk of pregnancy; however, no rapid cow-side test is currently available that limits the utility of this measurement on an individual animal-or herd-level basis.

Another parameter useful in assessing energy status is ketone body concentrations. At present measurement of â-hydroxybutyrate (BHB) concentration is most commonly used. However, BHB can come from dietary sources (poorly fermented silage) and not reflect aberrant metabolism. Serum BHB concentrations can be affected by energy and glucose balance, but it is less specific indicator of energy balance than NEFA concentrations. High values are associated with reduced milk production, increased clinical ketosis and LDA and reduced fertility. Concentrations of BHB < 26 mg/dl and > 14.5 mg/dl represent animals with subclinical ketosis. Those with concentrations e" 26 mg/dl are defined with clinical ketosis. Prior to calving, BHB concentrations generally do not exceed 6-8 mg/dl, unless the animal is in negative energy balance or consuming ketogenic silage. Following calving, BHB concentrations can become greatly elevated. Cows with BHB concentrations above 10 or 14 mg/dl are 3.2 and 4.3 times at greater risk for postpartum disease.

Plasma glucose is an insensitive measure of energy status because it is subject to tight homeostatic regulation. Blood glucose has more potential as an indicator of carbohydrate status and dietary starch content than as an indicator of energy balance. It has been demonstrated that at the same degree of negative energy balance, cows fed with a higher proportion of grain had higher blood glucose concentrations than those receiving a lower proportion of grain. A major problem with the use of blood glucose as a nutritional assessment variable is that postprandial or feeding-time effects introduce a large source of variability not associated with diet. In ruminants, in contrast to monogastric animals, blood glucose concentrations usually fall postprandially. This is because there is a volatile fatty acid-induced postprandial insulin surge in ruminants, but very little glucose is absorbed from the gut. The insulin surge tends to reduce blood glucose concentrations. An approach to removing postprandial effects on blood glucose interpretation is the measurement of serum fructosamine. Fructosamine represents the sum of glycosylated serum proteins and is an indicator of average serum glucose concentration over a period of days. It provides a long-term estimation of average blood glucose concentration. Fructosamine is a potentially more sensitive indicator of energy and carbohydrate status than blood glucose, because it removes variability associated with prandial fluctuations. Moreover, blood glucose concentrations are usually lower in early lactation and during the winter months. In early lactation, there is a heavy demand for glucose and during the winter, the energy intake is likely to be lower than necessary to meet requirements. Several factors may cause short-term changes in blood glucose. Blood glucose decreases at the time of milk secretion, which makes sampling time critical. Blood glucose may also be influenced by the chemical nature of the carbohydrate and physical form of the feed and the roughage content of the feed. In addition, elevation of blood glucose has been associated with excitement and low environmental temperature.

Metabolic Indicators of Protein Nutrition

Changes in major circulating proteins during the periparturient period are not well-characterized so far and relatively little is known about their sensitivity and specificity as potential diagnostic tools. Moreover, assessing protein status is a bit more difficult than energy balance because there is no single metabolite that can be measured to directly reflect protein status. Hence, multiple parameters are needed to assess protein status including serum urea nitrogen (SUN), creatinine, total protein, albumin and creatine kinase (Ck).

Urea nitrogen concentrations are influenced by a wide variety of inter-related parameters including: dietary protein intake and rumen degradability, dietary amino acid composition, protein intake relative to requirement, liver and kidney function, muscle tissue breakdown and dietary carbohydrate amount and rumen degradability. Milk urea nitrogen (MUN) can be used as a management aid to improve dairy herd nutrition and monitor the nutritional status of lactating dairy cows. Urinary nitrogen (UN) excretion has been shown to have a positive linear relationship with MUN. Elevated MUN indicates excess protein has been fed to the dairy cow for her given level of production. Serum urea nitrogen (SUN) is probably the blood metabolite best studied in relation to dietary protein status in ruminants. Serum urea nitrogen is influenced by protein status in all species, but in ruminants, it has a special relationship to protein digestion and metabolism by the rumen biomass. A large portion of most dietary protein is hydrolyzed and de-aminated by rumen microflora, resulting into increased levels of peptides and free ammonia in the rumen. A proportion of the free ammonia is absorbed and metabolized to urea, and the remainder is incorporated into microbial protein in the rumen. The amount of ammonia converted to urea in the body is a function of the total amount of protein degraded and the rate of ammonia incorporation into microbial protein. The incorporation of ammonia into the microbial protein is determinant of microbial growth rate. Therefore, microbial growth rate is substantially determined by the availability of energy to the rumen microbes. A high intake of degradable proteins, especially relative to rumen-available dietary energy, results in high SUN. The physiologic range of SUN is large, from less than 5 to more than 20 mg/dL, and most of this variability appears to be caused by nutrition in clinically normal animals. Increases in SUN concentration and ammonia occur primarily as a result of inefficient nitrogen utilization. An excess of rumen degradable protein results in an increase in the concentration of rumen ammonia, which is absorbed through the rumen wall and transported to the liver, where it is converted to urea. The catabolism of body protein for gluconeogenesis can also result in the production of ammonia, which is also converted to urea in the liver. Therefore, serum urea has been the most commonly used blood constituent for monitoring protein status and intake. But, nutrition has a substantial effect on SUN. Major non-nutritional variability factors affecting SUN values are postprandial and diurnal variation effects.

Urea moves passively from the blood into the milk and there is a close relationship between its concentrations in the two fluids. Hence, milk urea has been used as a non-invasive substitute for the measurement of the protein status and protein intake of ruminants. It is proposed to reduce postprandial and diurnal variation; however, some of this variation appears to exist in milk as well as in serum. To reduce the effect of non-nutritional variability on nutritional interpretation of SUN, it has been suggested that multiple samples should be taken from the same cows over a period of days, although this would not seem very practical for nutritional diagnostics in commercial herds. High milk yield in dairy cows is dependent on high intakes of dietary protein (17-19 % crude protein) and energy. Creatinine is used to assess renal function and its impact on BUN values. Creatine kinase is released from muscle, when it is catabolized or injured.

Additional blood variables related to protein status include serum and free amino acids. During protein catabolism, serum concentrations of non-essential amino acids tend to increase, whereas the concentrations of most essential amino acids diminish. This results in a reduction in the essential/nonessential amino acid ratio. This ratio has been used in humans as an indicator of protein status. Serum amino acid concentrations fluctuate broadly throughout the day, however, and are subject to prandial variation, making them relatively insensitive measures of protein status. In addition, with currently available analytic techniques, serum free amino acid concentrations are probably too expensive to determine for herd-level nutritional assessment. Serum proteins are probably better and more practical indicators of protein reserves. Serum proteins of hepatic origin are generally considered to be part of the visceral protein pool, which is a relatively labile portion of body protein. The major circulating visceral protein is albumin. Serum albumin concentration is influenced by protein status, but it is relatively insensitive because of the large pool size and long half-life of albumin (approximately 21 days in most species). In addition, fluid shifts associated with parturition and postpartum weight loss can alter the dilution of albumin in blood serum and interfere with nutritional interpretation of albumin concentration. Serum visceral proteins with short half-lives and small pool sizes, such as pre-albumin, retinol-binding protein, and transferrin, appear to be more sensitive indicators of protein status. In individual animals and humans, these proteins have been criticized as monitors of protein status because their serum concentrations can be depressed by inflammatory disease, during which the production of acute-phase reactant proteins appears to take precedence over that of visceral proteins; however, on a herd-level basis, in which only clinically normal animals are sampled, it seems unlikely that inflammatory conditions would be widespread. This would make the acute-phase versus visceral protein relationship less of an obstacle for the determination of herd-level protein status compared with protein status evaluation in individual animals.

Serum or urine concentrations of the amino acid 3-methylhistidine (3MI) have been extensively used in animal nutrition research for the estimation of protein catabolism rate. 3MI is an amino acid of skeletal muscle protein that is produced from histidine after protein synthesis is complete. As muscle proteins are catabolized, 3MI is released and cannot be re-incorporated into protein. It circulates in serum and is eventually excreted in urine. 3MI concentrations in serum or urine are a reflection of the rate of catabolism of skeletal muscle. Much of the 3MI testing that is done in experimental situations has involved quantitative urine collections. For practical application, means of interpreting concentrations in single urine samples or from blood serum would have to be developed. Other potential measures of protein status include rate of hair regrowth after clipping, milk components, lymphocyte count, and other general indicators of immune status.

Total protein and albumin reflect availability of protein and their concentration decline in the face of protein deficiency. However, this occurs over a period of time. Albumin has a relatively short half-life and can reflect protein deficiency problems over a period of a month or two. Concentrations of serum albumin are relatively stable during the periparturient period but increased slightly in the sample collected at or around the time of calving. Cows with elevated inflammatory response during the postcalving period had decreased serum albumin concentrations and changes in a variety of other serum and plasma components. Lactation stage has a substantial effect on serum albumin. Hence, animals should be grouped into: (a) dry cows (b) early lactation (1-10 weeks) and (c) later lactation. Minimal serum albumin values for dry cow are from 2.9 to 3.1 g/dl, for recently calved cows from 2.7 to 2.9 g/dl and 3.0 to 3.2 g/dl for cows in later lactation. Albumin is found to be associated with postpartum disease and can be used to predict disease risk in close-up and fresh periods. Fresh cows that could maintain serum albumin concentrations eH 3.5 g/dl were less likely to have postpartum disease. Serum albumin concentrations dH 3.25 g/dl in close-up dry cows resulted in a three-fold greater risk for postpartum disease. In spite of concerns about variables confounding albumin interpretation, it seems to be a good disease risk indicator, possibly reflecting availability of amino acids from the labile protein pool.

In most dairy herd dietary protein deficiency situations, BUN values will be low (<10 mg/dl) with normal albumin concentration (>3.5 g/dl) in the early dry cows. Close-up dry cows will have low to moderate BUN, lower albumin and elevated Ck values. Fresh cows generally have low BUN and low albumin (<3.0 g/dl). These fresh cows seemingly fail to properly respond to any disease insult. Protein deficient fresh cows may die from metritis, mastitis, foot rot, and anything else without antibiotic therapy.

Macro-minerals Estimations

Macro-minerals calcium (Ca), phosphorus (P), potassium (K), magnesium (Mg), sodium (Na), chloride (Cl) and sulphur (S) are of extreme interest because of their status relative to their role in milk fever, alert downer cows and weak cow syndrome. But, most of these minerals are tightly regulated in the body through a variety of homeostatic mechanisms. Therefore, blood concentrations of macro-minerals are not reflective of dietary status, when the homeostatic system is functioning properly. Hence, macro-mineral blood concentrations should be carefully interpreted in light of the operational homeostatic system. The concentrations of phosphorus, K, Mg and S in blood are somewhat sensitive to dietary intake. Following long-term insufficient dietary intake and cattle grazing on highly fertilized pasture, serum inorganic phosphate levels tend to fall and hypophosphatemia occurs. Serum magnesium levels are usually low during the winter months and subclinical hypo magnesaemia exists in many herds, especially in pregnant beef cattle. This can be converted into clinical hypomagnesaemia with a sudden deprivation of feed or a sudden fall in environmental temperature. Sodium and chloride concentrations are altered when renal or digestive function is compromised or in extreme dietary deficiency states.

Serum calcium levels vary only within narrow limits and are not sensitive indicators of input-output balance. However, assessment of Ca concentrations around the time of calving is a useful indicator of how well the Ca regulatory system is working and potential for clinical or subclinical hypocalcaemia problems. It is supposed that other than the 2 weeks prior to and following calving, blood Ca is not a very diagnostic value as a result of the intact regulatory system. Calcium status can be measured directly using either total Ca or ionized Ca concentrations in blood. Although ionized Ca is considered to be the more biologically active fraction, but recent research also suggests that the relationship between ionized Ca and total Ca varies in the days after calving and thus, cannot be used inter-changeably as indicators of Ca status. Most of the scientific studies used total Ca for relating Ca status with postpartum outcomes related to disease, milk production and reproduction. Whereas, ionized Ca has received limited evaluation as a predictor of these outcomes. On-farm tests for ionized Ca, although available, are expensive and have not been well validated for use with bovine blood. Due to the difficulty of handling samples to ensure accurate results and cost, ionized Ca is not commonly measured in research settings and is used even less for individual animal treatment or farm management decisions. The historical clinical impression of cold ears as an indicator of hypocalcemia has been recently evaluated using an infrared thermometer to determine ear skin temperature. Although cows with clinical hypocalcemia may have lower ear temperatures than cows with subclinical hypocalcemia, ambient temperature is a major confounder. Hence, ear temperature alone could not be recommended for accurate diagnosis of subclinical hypocalcemia.

Micro-minerals and Vitamins Assays

Assessment of trace mineral and fat-soluble vitamin status is routinely completed using direct blood concentration measurements. But there is an open question that, is there a predictive relationship between tissue and blood trace mineral or fat-soluble vitamin concentrations and presence of nutrient-specific deficiency disease? On superficial stance one would have to say yes, because we can document low nutrient concentrations in the presence of disease signs. But, how predictive mineral and vitamin concentrations are, and which ones are the best indicators is really questionable. To understand the issue here, we need to appreciate that trace minerals and fat-soluble vitamins are not confined in a single large pool in the body, but are distributed into a number of different pools, such as a storage, transport and biochemical function pools, which have different functions and availability. Therefore, due to the storage capacity for trace minerals and fat-soluble vitamins in the liver, moderate dietary deficiencies or short-term severe deficiencies can be overcome without any effect on the critical biochemical functions performed by the element in question. If the dietary insult is severe or prolonged enough to drain the storage pool, then some effects might be seen in the transport pool. Finally, when the transport pool has been compromised, the biochemical function pool will be compromised resulting in some dysfunction. It is only when the biochemical function pool reaches a critically low level that we see the overt clinical deficiency disease. Before we reach the clinical disease stage, we will see problems associated with subclinical disease including increased disease susceptibility as a result of compromised immune function. This is the prime pathway of the trace mineral and fat-soluble vitamin deficiency disease problems.

References

Baumgard, L. H., Collier, R. J., and Bauman, D. E. (2017). A 100-Year Review: Regulation of nutrient partitioning to support lactation. *J. Dairy Sci.*, 100(12): 10353–10366.

de Vries, M. A., Alipour, A., Klop, B., van de Geijn, G. J., Janssen, H. W., Njo, T. L., van der Meulen, N., Rietveld, A. P., Liem, A. H., Westerman, E. M., de Herder, W. W. and Castro, C. M. (2015). Glucose-dependent leukocyte activation in patients with type 2 diabetes mellitus, familial combined hyperlipidemia and healthy controls. *Metabolism*, 64: 213-217.

Drackley, J.K., Dann, H.M., Neil Douglas, G., Janovick Guretzky, N.A., Litherland, N.B., Underwood, J.P. and Loor, J.J. (2005).Physiological and pathological adaptations in dairy cows that may increase susceptibility to periparturient diseases and disorders. *Ital. J. Anim. Sci.*, 4(4): 323–344.

Esposito, G., Irons, P.C., Webb, E.C. and Chapwanya, A. (2014). Interactions between negative energy balance, metabolic diseases, uterine health and immune response in transition dairy cows. *Ani. Reprod. Sci.*, 144(3): 60-71.

Gelfert, C.C., Loeffler, L.M., Frömer, S., Engel, M., Männer, K. and Staufenbiel, R. (2010). Comparison of the impact of different anionic salts on the acid base status and calcium metabolism in non-lactating, non-pregnant dairy cows. *Vet. J.*, 185: 305–309.

Graugnard, D. E., Moyes, K. M., Trevisi, E., Khan, M. J., Keisler, D., Drackley, J. K., Bertoni, G. and Loor, J. J. (2013). Liver lipid content and inflammometabolic indices in peripartal dairy cows are altered in response to prepartal energy intake and postpartal intramammary inflammatory challenge. *J. Dairy Sci.*, 96: 918-935.

Grummer, R. R. (1993). Etiology of lipid related metabolic disorders in periparturient dairy cows. *J. Dairy Sci.*,76: 3882–3896.

Ingvartsen, K. L. and Moyes, K. M. (2013). Nutrition, immune function and health of dairy cattle. *Animal*, 7 (Suppl 1): 112-122.

Ingvartsen, L.K. and Moyes, K.M. (2015). Factors contributing to immunosuppression in the dairy cow during the periparturient period. *Jap. J. Vet. Res.*, 63(1): S15-S24.

LeBlanc, S. J. (2012). Interactions of metabolism, inflammation, and reproductive tract health in the postpartum period in dairy cattle. *Reprod. Domest. Anim.*, 47 Suppl 5: 18-30.

Lucy, M., Jiang, H. and Kobayashi, Y. (2001). Changes in the somatotrophic axis associated with the initiation of lactation. *J. Dairy Sci.*, 84: E113–E119.

Markusfeld, O., Galon, N., Ezra, E. (1997). Body condition score, health, yield and fertility in dairy cows. *Vet. Rec.*,141: 67–72.

Martinez, N., Sinedino, L. D., Bisinotto, R. S., Ribeiro, E. S., Gomes, G. C., Lima, F. S., Greco, L. F., Risco, C. A., Galvao, K. N., Taylor-Rodriguez, D., Driver, J. P., Thatcher, W. W. and Santos, J. E. (2014). Effect of induced subclinical hypocalcemia on physiological responses and neutrophil function in dairy cows. *J. Dairy Sci.*, 97: 874-887.

Moorby, J.M., Dewhurst, R.J., Tweed, J.K.S., Dhanoa, M.S., Bech, N.F.G. (2000). Effect of altering energy and protein supply to dairy cows during the dry period. 2. Metabolic and hormonal responses. *J. Dairy Sci.*, 83: 1795–1805.

Moyes, K. M., Graugnard, D. E., Khan, M. J., Mukesh, M. and Loor. J. J. (2014). Postpartal immunometabolic gene network expression and function in blood neutrophils are altered in response to prepartal energy intake and postpartal intramammary inflammatory challenge. *J. Dairy Sci.*, 97: 2165-2177.

Moyes, K. M., Larsen, T. and Ingvartsen. K. L. (2013). Generation of an index for physiological imbalance and its use as a predictor of disease in dairy cows during early lactation. *J. Dairy Sci.*, 96: 2161-2170.

Piccione, G., Messina, V., Marafioti, S., Casella, S.,Giannetto, C. and Fazio, F. (2012).Changes of some haematochemical parameters in dairy cows during late gestation, post partum, lactation and dry periods. *Vet Med Zoot.*, 58: 59-64.

Pithon-Curi, T. C., De Melo, M. P. and Curi, R. (2004). Glucose and glutamine utilization by rat lymphocytes, monocytes and neutrophils in culture: a comparative study. *Cell Biochem. Funct.*, 22: 321-326.

Radostits, O.M., Gay, C.C., HinchcliffK.W. and Constable, P.D. (2007). Veterinary Medicine: A Textbook of the Diseases of Cattle, Horses, Sheep, Pigs, and Goats, 10th edn, Elsevier Saunders, Edinburgh, pp. 1661–1667.

Roche, J.R., Friggens, N.C., Kay, J.K., Fisher, M.W., Stafford, K.J. and Berry, D.P. (2009). Invited review: body condition score and its association with dairy cow productivity, health, and welfare. J. Dairy Sci. 92: 5769–5801.

Seifi, H.A., Mohri, M., Farzaneh, N., Nemati, H., Nejhad, S.V. (2010). Effects of anionic salts supplementation on blood pH and mineral status, energy metabolism, reproduction and production in transition dairy cows. *Res. Vet. Sci.*, 89: 72–77.

Sordillo, L.M. and Raphael, W. (2013).Significance of metabolic stress, lipid mobilization, and inflammation on transition cow disorders. *Vet. Clin. North Am. Food Ani. Pract.*, 29(2): 267-78.

Spears, J.W. and Weiss, W.P. (2008). Role of antioxidants and trace elements in health and immunity of transition dairy cows. *Vet. J.*, 176: 70-76.

Stec, A., Kurek, L., Mochol and J., (2006). Selected elements of metabolic profile and condition state of dairy cattle on farms of different management systems and methods of fodder application. *Bull. Vet. Inst. Pulawy.*, 50: 199-203.

Tanritanir, P., Dede, S. and Ceylan, E. (2009). Changes in some macro minerals and biochemical parameters in female healthy siirthair goats before and after parturition. *J. Ani. Vet. Adv.*, 8: 530–533.

Taylor, V., Beever, D., Wathes, D., Kebreab, E. and Mills, J. (2004). Physiological adaptations to milk production that affect the fertility of high yielding dairy cows. Dairying: using science to meet consumers' needs. In: Conference Proceedings, University of Reading, UK, pp. 37–71.

Tilg, H., and Moschen, A. R. (2008). Insulin resistance, inflammation, and non-alcoholic fatty liver disease. *Trends Endocrinol. Metab.*, 19: 371-379.

Van Saun, R.J. (2016). Indicators of dairy cow transition risks: metabolic profiling revisited. *Tierarztl. Prax. Ausg. G Grosstiere. Nutztiere*. 44: 118–126.

Wathes, D.C., Cheng, Z., Chowdhury, W., Fenwick, M.A., Fitzpatrick, R., Morris, D.G., Patton, J. and Murphy, J.J. (2009). Negative energy balance alters global gene expression and immune responses in the uterus of postpartum dairy cows. *Physiol. Genomics*, 39: 1–13.

Chapter 23

Sustainable Economic model of Pig Farming

D.N. Singh, Yajuvendra Singh & Rajneesh Sirohi

Department of Livestock Production & Management, College of Veterinary Science and Animal Husbandry, Uttar Pradesh Pandit Deen Dayal Upadhyaya Pashu Chikitsa Vigyan Vishwavidhyalaya Evam Go Anusandhan Sansthan, Mathura

The term "sustainability" entered the mainstream of public discourse in 1987 with the publication of the Brundtland Commission report. That report defined sustainability as development that "meets the needs of the present without compromising the ability of future generations to meet their own needs." The use of pigs as converters, rather than scavengers, to transform farm left-over or kitchen swill to favourable animal products not only provides organic fertilizer for crops, but also beneficial for nutrient management, and undoubtedly constitutes husbandry. Pigs under such a minimum waste system of conventional agriculture are traditionally kept in small herds as a sideline source of farm revenue.

Pig rearing is one of the most important occupation of rural society, especially the tribal masses of India. Pig farming constitutes the livelihood of rural poor belonging to the lowest socio-economic strata and they have no means to undertake scientific pig farming with improved foundation stock, proper housing, feeding and other management. As per 19th Livestock census, India's pig population is 10.294 million which amounts to about 2 % of the country's entire livestock. Total population of exotic/crossbred was 2.456 million, while indigenous pigs were 7.837 million. Total population of exotic/ crossbreds in rural areas was 2.126 million, while it was 0.329 million in urban areas. In case of indigenous pigs, population in rural areas was 7.099 million, while it was 0.737 million in urban areas. Highest share of country's pig population was found in Assam (15.89%)

followed by Uttar Pradesh (12.96%), Jharkhand (9.35%), Bihar (6.31%) and West Bengal (6.30%). Pig farming have attains more popularity and acceptance in North-Eastern hilly region of India.

Pigs are potential source of animal proteins and avenues for additional income and employment that can improve the livelihood in a sustainable manner. Presently, our pig production system has many lacunae namely absence of sufficient number of breeder farmers, tendency of the pig grower to raise pig to marketable age on negligible inputs and lesser preference of the consumers for pork from the local pigs, etc. Absence of sufficient number of breeder farmers throughout the country is also a major constraint leading to lesser availability of quality pigs for fattener farmers and market. Therefore, genetic improvement of indigenous pigs must be undertaken on priority for production of superior germplasm. Selective breeding and cross-breeding has to be expanded for improving production and productivity. There is need for strengthening the pork marketing mechanisms at the local level to the marketing channels, and integrate production programme with slaughter houses to ensure better sustainability. Given its prospects, piggery has the potential to have a positive impact on the livelihood of millions of resource poor, under-privileged, landless and marginal farmers.

Salient features of Pig production system in India

- Pig farming has been adopted by small and landless farmers, and in tribal areas.
- Production is small-scale, backyard, marketed-oriented enterprise.
- Pigs are mainly dependent on locally available feed resources/ vegetations, crop residues and kitchen waste which are of low or no cost.
- It is low-external input activity relying mainly upon women's labour for rearing
- There is lack of proper housing and shelter under low-input traditional system thus exposing pigs to adverse weather conditions like high temperatures and rain.
- Most of pig sty are located in backyard of house and the unhygienic conditions of these building predispose pigs to diseases.

- Best breeding stock rarely goes to the market, resulting in the use of a foundation stock with poor breeding qualities.
- There is non-utilization of improved breeds from government farms and increased use of own stock and that of neighbors, which gives rise to inbreeding and consequently low productivity (Nath *et al.*, 2013).
- A wide gap still exists between the need/demand and availability of pork. The major reason is that the pigs reared by the farmers are of the nondescript local breed, whose growth rate is claimed to be poor, and hence, their production is hardly adequate.
- Producers have inadequate knowledge about feeding, health care and breeding management
- The commercial pig production system in India is characterized by improved crossbred/exotic breeds of pigs that are bred and reared under confinement.

Inherent merits of Pig farming

In comparison to other livestock species, pig rearing has higher potential to contribute to more economic gain for small, marginal farmers or rural poor belonging to the lowest socio-economic strata due to its following advantages:

- Better feed conversion efficiency of pigs i.e. they attain more unit weight gain per kg of feed consumed as compared to other meat producing animals except broilers.
- Higher fecundity in pigs - Sows produce 6-12 piglets in each farrowing.
- Pigs reach sexual maturity at an early age. A sow can be bred as early as 8-9 months of age and can farrow twice in a year under optimal management conditions.
- Pigs have shorter generation interval as compared to other classes of livestock offers quick returns since the market weight of 60-90 kg can be achieved in a period of 7-10 months.
- One of the few livestock animals where nearly all parts of the animal can be consumed by the farm family and/or sold
- Converts damaged feeds which are either not edible or not very palatable to human beings into valuable nutritious meat.

- Apart from providing meat, it is also a source of bristles and manure can survive and grow on wide variety of feed stuff viz. grains, vegetables, fruits, fodder, sugarcane, kitchen waste offers employment opportunities to seasonally employed rural farmers and supplement income to improve their living standards
- Require little initial investment on building and gear.
- Pigs can raise for their entire lifetime in enclosure as they do not contribute to loss of grazing lands (Mpofu and Makuza, 2003).
- Pig products range from primary commodities, such as pork, to processed food products such as sausages and smoked hams to cooked salted ears, eaten as snack foods.
- Demand for pig's fat in poultry feed, soap, paints and other chemical industries.
- The small scale pig sector has seemingly greater potential to reduce poverty (Lanada *et al.*, 2005).

To make the pig farming for sustainable livelihood we should adopt different technologies for attaining more income for the farming community:

1. Genetic improvement of Indigenous pig

Different pig breeds have been adapted to the most diverse climatic conditions in our country, however, they are low producers. The indigenous pig breed Ghungharoo, Ankamali, Ghori, Niang megha has been used for pig production for a long period of time. The major reason is that the pigs reared by the farmers are of the non-descript local breed, whose growth rate is claimed to be poor, and hence, their production is hardly adequate for the fast-growing population (Nath *et al.*, 2013). Exotic breeds are now being utilized for crossbreeding to augment genetic base for pig production in the rural areas. Several exotic pig breeds are available in India are as follows:

i) **Large white Yorkshire :** It is most extensively used exotic breed in India. White coat colour with occasional black pigmented spots, erect ears, snout of medium length and dished face are typical characteristics of this breed. Mature body weight ranges from 300 to 500 kg.

ii) **Middle White Yorkshire :** Typical characteristics of this breed include white coat colour, long muscular neck and long back with a mature body ranging from 270 to 360 kg.

iii) **Landrace :** Pigs of this breed are typically white coloured with black skin spots. They have a long body, large drooping ears and long snout. Mature body weight ranges from 250-350 kg.

iv) **Berkshire :** Black coloured animals with white patches on feet, snout and tail. Small head, face depressed in middle and saucer shaped body with flexible ribs are typical characteristics of this breed. Mature body weight ranges from 280-350 kg.

v) **Hampshire :** Animals are black with white strip across forelegs to shoulder. Typical characteristics include small and erect ears, small and compact body. Sows have good mothering ability.

Crossbreds

Under All India Co-ordinated Research Programme (AICRP) on Pigs, breeding programmes were developed to generate the following genotypes/genetic groups:

- Improved indigenous pigs
- Crossbreds having 50:50 inheritance from Landrace and indigenous pigs
- Large White Yorkshire crossbreds having 50% indigenous inheritance
- Crossbreds having 75% Large White and 25% indigenous inheritance
- Landrace crossbreds having 25% indigenous inheritance
- Hampshire crossbreds carrying 25% and 50% indigenous inheritance
- Landrace X indigenous half-breds from reciprocal crosses

Breeding Strategies

Farmers should always taken in consideration about the breeding strategies of their breedable animals to gain more profit in least duration. Farmers must be consider for selection of breeding stock on the basis of breed characters, type & appearance, health, transmitting ability, performance, litter size, strength & vigour of litters, milking ability, temperament, body weight gain & feed conversion efficiency, fertility & prolificacy basis.

Provision of more emphasis on grading-up breeding programme for continuous improvement of non-descript indigenous pigs from the bulk of pig population in the country. It will be advantageous to grade-up of indigenous hogs by successive use of boars of Indian Large White Yorkshire or landrace breed. These two breeds were used in All India Co-ordinated Research Projects in the country:

a) **Selection criteria for Boar :** It should be true to the breed, masculine appearance, strong limbs, smooth soldier, long deep body, free from disease, no-crypt-orchid condition and sound health records.

b) **Selection criteria for Sow**

    i) Sow must be from a litter whose litter size, birth weight and weaning weight is maximum.

    ii) Sow must be have well-developed udder with 12 teats.

    iii) Minimum back fat thickness

    iv) Sow must have good mothering ability.

    v) High fertility & prolificacy.

Reducing Feed cost & Feeding Schedule

Feeding constitutes the greatest cost (about 70%) in raising pigs and affects the pig's performance and sustainability of the sector. More than 60% deficiency in concentrate feed sources is a threat to the pig industry, which compete directly with human for grains. Feed manufacturers and livestock producers are facing problems as prices of grains and oilcakes are increasing day-by-day. Therefore, researchers always search for alternate feed resources to replace the conventional ingredients used for the animal production. Alternate feed resources include various organic by product from the food processing industry, feeding of food, kitchen waste or garbage and bread waste to swine is a common practice throughout the world.

The growth and mortality of pigs largely depend on their feeding regime. Pig is the most efficient animal in converting feed to meat. Generally, farmers want to rear pigs with zero ,like kitchen waste as well as vegetable waste mixed with rice polish/ wheat bran only. However, with this feed it is not possible to get desired body weight and other production norms. It is, therefore, very much important to feed the animals with economical but balanced feed which will contain all the nutrient requirements for growth and to support the life.

Feeding Schedule for Pig

i) **Suckling pig :** Upto one week, piglets nourished on sow's milk. They should be assisting to suckle about 8-10 times a day.

ii) **Creeper Pig :** The pigs usually start nibbling at feed at 1 week of age. Pre-starter ration increases growth rate and reduces demand on sow's milk. Since milk production starts to decline after 3 weeks of lactation. It is necessary that piglets start on feeding solid food to meet nutritional requirements. Creeper ration containing 20 % crude protein is fed upto 2 months of age. The creeper ration should be fed at the rate of 250-750 g per day between 15 to 60 days of age.

iii) **Grower Pig :** The grower pig between 3- 6 months of age should be offered grower ration containing 18% of crude protein. The daily amount varies from 0.75 -1.5 kg.

iv) **Finisher Pig :** The finisher pig after 6 months of age should be offered 1.5 to 2.5 kg finisher ration containing 16% of crude protein.

Housing of Pigs

Pigs are reared under following two housing systems: 1.Outdoor System/Open air system/Extensive System 2. Indoor System/ intensive System.

Ideal Pig Housing Environment Parameters

i) Temperature : For new born pigs- 75- 85 ^{0}F

Farrowing sow- 60-70 ^{0}F

Weaners- 70-75 ^{0}F

Growing fattening pig : 62-65 ^{0}F

Finisher : 50-60 ^{0}F

ii) **Relative humidity :** Ambient relative humidity should not be more than 75%. While optimum R.H. varies between 60-70%.

iii) **Ventilation :** The level of purity of air in pig house should not be less than 96.7%. Per pig requires 28 cubic meter of fresh air/ hour. If the wind is blowing in normal speed of 5 Km/hour, then 6-15 square meter of inlet and outlet area will be sufficient for one pig. Accordingly, inlet and outlet area can be determined after considering wind speed in locality and number of pigs to be housed.

iv) **Light :** In addition to disinfection and cleanliness of houses, light also plays an important role in ovarian cyclicity. Increase in light period, improves milk production and ovulation rate in sows, whereas, darkness improves feed intake. So, breeding pigs should be exposed to more light intensity and duration. Whereas, fattener, for more feed intake and growth rate, should have less light intensity and duration.

Building for different categories of pigs A pig farm posses following types of buildings:

i) **Boar sty :** Each boar sty should not have more than 24 pens under one roof and each pen should not have more than one boar.

ii) **Dry sow and gilt sty :** Each sty should not have more than 40 pens under one roof and each pen accommodate 3-10 pigs.

iii) **Farrowing/Nursing sty :** Each sty should not have more than 40 pens and one pen may accommodate one sow with its litter.

iv) **Weaning sty :** In this case each weaning sty should not have more than 20 pens, each must not contains more than 30 pigs.

v) **Sick animal sty :** Should be constructed in 5% space required for the whole stock.

Table 1: Optimum Space Requirement for Pigs

Type of Pig	Covered area (square meter)	Open area (square meter)	Number per pen
Boar	6-7	8.8-12	1
Farrowing sow	7-9	8.8-12	1
Weaner /fattening	0.9-1.8	0.9-1.8	30
Dry sow/gilt	1.8-2.7	1.4 -1.8	3-10

Table 2: Feeding and Watering Space Requirement of Pigs

Type of animal	Space per animal (cm.)	Total manger length (cm..100 pigs)	Total watering trough length (cm.100 pigs)	Dimensions of water trough or manger (cm)		
				Width	Depth	Height
Adult Pig	60-75	60000-7500	600-750	50	20	25
Growing Pig	25-35	2500-3500	250-300	30	15	20

Adopt Scientific Managemental Techniques

Care and Management during Breeding : Gilt is the power house of all pig enterprises for sustainable optimum production. The consistent achievement of maximum output depends upon devising and following a sensible plan of action to have gilt ready for breeding at right time in right numbers in right conditions. For successful pig farming, annual replacement rate and mortality of breeding sow should not be more than 38-40 % and 5-6 %.

1. Selection of breeding stock

a) **Breeding sow :** Gilt supposed to be use as future breeding sow should be from uniform herd, largest litter, having minimum 6 pairs of functional teats, posses breed characteristics, straight back, not pot belly, deep and long body, fine and well set shoulder, well sprung ribs, no hanging jowl, good temperament and 6 monthly body weight should not be less than 30-35 Kg for indigenous, 45-50 for crossbred and 60-70 kg for exotic.

Provision of flushing have a better results for attaining maximum profit from the swine farming. Feeding of extra allowances of grains by about 0.5 to 0.70 kg before breeding season is called flushing.

Advantages of flushing

i) Improvement in physical condition of female

ii) Production of more number of viable ova

iii) Increased litter size

iv) Increased conception percentage

v) Minimize embryonic loss

b) **Breeding Boar :** As per standards of advanced countries, at 6 month of age, the body weight of breeding boar should be 90 kg and body length 100 cm. This standard can be relaxed for crossbred and indigenous boar. Although, breeding boar should be selected from largest and heaviest litter at the time of weaning. The breeding boar should be active alert and with good libido.

2. Feeding of breeding stock

In order to improve ovulation rate, breeding sow around 2 weeks before breeding should be fed a concentrate ration in such away that body weight gain should be between 450-670 g/ day but should not allow to fatten.

3. Mating

Sow is polyestrous animal, regular cycle throughout the year and duration of estrous cycle is 21 days with a normal range of 18-24 days. Duration of estrus varies 48-72 hours and normally ovulation occurs 38-40 hours after starts of estrus. Normally upto 20 ova are released at a single ovulation. Best time of mating is 30 hrs after onset of estrus or 10-12 hours before ovulation. Estrous is characterized by following gradual behavioural and physiological signs. Swelling and reddening of vulva, mounting over other females or allowing mounting by other females, standing reflex (Showing interest in boar and adoption of immobile posture, when pressure is applied on back, normally, at the starts and end, the standing reflex is shown by sow only in presence of boar, but at the height of estrus sow show standing reflex, when pressure is applied on back even in absence of boar), ear pricking, grunting, etc. Many a times lactation hinders the expression of estrus signs. Normally first three heats after puberty is missed as poor conception rate in these decreases litter size. So, in gilts first mating is allowed in at 4th estrus. Boar and gilt should be kept separately to avoid accidental mating for further ease of managemental practices. To bring the gilt in to heat leave the boars with gilts for 4-5 days until first gilt sows sign of heat. Allow boar for 15-20 minutes in the pen of sows under close supervision. To increase the litter size, sow should be served two times at an interval of 8-10 hrs.

4. Pregnancy diagnosis

Three weeks after mating sow should be checked for estrus Pregnancy diagnosis should be carried out about 3 weeks after service with the objective of separating pregnant and non-pregnant and to rebred the non-pregnant or cull them to avoid feed wastage. Pregnancy diagnosis is done by non-return in estrus, rectal palpation for enlarged uterine artery after 45 days of gestation, vaginal biopsy, blood progesterone or estrogen assay. Pregnant should be separated and fed accordingly. Increase the amount of ration in last 3 weeks.

Care and management of sow at farrowing : Since the sow is polytoccus animals (gives birth to many offspring at a time), so piglets are prone to injury during the first few days of their lives, a separate pen is needed for each sow and her litter at farrowing time and for at least 3-5 days following farrowing :

1. ***Disinfection of pregnant sow*** : Before transferring the sow in to farrowing pens, sow should be thoroughly scrubbed with soap and warm water, especially in the region of sides and undersurface of the body. This will remove ectoparasites and their eggs and other disease germs. The sow should be transferred to farrowing pen in around 3-4 days prior to farrowing date.
2. ***Disinfection of farrowing pen*** : The farrowing pen should be thoroughly cleaned disinfected to reduce possible infection. This may be done by scrubbing the walls and floors with phenyl water. As a precaution, apply a 4% standard disinfectant, using a pump spray to force it into all the cracks and crevices and angles. In case of katcha floor, 2-3 inches of the top layer should be removed and replace it with fresh earth.
3. ***Bedding of farrowing pen*** : When the pens are thoroughly dry, any soft, dry, absorbent material should be bedded on the floor of farrowing pen. Paddy or wheat straw and say dust is a suitable material.
4. ***Housing*** : Pigs are more sensitive for extreme hot and cold, particularly at the time of farrowing. The types of farrowing pen which seems best adapted to the weather and other conditions should be used. The main requirements of the satisfactory housing are that the quarters be dry, sanitary and well ventilated and that they provides good protection from heat, cold and winds. The guard rail around the farrowed pen is an effective mean of preventing sows from crushing their piglets.

5. Clean the sow with luke warm water and allow her to suckle piglets.
6. Check the udder for agalactia, mastitis and patency of teats.
7. Spray the sow udder with saturated solution of ferrous sulphate (50 g/litre of water) to prevent piglet anemia.

Care and management of Young Piglet

Mortality rate in young piglet varies from 20-25%. In first 2 months of age. Especially the high mortality 80-90% of mortality occurs in the beginning of life and most of the mortality is due to starvation, Crushing and chilling. So, following care should be taken to minimize those:

1. ***Induced Respiration :*** At farrowing time observe each and every piglet. The piglets which are encased in placenta should be removed immediately to avoid death due to suffocation. Be sure the piglets are respiring properly. Give artificial breathing, in case of any difficult breathing. This is achieved by plastic funnel by keeping its large end up over the nostrils and blowing the air from the other broader end. Vigorous Shaking of piglets by holding them by hind legs and opening mouth with thumb and fingers of other hand, messaging and rubbing of each side of rib cage. Clean the mucous membrane from mouth and nostrils with sterilized piece of cloth or cotton.
2. ***Assisted Suckling :*** Weak and small chilled piglets should be assisted to suck their share of colostrum and milk. Additional warmth should be provided to the young piglets, especially in winter by means of heater or infrared lamp. The temperature inside the creep during eight hours should be maintained between 80-85 ^{0}F .
3. ***Bedding :*** Piglet should be provided good bedding of about 2" chaffed straw of hay, etc. But saw dust should not be used as they can ingest it leading to death.
4. ***Removal of Naval cord :*** Normally the length of naval cord ifs 1' but it should be cut 4-5 cm below the belly by ligating it with silk thread. Apply weak iodine solution to avoid infection.
5. ***Cutting of needle teeth :*** At the time of birth piglets have 8 black coloured wolf teeth (4 incisors and 4 canines). They are of no use rather causes injury to sow teats at the time of suckling leading

to udder infection and injury to other piglets due to biting. Due to pain caused by teat injury and udder infection sow may not nurse piglet properly leading to starvation and death. Therefore, at the time of birth these needle teeth should be cut near to their top. Care should be taken to not to cut too close to gum because tooth may be shattered and gum infection may occur.

6. ***Cross-Fostering*** : Equalization of litter may be practised in large herd, where many sows farrow at a time. Piglets from larger litter may be transferred to small litter with small number. It should be done after 3 days so that all piglets receive colostrum from their mother. Rub the piglets with each other or strong pungent smell like garlic onion before fostering. The orphan pig, due to death of sow after farrowing, should be allow to suckle foster mother or cowmilk is used as replacer, but take care that if possible, colostrum is available from sow.

Care and management of lactating sow

1. Do not offer full amount of feed to recently farrowed sow.
2. Increase amount of feed gradually every day.
3. Amount of feed should be determined at the rate of 500 g per piglet in the litter.

Care and management of fattening pig

1. Provide dry, well-ventilated, draft free housing. Extra bedding during cold and adequate shed during cold is necessary. Spraying and wallowing can also reduce the heat stress.
2. To prevent indiscriminate breeding, improve meat quality, growth rate and mask boar odour in cooked meat, piglets for fattening purpose should be castrated before 3-4 weeks of age, so that wound heals up before weaning.
3. Separate the pigs in groups according to size, age and body weight. In no case, there should not be more than 40 pigs in one group.
4. Offer well balanced ration fortified with additives and fresh and clean water should be available for 24 hours.
5. Control the internal parasites, especially round worms and Ascarids through sanitation, pasture rotation and use of anthelmentics drugs.

6. Follow lice and tick control program, routinely by malathion and lindane.
7. Follow standard vaccination program.
8. Isolate sick pig immediately and give treatment as per veterinarian's advice.

Adopt Integrated Pig Farming Model

It has been accepted across the globe that sustainable development is the only way to promote rational utilization of resources and environmental protection without hampering economic growth. Integrated farming systems (IFS) are a viable option in this regard as waste is minimized, the by-product of one system becoming an input for others and thus, optimizing the use of resources, while reducing pollution. IFS can provide a reasonable rural livelihood, a clean environment and adequate food and products with a greater degree of stability in the production process by spreading the risk of production over several activities.

i) Pig-Fish integration model: In the north-east hill region, integrated fish farming is one of the best alternatives for improving livelihoods as most of the houses in rural areas have access to ponds and livestock. The advantages of this systems:

ii) Pig-Duck-Fish Integration model.

iii) Pig-poultry integration model.

Advantages

1. The fish utilize the food spilled by pigs and their excreta, which is very rich in nutrients.
2. The pig dung acts as a substitute for pond fertilizer and supplementary fish feed. Hence, the cost of fish production is greatly reduced.
3. No additional land is required for piggery operations.
4. Cattle fodder required for pigs and grass are grown on the pond embankments.
5. Pond provides water for washing the pig - sties and pigs.
6. It results in high production of animal protein per unit area.

7. It ensures high profit through less investment.
8. The pond muck which gets accumulated at the pond bottom due to constant application of pig dung can be used as fertilizer for growing vegetables and other crops and cattle fodder.

Pig Breeds suitable for integrated pig cum fish farming

1. Large and Middle White Yorkshire
2. Barkshire
3. Duroc
4. Hereford
5. Landrace
6. Chesterwhite
7. Tamworth

Crosses between exotic and indigenous pigs and pure local breeds are also available, however, in Indian condition Large and Middle White Yorkshire and their crosses are most adaptable.

Conclusions

Absence of properly defined production practices and organized breeding programmes are among main hurdles in improvement. In subsistence-driven systems, Lack of knowledge about Integrated farming systems, improper feeding, ineffective health care and inbreeding are the major hindrance to pigs expressing their full performance. In order to effectively address constraints in pig production systems, holistic approach involving feeding, breeding, health, management and marketing infrastructure is the need of hour. Smallholder livestock production systems improve livelihood and food security for the poorest people, in addition to providing protein for human consumption, pigs are often one of the main sources of cash income in rural areas and provide manure for cropping.

References

1. Ajala, M.K., Adesehinwa, A.O.K. and Mohammed, A.K. (2007). Characteristics of smallholder pig production in Southern Kaduna area of Kaduna state, Nigeria. American–Eurasian Journal of Agriculture and Environmental Science, 2: 182–187.

2. Deca, R., Thorpe, W.M., Lapar, L. and Kumar, A. (2007). Assam's pig sub-sector: current status, constraints and opportunities. Project Report. Nairobi (Kenya): ILRI
3. Kagira J.M., Kanyari P.W.N., Maingi N., Githigia S.M., Ng'ang'a J.C. and Karuga J.W. (2009). Characteristics of the smallholder free-range pig production system in western Kenya. Tropical Animal Health and Production 42(5): 865-873.
4. Kumaresan, A., Bujarbaruah, K.M., Pathak, K.A., Das, A. and Bardoloi, R.K. (2009). Integrated resource-driven pig production systems in a mountainous area of Northeast India: Production practices and pig performance. Tropical Animal Health and Production, 41(7): 1187–1196.
5. Lanada, E.B., Lee, J.A., More, S.J., Basito, S. and Taveros, A. (2005). A longitudinal study of sows and boars raised by smallholder farmers in the Philippines. Preventive Veterinary Medicine 70: 95-113.
6. Moanaro, Ngullie, E., Walling, I., Krose, M. and Bhatt, B.P., 2011. Traditional Animal Husbandry Practices in Tribal States of Eastern Himalaya, India: A Case Study. Indian Journal of Animal Nutrition, 28(1): 23–28.
7. Mpofu I. and Makuza S.M.M. (2003). Pig Production Science and Technology, 1st edition, Ed: A. Shonhiwa, Upfront Publishing, UK.
8. Nath B.G. & P.K. Pathak & S.V. Ngachan & A.K. Tripathi and A.K. Mohanty Characterization of smallholder pig production system: productive and reproductive performances of local and crossbred pigs in Sikkim Himalayan Region. Tropical Animal Health and Production (2013) 45: 1513–1518.
9. Njuki, J., Pali, P., Mburu, S., and Poole, J. (2010). Pig Production, Management and Marketing in the North East Indian State of Nagaland. International Livestock Research Institute, Nairobi.
10. NRC on Pig. (2011) Annual Progress Report. National Research Centre on Pigs, ICAR, Rani, Guwahati, Assam. 1-4.
11. Nsoso, S.J., Mannathoko, G.G. and Modise, K. (2006). Monitoring production, health and marketing of indigenous Tswana pigs in Ramotswa village of Botswana. Livestock Research for Rural Development. 18(9): 125.
12. Patr, M.K., Begum, S. and Deka, B.C. (2014). Problems and Prospects of Traditional Pig Farming for Tribal Livelihood in Nagaland. Indian Research Journal of Extension Education 14(4):6-11.

13. Prasad, J. (2014). Pig production & management. A text book on Goat, Sheep and Pig production & management. 5th edn. Kalyani Publishers.

14. Sastry, N.S.R. & Thomas, C.K. (2015). Swine Production. A textbook of Livestock production management.5th revised edition. Kalyani Publishers.

15. Westendorf, M.L., Schuler, T. and Zirkle, E.W. (1999) Nutritional quality of recycled food plate waste in diets fed to swine. Prof. Anim. Sci., 15(2): 106-111.

❑❑❑

Chapter 24

Promotion of Value Addition Techniques in Poultry Sector

V.P. Singh
Department of Livestock Products Technology, College of Veterinary Science and Animal Husbandry, Uttar Pradesh Pandit Deen Dayal Upadhyaya Pashu Chikitsa Vigyan Vishwavidhyalaya Evam Go Anusandhan Sansthan, Mathura

Poultry industry in India is a mega billion industry having third position in egg production and fifth position in broilers in the world. The total egg production accounts to 68 billion and broilers 2.8 billion. The average cumulative growth rate in layer and broiler is 8% and 12 % respectively. Even though production is in accelerated trend still processing and marketing strategies are not in a well defined manner which leads to overall moderate profitability and less export promotion. This sector is responsible for 0.45% of India's Gross Domestic Product (GDP) and 10% of livestock GDP. Poultry production in India contributes to 5% of meat and 2.5 % egg of total global output. Even though production is in faster rate, the per capita consumption of egg and poultry meat is 52 eggs and 2.4 Kg of meat. In India the consumption pattern varies between urban and rural areas. In urban areas one third of the population consumes two third of the poultry products due to increased farm size, increased income and better knowledge on health and nutritional benefits of poultry meat. But in rural areas due to decreased knowledge on nutritional benefits of poultry meat and poor families their consumption is lower than urban people.

Marketing Trend of Poultry Sector

Currently the bulk (80-85%) of broilers are either sold alive or as deskinned carcasses in retail markets, 10 to 15% are dressed in numerous small poultry processing units in an unscientific manner to be sold as freshly dressed whole chicken, cut-up parts and only about

5% of them are processed scientifically in about a dozen modern, mechanized processing plants (2000-6000 chickens/hr) established in our country over the last one and a half decades. Some new poultry processing plants are in the pipeline, which together with the increased capacity utilization of the existing plants would increase the proportion of chicken processed in automated/semi-automated plants to over 10% in coming years.

Of the dressed chickens, approximately 75% are sold as hot dressed, chilled or frozen whole carcass while the raw or marinated cut-up portions, deboned meat, fillets and further-processed, value-added products (VAP) such as tandoori chicken, sausages, patties/ burger, nuggets, fillets, chicken samosa and kababs, etc. constitute the remaining 25% of product segment. Moreover, all these product mix cater mainly to urban population, constituting about 30% of total population, leaving a vast (70%) rural population untapped for whom desi chicken, spent hens, ducks and to a limited extent broilers are the source of poultry meat. Opening of retail outlets and fast food restaurants by some vertically integrated broiler producers in metros/ big cities is a welcome development for promoting processed products and avoid dependence on middlemen. In contrast, only about 10-20% of broilers are being sold as whole carcass and the remaining as portions, deboned meat and further-processed products in the USA and some other economically developed countries.

The current international trade in poultry products is around 8% of the global output of about 65 million tons chicken meat. Although, India has emerged as a leading exporter of both frozen and dried egg products in recent years but her share in export of frozen broiler and further- processed poultry meat products is still negligible. The poultry-processing sector in India has to go a long way to catch-up with some developing countries such as Brazil and Thailand which have modernized and expanded their processing sector to emerge as major exporters of processed poultry products to developed and high economy developing countries. However, the upcoming horizontal and vertical integrations in poultry production and processing, expected large investment in processing technologies and equipments, creation of cold-chain and launching of sales promotion by some domestic and multinational food chains would promote the growth of this vital sector of poultry industry and thereby offer convenience, quality and sufficient value for money for VAP to domestic consumers and also expand the export potential of Indian poultry products.

Furthermore, trade restriction imposed on chicken products from countries affected by avian influenza epidemics and quality approval of Indian chicken products processed at modern processing plants by the European Union team recently would boost the export prospects.

Value addition and its prospects

Value addition is a process in which for the same volume of a primary product, a high price is realized by means of processing, packing, upgrading the quality or other such methods.

Need for value addition

1. To improve the profitability of farmers
2. To empower the farmers and other weaker sections of society especially women through gainful employment opportunities and revitalize rural communities.
3. To provide better quality, safe & branded foods to the consumers.
4. To emphasize primary and secondary processing.
5. To reduce post harvest losses.
6. Reduction of import and meeting export demands.
7. Way of increased foreign exchange.
8. Encourage growth of subsidiary industries.
9. Reduce the economic risk of marketing.
10. Increase opportunities for smaller farms and companies through the development of markets.
11. Diversify the economic base of rural communities.
12. Overall, increase farmers' financial stability.

Market forces for product differentiation and value addition

1. Increased consumer demands regarding health, nutrition and convenience.
2. Efforts by food processors to improve their productivity.
3. Technological advances that enable producers to produce what consumers and processors desire.

Producers have a challenge to be responsive to consumer demands by producing what is desired. Attentiveness to consumer demands in quality, variety and packaging are important because demographic trends show growth in the convenience-oriented, health conscious and environmentally concerned sectors where price is not as important as quality.

Value addition as new product development

To be unique and novel new product development should be attempted and this can be approached through various ways.

1. A product entirely new in character.
2. A product apparently similar in character in many respects to some existing brands but with distinguishing features.
3. A product similar to one already in the market but new form of manufacture
4. A product novel in kind, made by novel process or through novel ingredient.
5. A product resulting from substantial modifications of the characters with change in nature/proportion of ingredients or processing methods or conditions or packing system.

Choice for value addition

Any attempt for value addition should focus for following parameter for deriving maximum benefit :

1. *Unique* - The product we develop should be one of its own kinds for which crop and variability indigenous to our country should be exploited.
2. *Novelty* - The product should be new and unusual like blue or black rose and likewise so that no one can compete.
3. *Export potential* - The product developed should have demand in international market for higher return and appreciation of benefit of global trade.
4. *High value* - The product should have high value for low volume for ease of trading and distribution and the extracts from Indian spices and herbal medicinal plants can fulfill this requirement.
5. *Availability* - Consistent availability of the product in required quantity should be ensured for stable market and faith.

6. *Market* - Any product that is developed must have market because market is the key for success of any product.

Values added poultry products

Emulsion based meat products : Development of emulsion based meat products facilitate better utilization of meat and byproducts from different spent animals including spent hens. Tough meat is minced in a mincer and emulsion is produced in bowl chopper adding meat, fat, salt, phosphate, spices, condiments, binders, ice flakes, etc. in correct proportion and sequence and chopping to a desired consistency. Emulsion quality contributes to product yield and palatability to a large extent. A large variety of palatable products such as sausages, patties, nuggets, kababs, meat balls, meat pakoda, etc. could be produced from the same emulsion. Emulsion technology is more relevant in Indian situation with availability of tough meat and desire to incorporate a number of spices, condiments and non-meat extenders such as eggs, milk solids, potato, soya pulses, etc.

Restructured meat products : These are meat products having made by restructuring dark and white meat from heavy broilers. Excessive fat is trimmed off and other connective tissues are chunked out and formed. Blade tenderization, flaking and bay tumbling are modern methods available to produce tender products. Prepared meats can be used as steaks, cutlets, chops and roasts or they can be freezing stored.

Cured and Smoked Products : Curing process involves addition of curing agents like salt, sugar, sodium nitrite, sodium ascorbate and sodium polyphosphate to the primal chicken cuts for enhancement of colour, flavour and preservation. Chicken is injected with pickle and dipped in it for faster curing giving a juicy texture. Smoking involves heating, drying, smoking, steaming/cooking showering, chilling and packaging which give a distinctive flavour.

Enrobed/ Coated Products : Enrobing involves applying an edible coating to the products for improving their texture, flavour, nutritive value, juiciness and tenderness. They act as sealing agents to prevent excess oil absorption. Chicken parts can be enrobed using whole egg liquid, curd, flours, corn flakes and bread crumbs which give crispy taste.

Retort Pouched Products : Thermal processing of meat destroys microorganisms and enzymes responsible for food spoilage. Thermal processing in metal cans or retort pouches increases shelf life of products and decreases 50% processing time. Some products include traditional Indian curries, soups, Keemas etc. Retort packaged products could be stored for a period of 6 to 12 months.

Incorporation of vegetables in meat products : Incorporation of seasonal vegetables such as cabbage, cauliflower, carrot, bottle guard, pumpkin, etc. in meat products would be advantageous to reduce cost of meat products, to provide fiber and flavonoids in meat products, to facilitate consumption of vegetables and to provide balanced and healthful diet meat products. Meat products added with vegetables may find wide popularity among Indian consumers.

Heritage Products : Heritage chicken products include traditional fast foods such as meat balls, kebabs, tikka, chicken tandoori, haleem, curries, enrobed and battered products and pickles which are prepared from chicken breast, thigh, drumstick and gizzard muscles. Pickles preserved with vinegar are stable up to 3 months.

Value Addition to Edible by Products : Edible poultry by products like dressed whole chicken carcass and giblets such as liver, heart, gizzard and neck have good marketing values which are sold as package stuffed into cavity of carcass. Minced skin, gizzard and heart are used in emulsion of chicken products. Ova collected during dressing of layer chickens are used in sausage formulations, patties and kebabs. Chicken soup is another nutritious food that is categorized as low fat food.

Commercial Egg Products

USDA classification of egg products

Class	Egg products
Refrigerated as liquid	Whole eggs, whites or yolks, sugared egg yolks, salted egg yolk, scrambled egg mix, extended shelf life whole eggs
Frozen	Whole egg, white or yolk, scrambled egg mix, salted whole egg, sugared egg yolk and whole egg mix
Dried	White egg or yolk solids, dried egg, whole egg
Specialty products	Dried hard cooked, peeled egg, whole hard cooked peeled egg, egg yolk, long egg quiche mix, and ultra-pasteurized liquid egg products.

Certain commercialized egg product preparations are as follows:

1. *Pickled eggs* : A simple, cost-effective and efficient technology developed for ready to eat pickling of quail eggs/chicken eggs for storage and marketing at ambient temperature.
2. *Salted chicken eggs* : Preparation of salted chicken eggs technology is so simple to be used by unskilled people.
3. *Albumen rings* : Albumen rings are egg snack food, prepared by cooking blended egg albumen in ring moulds and battering and breading the coagulated albumen prior to deep fat frying.
4. *Egg roll* : It is a nutritious, tasty and convenience egg product suitable for meals or as snack foods.
5. *Egg crepe* : Egg crepe is a thin, fat, circular product and may be filled with meat or vegetables and rolled or folded.

Value added poultry product may be helpful in set up of new trend in meat sector but the need is of continuous research and development leads to the development of low cost and efficient poultry processing technologies and well established quality control norms. Poultry marketing system in India dominated by private traders and commission agents needs to be transformed into an organized system for uniform sharing of profits by all players in the industry.

References

1. Deogade A. H., Zanjad P.N. and Raziuddin M. (2008). Value Added Meat Products. Veterinary World, 1(3): 88-89.
2. Kondaiah, N. (2004). Value added meat products and development of processed meat sector. Natural Product radiance, 3(4): 281-283.
3. Thyagarajan D. and Barathi M. (2014). Prospects of value-added poultry products marketing in India. Animal and Veterinary Sciences, 2(4): 118-123.
4. Wildes D. (1988). Value added developments for poultry. Journal of Food Distribution Research, Feb: 12-16.

❑❑❑